New Clinical Genetics

2nd Edition

Other titles from Scion

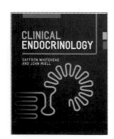 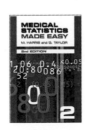 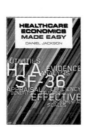 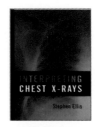 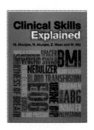 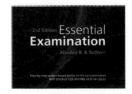

9781904842859   9781904842552   9781904842941   9781904842781   9781904842774   9781904842842

For more information see www.scionpublishing.com

New Clinical Genetics

Genetics

2nd Edition

Andrew Read and Dian Donnai

Genetic Medicine
Manchester Academic Health Sciences Centre
University of Manchester
St Mary's Hospital, Manchester, UK

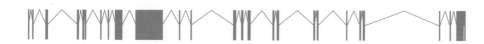

© Scion Publishing Ltd, 2011

First published 2011, reprinted 2012

First edition published 2007, reprinted 2009, 2010

A CIP catalogue record for this book is available from the British Library.

ISBN – 978 1 904842 80 4

Scion Publishing Limited
The Old Hayloft, Vantage Business Park, Bloxham Road,
Banbury OX16 9UX, UK
www.scionpublishing.com

Important Note from the Publisher

The information contained within this book was obtained by Scion Publishing Limited from sources believed by us to be reliable. However, while every effort has been made to ensure its accuracy, no responsibility for loss or injury whatsoever occasioned to any person acting or refraining from action as a result of information contained herein can be accepted by the authors or publishers.

Readers are reminded that medicine is a constantly evolving science and while the authors and publishers have ensured that all dosages, applications and practices are based on current indications, there may be specific practices which differ between communities. You should always follow the guidelines laid down by the manufacturers of specific products and the relevant authorities in the country in which you are practicing.

Although every effort has been made to ensure that all owners of copyright material have been acknowledged in this publication, we would be pleased to acknowledge in subsequent reprints or editions any omissions brought to our attention.

Illustrations by Matthew McClements at Blink Studio Ltd, www.blink.biz
Typeset by Phoenix Photosetting, Chatham, Kent, UK
Printed in India by Imprint Digital Ltd.

Contents

Chapter 3 – How do genes work?

Chapter 4 – How can a patient's DNA be studied?

Chapter 5 – How can we check a patient's DNA for gene mutations?

Chapter 6 – What do mutations do?

Chapter 7 – What is epigenetics?

Chapter 8 – How do our genes affect our metabolism, drug responses and immune system?

Chapter 9 – How do researchers identify genes for mendelian diseases?

Chapter 10 – Why are some conditions common and others rare?

Chapter 11 – When is screening useful?

Chapter 12 – Is cancer genetic?

Chapter 13 – Should we be testing for genetic susceptibility to common diseases?

Chapter 14 – What services are available for families with genetic disorders?

Guidance for self-assessment questions

Glossary

Index

Case notes – Summary of cases and their page references

| CASE 1 | Ashton family | 1 | 7 | 65 | 106 | 154 | 389 |

- John – 28-year-old son of Alfred Ashton
- ? Huntington disease
- Other family members with similar symptoms
- Autosomal dominant inheritance shown in pedigree
- Diagnostic test ordered – *Chapter 1*

| CASE 2 | Brown family | 2 | 8 | 66 | 132 | 154 | 281 | 389 |

- Girl (Joanne) aged 6 months, parents David and Pauline
- ? Cystic fibrosis
- Order molecular test? – *Chapter 1*
- Define mutations in *CFTR* gene – *Chapter 5*
- Universal newborn screening? – *Chapter 11*

CASE 9 — Ingram family — 26 | 41 | 69 | 104 | 187 | 389

- Isabel – first daughter of Irene and Ian
- Small stature despite tall parents
- ? Turner syndrome – *Chapter 2*
- Diagnosis confirmed by karyotyping – *Chapter 7*

CASE 10 — Johnson family — 55 | 65 | 389

- Marfan syndrome – *Chapter 3*

CASE 11 — Kavanagh family — 81 | 97 | 156 | 389

- Healthy first baby boy
- Second child, Celia, pale with low hemoglobin levels
- Sickle cell disease – *Chapter 4*
- Single nucleotide mutation, Glu→Val – *Chapter 6*

CASE 12 — Lipton family — 82 | 98 | 389

- Family history of learning difficulties
- Baby boy, Luke, with poor head control
- ? Fragile X syndrome – *Chapter 4*
- Diagnosis confirmed by Southern blotting

CASE 13 — Meinhardt family — 83 | 102 | 389

- Baby girl, Madelena, with a small head, large ears and needing to be tube fed
- Normal 46,XX karyotype
- ? Underlying chromosome problem
- *De novo* 2.8 Mb deletion of chromosome 16 found by SNP chip analysis – *Chapter 4*

CASE 14 — Nicolaides family — 117 | 135 | 157 | 389

- ? β-thalassemia carriers
- Check mutations – *Chapter 5*
- p.Gln39X nonsense mutation for Spiros
- c.316–106C>G mutation for Elena – *Chapter 6*

CASE 15 — O'Reilly family — 145 | 158 | 389

- Family history of myopia and hip problems
- Orla has severe myopia, is short, and has hip problems
- ? Stickler syndrome
- Frameshift mutation in *COL2A1* – *Chapter 6*

CASE 16 — Portillo family — 177 | 188 | 216 | 389

- Sickly boy, Pablo
- Family history of similar symptoms
- Blood tests suggest X-linked severe combined immunodeficiency – *Chapter 7*
- Check that bone marrow transplantation is appropriate – *Chapter 8*

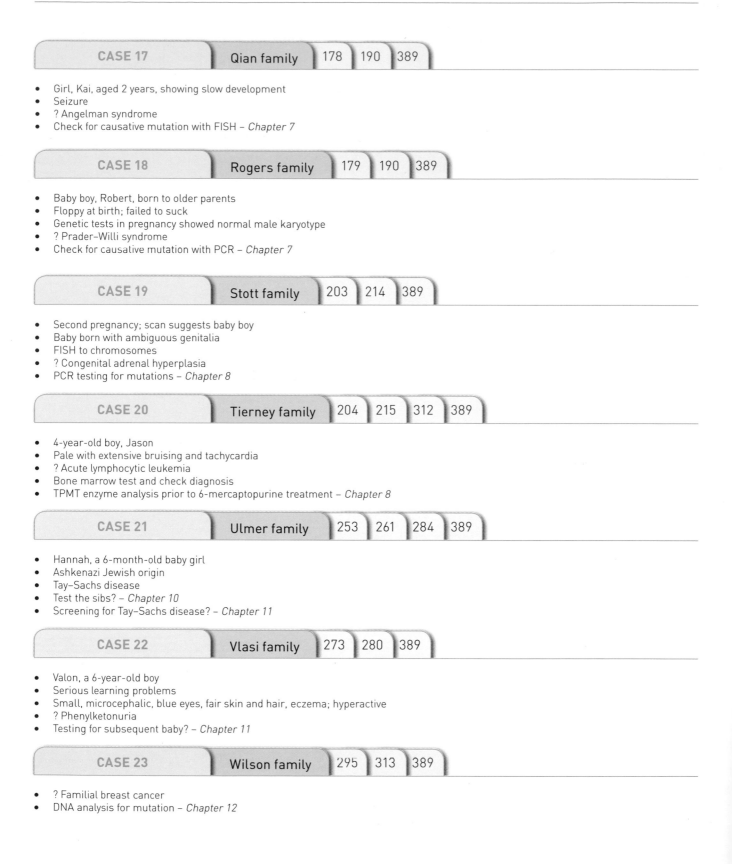

- Family history of bowel problems
- ? FAP – *Chapter 12*

- Family history of dementia
- ? Alzheimer disease
- Test for ApoE4? – *Chapter 13*

- Woman aged 52 years, Zafira
- Overweight; sedentary lifestyle; insatiable thirst
- Type 2 diabetes
- Test son – *Chapter 13*

Preface to the first edition

This book is the result of a collaboration between a scientist (Andrew Read) and a clinician (Dian Donnai). As such, it represents the way clinical genetics operates. We have been fortunate to work in an integrated genetics unit where clinicians, counselors, diagnostic scientists and researchers all work closely together and strike sparks off each other. When we both arrived in the Department of Medical Genetics at St Mary's Hospital, Manchester one day in 1977, we were assigned adjacent desks in a corridor, the department having as usual outgrown its accommodation. We were both there because we thought this was the most exciting and dynamic area in all biology and medicine. The ensuing years have more than vindicated that judgement.

Our primary audience for this book is medical students, but we hope it will also be useful to counselors and scientists, and indeed established clinicians, who want an introduction to the place of clinical genetics in medicine and biology. Only a few of today's medical students will specialize in genetics. All, however, need to understand genetic principles and their application since, in the future, genetic knowledge will underpin much of medical practice. We have tried to produce a book that will make learning interesting by focusing on patients and real clinical situations, without losing sight of the strong underlying conceptual framework of genetics. As explained in the section, *How to Use this Book*, we have designed the book so that it can be used either for a case-based course of study, or in a more traditional way focusing on the science.

We have based the content of the book around the curriculum of the American Society of Human Genetics and the *List of Competencies* for undergraduate medical students being developed by the UK NHS Genetics Education Centre. Annotated versions of these two documents, showing the main places in the book where the relevant material can be found, are available to download at http://www.scionpublishing.com/newclinicalgenetics

We are grateful to David Cooper, Susan Hamilton, Lauren Kerzin-Storrar, Helen Middleton-Price, Rehat Perveen and Alison Stewart, who read through various sections and provided ideas and suggestions. Susan Hamilton also provided most of the cytogenetic pictures. We also thank the many colleagues who we pestered for photos or data, for their kindness and forbearance, and the families who generously agreed to our use of their photos. We hope we have duly acknowledged the sources of all our illustrations, but if anybody notices a picture of theirs used without due acknowledgement, they should please contact us. Finally, we would like to thank Jonathan Ray of Scion Publishing Ltd for his good ideas, hard work and unfailing patience, without which this book would never have come to fruition.

Andrew Read and Dian Donnai
August 2006

Preface to the second edition

The first edition of a new book is always a bit of a leap in the dark, and we were gratified by the warm reception our book met in many quarters. We were also pleased to receive quite a few suggestions for improvement. In the light of these, and of our own more mature thoughts, we have corrected several errors and made a number of other changes. In particular we have expanded the final chapter to give an overview of how genetics services are delivered to patients and their families and added sections on teratogenesis and reproductive problems. There is a much expanded section on dysmorphology, and Fragile X syndrome now has its own case study and detailed explanation. Other changes have been mandated by scientific progress and the continuing rapid developments in technology. SNP chips and next generation sequencing are now covered, with some examples of what these techniques can do. We have removed some biochemical detail that in retrospect went beyond the level appropriate for this book. In the time since the first edition, the strengths and limitations of genome-wide association studies have become apparent, and we can now form a clearer view of their potential to provide clinically useful information. The basic structure, with its dual tracks of case studies or expository material, remains unchanged.

As always, we are indebted to the many colleagues who have made suggestions, provided material and criticised drafts. Our particular thanks go to Jonathan Ray of Scion Publishing, who has bullied us with great tact and charm, and turned our drafts with admirable efficiency into an attractively designed book. Thank you Jonathan.

Andrew Read and Dian Donnai
September 2010

Abbreviations

ACTH	adrenocorticotrophic hormone		MHC	major histocompatibility complex
AFP	alpha-fetoprotein		ML	mucolipidosis
AIS	androgen insensitivity syndrome		MLPA	multiplex ligation-dependent probe amplification
ALAS	amino levulinic acid synthase		MMR	mis-match repair
ALL	acute lymphocytic leukemia		MODY	maturity-onset diabetes in the young
APP	amyloid precursor protein		MSAFP	maternal serum alpha-fetoprotein
ASO	allele-specific oligonucleotide		MZ	monozygotic
ASP	affected sib pair		NK	natural killer
CAH	congenital adrenal hyperplasia		NSC	National Screening Committee
CDK	cyclin-dependent kinase		NTD	neural tube defect
CGH	comparative genomic hybridization		OLA	oligonucleotide ligation assay
cM	centiMorgan		OMIM	Online Mendelian Inheritance in Man
CNVs	copy number variants		PCR	polymerase chain reaction
dHPLC	denaturing high performance liquid chromatography		PKU	phenylketonuria
DMD	Duchenne muscular dystrophy		PWS	Prader–Willi syndrome
DNA	deoxyribonucleic acid		QTL	quantitative trait locus
DSH	dyschromatosis symmetrica hereditaria		RB	retinoblastoma
DTDST	diastrophic dystrophy sulfate transporter		RFLP	restriction fragment length polymorphism
DZ	dizygotic		RNA	ribonucleic acid
FAP	familial adenomatous polyposis		RSTS	Rubinstein–Taybi syndrome
FDA	Food and Drug Administration		SNP	single nucleotide polymorphism
FH	familial hypercholesterolemia		SSCP	single strand conformation polymorphism
FISH	fluorescence *in situ* hybridization		SUMF	sulfatase modifying factor
GvH	graft versus host		T2D	type 2 diabetes
GWAS	genome-wide association studies		TDT	transmission disequilibrium test
HLA	human leukocyte antigen		TGFβ	transforming growth factor β
HNPCC	hereditary non-polyposis colon cancer		TPMT	thiopurine methyl transferase
Ig	immunoglobulins		TS	tumor suppressor
IRT	immunoreactive trypsin		UPD	uniparental disomy
IVF	*in vitro* fertilization		VKOR	vitamin K epoxide reductase
LDL	low density lipoprotein		X-SCID	X-linked severe combined immunodeficiency
LHON	Leber hereditary optic neuropathy			
MAPK	mitogen-activated protein kinase			
MCAD	medium chain acyl-CoA dehydrogenase			

How to use this book

Each chapter addresses a specific question that students may have about genetics, e.g. How can we study chromosomes? Is cancer genetic? etc. Chapters follow a common structure:

- *Learning points* – summarizing what the chapter should enable the student to achieve. These are chosen to cover the curriculum published by the American Society of Human Genetics and the list of competencies being developed by the UK NHS Genetics Education Centre.
- *Case studies* –all chapters except the last one have this section, which introduces a series of short clinically oriented descriptions of a family and the reasons they sought genetic counseling or testing. The cases are all fictional and the photographs illustrate the condition rather than the patients described; but they are based on our long experience of dealing with real families.
- *Science toolkit* – an explanation of the methods and concepts that are necessary to understand the next section.
- *Investigations of patients* – using the case studies to illustrate the application of the methods and concepts in realistic scenarios. These form running stories that develop over several chapters.
- *Going deeper …* – summarizes and extends the relevant science.

Students can choose different routes through the material:

| CASE 1 | Ashton family | 1 | 7 | 65 | 106 | 154 | 389 |

- John – 28-year-old son of Alfred Ashton
- ? Huntington disease
- Other family members with similar symptoms
- Autosomal dominant inheritance shown in pedigree
- Diagnostic test ordered

- Those who prefer a problem-based approach would move from the initial *Case studies* to the *Investigations of patients* sections. They should treat the other sections as reference material. The page design includes page references to enable students to follow cases that run through several chapters. For example, the Ashton family case is covered on pages 1, 7, 65, 106, 154 and 389. In addition, the bullets associated with each case serve as reminders as to what has been covered previously

- Students who prefer a more didactic approach can concentrate on the science in the *Background* and *Summary and extension* of sections. The other sections provide illustrations and examples.

Chapters finish with self-assessment questions so that students can check that they have mastered the material, regardless which route they chose to take through it.

The book is not intended as a diagnostic manual and so does not aim to describe all the major mendelian and chromosomal disorders. However, the cases and the *Disease boxes* help to show the range and variety of genetic conditions. More details of the diseases most commonly encountered in clinical genetic practice can be found at www.scionpublishing.com/newclinicalgenetics. For specific information you should refer to the reliable websites listed in the *References* section of relevant chapters. The first place to look should be the OMIM database: http://www.ncbi.nlm.nih.gov/omim – OMIM reference numbers are given throughout the book.

01 | What can we learn from a family history?

After working through this chapter you should be able to:

- Take a family history

- Draw a pedigree using correct symbols

- Identify the most likely mode of inheritance, given a straightforward pedigree

- Describe how genes segregate in autosomal dominant, autosomal recessive, X-linked dominant, X-linked recessive, Y-linked and mitochondrial conditions

- Define penetrance and expressivity

- Show appreciation of the human and scientific issues raised by the conditions described

1.1. Case studies

| CASE 1 | Ashton family | **1** | 7 | 65 | 106 | 154 | 389 |

- John – 28-year-old son of Alfred Ashton
- ? Huntington disease
- Other family members with similar symptoms

Alfred Ashton, aged 52, had been getting forgetful and was thought to be depressed following losing his job. He has been seeing a psychiatrist, who noted that Alfred was restless and had some choreiform movements (involuntary jerky movements of his fingers and shoulders and facial grimacing). Alfred had told the psychiatrist that he thought he was developing 'the family disease', though he was vague as to what this was. The psychiatrist suspected that Alfred had Huntington disease (OMIM 143100). His 28-year-old son John has been referred to the genetic clinic by his family doctor at the suggestion of the psychiatrist. John knows nothing about Huntington disease; he is preoccupied with other things, having recently married and bought a house.

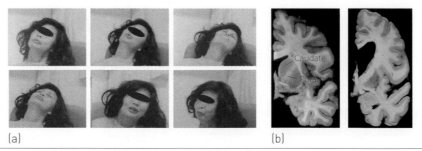

(a)   (b)

Figure 1.1 – Huntington disease.
(a) A patient in the advanced stages of the disease showing involuntary movements of the head and face. (b) Post mortem sections comparing normal brain (left) with brain from Huntington disease patient (right); note the loss of tissue in the Huntington disease brain. Photos courtesy of Dr David Crauford, St Mary's Hospital, Manchester.

CASE 2	Brown family	**2**	8	66	132	154	281	389

- Girl (Joanne) aged 6 months, parents David and Pauline
- ? Cystic fibrosis

Joanne is the second child born to David and Pauline Brown. Her older brother Jason is now 4 years old and very healthy, in fact his parents have to buy age 6 clothes for him. Joanne, however, is a different matter. She has worried her parents from the start. Although she took her bottle well she was very slow to put on weight and in her first few months seemed constantly to have a cold and a cough. At first Pauline and the doctor put this down to the fact that Jason had just started nursery and had a few colds himself. When she was 5 months old Joanne was really ill and was admitted to hospital with a chest infection. The nurses commented that her bowel motions were very bulky and offensive, and when her weight and height were plotted on the charts they were on lower centiles than they had been at birth and in her first month. The doctors suspected she might have cystic fibrosis (OMIM 219700) and therefore arranged for her to have a sweat test. This confirmed their suspicion (Na^+ level of 87 mmol/l, well above the normal upper limit of 60 mmol/l). The diagnosis came as a complete bombshell to Pauline and David. At their request, Joanne's pediatrician arranged for them to see a geneticist to talk things through.

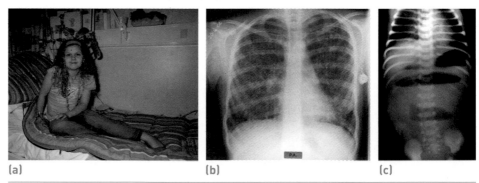

(a)   (b)   (c)

Figure 1.2 – Cystic fibrosis.
(a) The outlook for cystic fibrosis patients has improved over the years but they still need frequent hospital admissions, physiotherapy and constant medications. (b) Chest X-ray of lungs of cystic fibrosis patient. (c) Erect abdominal film of newborn with meconium ileus showing multiple fluid levels. Photos (a) and (b) courtesy of Dr Tim David, Royal Manchester Children's Hospital.

BOX 1.1

The pleiotropic* effects of cystic fibrosis

- **Lung** — Abnormal mucus leading to infection and lung damage
- **Gastrointestinal tract** — Meconium ileus
  Distal intestinal obstruction
  Rectal prolapse
- **Pancreas** — Exocrine pancreas dysfunction
  Malabsorption
- **Hepatobiliary tract** — Biliary cirrhosis
  Gallstones
- **Sweat glands** — Elevated chloride and sodium in sweat
- **Reproductive tract** — Congenital bilateral absence of vas deferens (CBAVD)
  Thick cervical secretions

*Pleiotropic = having many effects.

CASE 3	Choudhary family	3	9	66	242	262	389

- Girl (Nasreen) aged 8 months, parents Aadnan and Mumtaz
- Deaf
- Parents are first cousins

Nasreen is the first child born to young parents (Aadnan and Mumtaz Choudhary) who are first cousins. The pregnancy and birth were normal and Nasreen thrived. She smiled, lifted her head and rolled over all at the normal times. She was taken regularly to the routine baby clinic. When she had her hearing test at 8 months she didn't seem to react normally to sound. Her mother hoped it was just because she was sleepy but her audiograms showed that she had profound bilateral hearing loss.

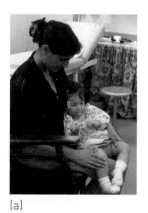

(a)

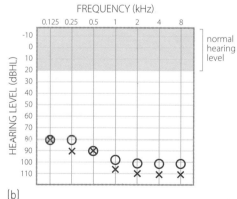

(b)

Figure 1.3 – Result of a hearing test.
(a) Testing a baby's hearing by checking the auditory brain stem response.
(b) Audiogram showing bilateral severe–profound hearing loss. The horizontal axis shows the frequency and the vertical axis the hearing threshold in decibels. Different symbols are used for readings from the two ears. 0–20 dB is normal hearing; hearing loss is defined as 20–40 dB (mild), 40–70 dB (moderate), 70–95 dB (severe), over 95 dB (profound).

| CASE 4 | Davies family | **4** | 10 | 67 | 104 | 155 | 186 | 281 | 389 |

- Boy (Martin) aged 24 months, parents Judith and Robert
- Clumsy and slow to walk
- Family history of muscular dystrophy

Martin is the first son born to Judith and Robert Davies; they already have two daughters Leanne and Kathryn. The girls were very quick with their motor milestones and both were walking just before their first birthdays. Martin seemed slower in many ways and his mum thought it was just that he was a boy. However, when he still wasn't walking at 18 months she asked the doctor at the clinic for advice. The doctor didn't find anything when he examined Martin and arranged for another assessment in 6 months' time. Meanwhile Martin did take his first steps at 20 months but the doctor, at the next appointment, noticed Martin was very clumsy and that when he got up from the floor he had to hold on to a chair or push himself up by propping his hands on his legs. Both the doctor and Judith were very worried at this point because they knew that there was a family history of muscular dystrophy, and although there are many reasons why a little boy might be slow to walk and clumsy, these can also be early signs of that disease. They agreed that Martin needed to be referred to a neurologist, and Judith and Robert needed to see a geneticist.

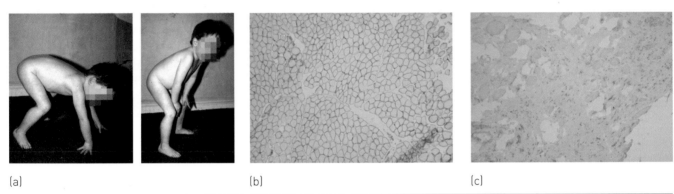

(a) (b) (c)

Figure 1.4 – Duchenne muscular dystrophy.
(a) Affected boys stand up by bracing their arms against their legs (Gower's maneuver) because their proximal leg muscles are weak. (b) and (c) Muscle histology (Gomori trichrome stain). Normal muscle (b) shows a regular architecture of cells with dystrophin (brown stain) on all the outer membranes. (c) Shows muscle from a 10-year-old affected boy. Note the disorganization, invasion by fibrous tissue and complete absence of dystrophin. Histology photos courtesy of Dr Richard Charlton, Newcastle upon Tyne.

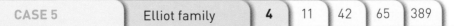

| CASE 5 | Elliot family | **4** | 11 | 42 | 65 | 389 |

- Miscarriage
- Very small dysmorphic baby girl (Elizabeth), parents Elmer and Ellen
- Heart problems

Elmer and Ellen decided they wanted to start a family soon after they came back from their honeymoon in Jamaica where Elmer's parents were born. It wasn't long before Ellen became pregnant but 8 weeks after her last period she started bleeding and after that the pregnancy test was negative. The next pregnancy 5 months later seemed to go well at first but at 30 weeks' gestation a scan showed the baby to be small. This didn't worry the couple since Ellen was petite herself.

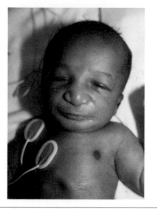

Figure 1.5 – **A baby with multiple congenital abnormalities and dysmorphic features.**

However, when Elizabeth was born at 37 weeks' gestation it was clear that all was not well. Elizabeth was overall a small baby (her length and weight were on the 3rd centiles) but her head circumference was significantly below the 3rd centile. She needed tube feeding and seemed to get breathless very easily. A heart murmur was detected and an echocardiogram showed she had a ventricular septal defect and a narrowing of her aortic valve. The pediatrician asked the geneticist to see Elizabeth and her parents and advise which investigations might be helpful. Ellen told the geneticist her sister had had two early miscarriages and her aunt who lives in Trinidad had a baby who died with a congenital heart defect and a stillborn baby before she had two healthy children.

| CASE 6 | Fletcher family | **5** | 12 | 67 | 137 | 156 | 389 |

- Frank, aged 22, with increasingly blurred eyesight
- Family history of visual difficulties

Frank was an electrician who, at 22 years old, had just finished his college course. He enjoyed going out with his friends and he tended to drink quite a lot of alcohol at weekends. He had always had good eyesight but one week he noticed that his vision was blurred and the colors of the wires he was working on seemed paler than usual. When this didn't improve he went to the optician who noticed changes in Frank's retina and made an urgent referral to the Eye Hospital. There they found he had disk swelling (pseudoedema of the nerve fiber layer), and increased tortuosity of the retinal vessels. Gradually over the next few months his central vision became much worse and he had to give up his job. His mother, Freda, was a healthy woman but her only brother had been registered blind since 28 years of age with what she remembered to be optic atrophy. Her sister Doreen also has serious visual difficulties which came on when she was around 45 years old. The ophthalmologist referred Frank to the genetic clinic because of this family history.

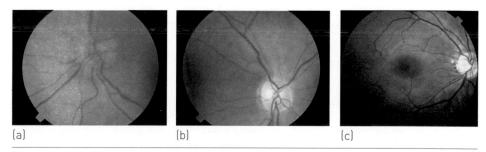

(a) (b) (c)

Figure 1.6 – **Leber hereditary optic neuropathy.**
(a) Optic disc 3 weeks after patient noted reduction in vision; note hyperemia of disc with blurred margins. (b) Retina of uncle; vision lost several years previously. Note pallor of disc particularly temporally corresponding to optic atrophy. (c) Normal retina. Photos courtesy of Mr Graeme Black, St Mary's Hospital, Manchester.

1.2. Science toolkit

The first thing to do with any of these patients is to take a family history. Even when the referral letter gives a family history, it is important for the geneticist to go carefully through, following the protocol in *Box 1.2*. The family history can give important clues about the genetic diagnosis; it also forms a necessary background for genetic diagnosis and counseling.

BOX 1.2

How to take a family history and draw a pedigree

Take a special pedigree proforma or a sheet of blank paper and rule four lines across the long dimension. Start with the **consultand** (the person who is referred to the clinic) in the middle of the next-to-bottom line. Draw in the appropriate symbol (see below) and note his or her name, date of birth and any relevant clinical features. Next record details of the spouse(s) or partners, if any, then proceed systematically through their children, parents, and brothers and sisters (sibs). For each sib record their partners and children. Next ask about the sibs of each parent and their partners and children. Finally document all four grandparents and their sibs. Unless there is some reason to do so, it should not be necessary to go beyond that. Be careful to ask systematically about each person, and for each person note their name, date of birth, if dead the date and cause of death, and any relevant clinical information. Ask about miscarriages or reproductive problems and, if appropriate, about the place of origin of each person. Even if the consultands are convinced that they know which side of the family is the source of the problem, it is wise to collect full details of both sides – family myths can be very misleading.

Some institutions use computerized systems that take you through a series of questions similar to those above, and draw the pedigree for you.

Build up the pedigree as you go along, keeping each generation on one horizontal line. List sibs in the order of their birth if this can be done without too many lines crossing on the drawing. If the pedigree is at all complicated you will probably need to re-draw it neatly later. You can use the pedigrees in this chapter as models. The appropriate symbols to use are:

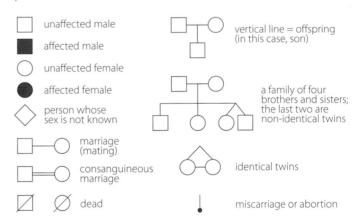

1.3. Investigations of patients

In each of our cases the initial investigation was to construct a detailed pedigree. The pedigrees below illustrate some of the typical features of autosomal dominant (Huntington disease), autosomal recessive (cystic fibrosis and Nasreen's deafness) and X-linked recessive (Martin's muscular dystrophy) conditions. The final two pedigrees (for the Elliot and Fletcher families) raise issues of interpretation that will be considered towards the end of this chapter.

| CASE 1 | Ashton family | 1 | **7** | 65 | 106 | 154 | 389 |

- John – 28-year-old son of Alfred Ashton
- ? Huntington disease
- Other family members with similar symptoms
- Autosomal dominant inheritance shown in pedigree
- Diagnostic test ordered

John's mother comes to the clinic with John to help construct a family tree. As well as John, she has a daughter who has two young sons. Alfred Ashton's father Frederick (John's grandfather) was killed in an industrial accident aged 38 years but Alfred's mother is alive and well at 77 years. Alfred's paternal grandmother became demented in her 50s and needed institutional care, as did one of her two brothers and her only sister. Although the family have lost touch with the extended family, since they became aware of the diagnosis in John's father they have heard that other people in the family have Huntington disease. They are very worried about Alfred's sister who lives in Australia and who has been demonstrating jerky movements like her brother.

This pedigree shows autosomal dominant inheritance. The child of somebody affected by Huntington disease has a 1 in 2 chance of having inherited the Huntington disease gene. If they do inherit the gene, they will inevitably develop Huntington disease unless they die of something else first, like Alfred's father did. The disease may develop at any age from childhood to 70+, but most usually when the person is in their 40s.

Severe late-onset genetic conditions like Huntington disease cause agonizing dilemmas for at-risk people. John has just got married and bought a house. His wife and he are thinking of starting a family. Although he shows no symptoms of the disease, if he does carry the Huntington disease gene he will inevitably develop this severe disease later in his life, and any child he has would be at a 1 in 2 risk. A DNA test is available that could tell John definitively whether or not he carries the mutation. Deciding whether or not to take the test will be one of the biggest decisions of his life. In the UK about 70% of people in this situation

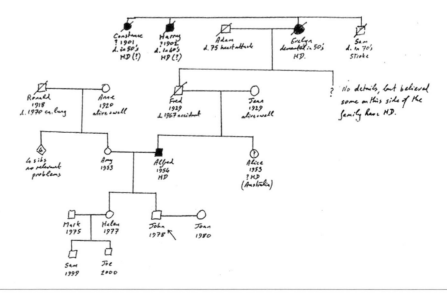

Figure 1.7 – Pedigree of John Ashton's family.
This is shown as it might be recorded in the clinic but because the cases and families in this book are fictional, all subsequent pedigrees show only information that is relevant to following the case and understanding the genetics.

opt, after full counseling, not to take the test. Genetic counselors must always respect a patient's right *not* to know, in this or any other situation, if that is their choice. Before embarking on this whole process, it is crucial to confirm that the family disease really is Huntington disease and not either an unrelated neurodegenerative condition or one of the rare autosomal dominant diseases that can resemble Huntington disease. In this case the psychiatrist is confident of the diagnosis for Alfred, but a test of Alfred's DNA (see *Chapter 4* for a description of type of test) is used to make sure. Note that testing somebody who is already ill constitutes a **diagnostic test** which is not as ethically sensitive as a **predictive test** on a healthy person like John, although a positive result in Alfred would confirm the poor prognosis.

| CASE 2 | Brown family | 2 | **8** | 66 | 132 | 154 | 281 | 389 |

- Girl (Joanne) aged 6 months, parents David and Pauline
- ? Cystic fibrosis
- Order molecular test?

The pedigree shows that there is no family history of cystic fibrosis or other evident genetic problems. "How can it be genetic, when nobody in either family has ever had it?" Pauline asked. In fact this pedigree is typical of the way autosomal recessive diseases present in societies where consanguinity is not common. The affected child is usually the only affected case born to a non-consanguineous couple with no relevant family history. Thus the pedigree gives no clue that the condition is genetic. Identifying the cause usually starts with making a clinical diagnosis. Sometimes the condition is so unmistakable, and the genetics so unambiguous, that a clinical diagnosis provides an adequate degree of certainty. More often the clinical diagnosis is really a hypothesis, more or less plausible. Ideally it would be confirmed by a molecular test demonstrating a mutation.

In most cases of cystic fibrosis the clinical history and a positive sweat test (showing characteristically raised sodium) make the diagnosis fairly secure. Genetically, cystic fibrosis is always autosomal recessive, and always caused by mutations in the *CFTR* gene on chromosome 7 (see *Chapter 3*). A molecular test to demonstrate the mutation is needed for advising relatives about their carrier status, for prenatal testing, and to confirm the diagnosis in atypical cases.

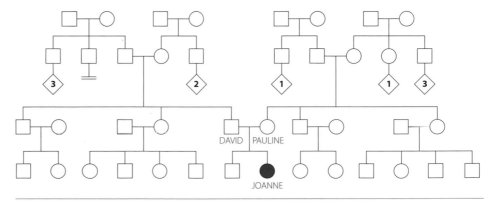

Figure 1.8 – **Pedigree of Joanne Brown's family.**
Note the complete absence of any family history of cystic fibrosis. Autosomal recessive conditions commonly present as a single isolated case.

| CASE 3 | Choudhary family | 3 | **9** | 66 | 242 | 262 | 389 |

- Girl (Nasreen) aged 8 months, parents Aadnan and Mumtaz
- Deaf
- Parents are first cousins
- Pedigree suggests autosomal recessive deafness

The clinic visit turned out to be a family affair because Aadnan's sister Benazir and Mumtaz's brother Waleed also asked to come, together with Aadnan, Mumtaz and Nasreen. Waleed was deaf, but was skilled at lip-reading, and with careful attention to seating and lighting he was able to play his full part in the consultation. The pedigree revealed an extensive family with several consanguineous marriages. In the UK pedigrees of this type are most often seen in people originating from the Middle East or the Indian subcontinent. Aadnan and Mumtaz are first cousins (see *Box 1.3*). Mumtaz's parents (who are also first cousins) have four children in addition to Mumtaz. Two boys, Waleed and his brother Mohammed, are deaf and attend a college for deaf students where they are doing well academically. Aadnan and Mumtaz want to know the risk of deafness in any children they might have in the future. Mumtaz has had two miscarriages, and she fears that she will never have healthy children.

Congenital deafness can be due to environmental factors such as maternal rubella or birth trauma. The geneticist had checked Mumtaz's notes to make sure there was no evidence of such problems, but she noted the need to check with Mumtaz's mother and her family doctor that there was no evidence of such factors with Waleed or Mohammed. The pedigree is most simply interpreted as showing autosomal recessive deafness. About two-thirds of congenital deafness has such a cause. If this interpretation is correct, then each subsequent child of Aadnan and Mumtaz has a 1 in 4 risk of being deaf. The extensive inbreeding is an additional pointer to a recessive condition. Although consanguineous marriage roughly doubles the risk of abnormal children (depending on the degree of consanguinity - see *Chapter 10*), the increase is only from 2% to 4%. In other words, the chance of a healthy child is only reduced from 98% to 96%. In many traditional societies there are good social reasons to marry a relative rather than a stranger. Mumtaz's two miscarriages are very unlikely to be related to the deafness. They might

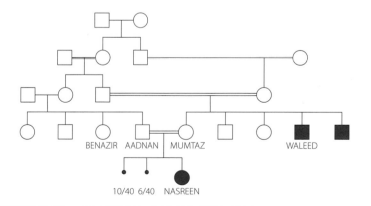

Figure 1.9 – Pedigree of Nasreen Choudhary's family.
Note the use of double marriage lines to highlight consanguineous marriages. Two early miscarriages are indicated. In a real family you would mark the dates of birth of Aadnan's and Mumtaz's sibs, because arranging them in birth order would probably make it difficult to draw a clear pedigree.

be evidence of another, much more severe recessive condition in the family, but there are many non-genetic causes of miscarriage. The geneticist reassured Mumtaz that two early miscarriages is quite a common history that usually has no sinister import.

The presence of Waleed and Benazir at the clinic visit was explained by the fact that they have been introduced and a wedding is planned. Benazir was worried that if a child of theirs was deaf, it might relate exclusively to Waleed and she would be cut out of the family circle. Waleed, however, took a much more relaxed view. The geneticist had to be sensitive to the undercurrents and careful not to try to impose her own views. Consanguineous marriage within a family with a known recessive condition does carry specific risks. In *Chapter 10* we will see how the geneticist calculated the risk for Waleed and Benazir. However, that calculation would only be valid if Waleed's and Nasreen's deafness was confirmed to be autosomal recessive. The family were keen to know if a DNA test was available to confirm the interpretation. This is discussed in *Chapter 3*.

BOX 1.3

Relationships

Sibs means brothers or sisters, regardless of sex

Cousins: Jack and Jill are **first cousins** if one of Jack's parents is a sib of one of Jill's parents. They are **second cousins** if one of Jack's parents is first cousin of one of Jill's parents.

In some cultures the word 'cousin' is used much more loosely to mean 'kinsman'. For genetic purposes it should be used in the strict sense defined above. More complex relationships such as in the **Choudhary family (Case 3**, *Figure 1.9*) are best defined by drawing or describing the pedigree details. We will see in *Chapter 10* how to calculate exact degrees of relationship and inbreeding.

| CASE 4 | Davies family | 4 | **10** | 67 | 104 | 155 | 186 | 281 | 389 |

- Boy (Martin) aged 24 months, parents Judith and Robert
- Clumsy and slow to walk
- Family history of muscular dystrophy
- Pedigree shows X-linked recessive inheritance
- Order diagnostic DNA test

The pedigree shows that Judith's aunt (her mother's sister) had had two boys who died in their teens having had a progressive muscle disease. There were no other affected relatives in the family. The pedigree is consistent with X-linked recessive inheritance. If Martin does indeed have the same condition as his two dead relatives, then X-linked inheritance is highly likely, but at this stage this is still not certain.

It was crucial to check the exact diagnosis of these two boys. There are many different degenerative muscle diseases. While these might have roughly similar implications for management of the patient, the implications for the wider family depend critically on a precise genetic diagnosis. The geneticist will request the case notes, paying particular attention to the detailed course of the boys' decline and to any reports of muscle histology. Given the dates of their deaths it is unlikely that any DNA test results would be available. As described in *Chapter 4*, testing Martin's DNA will play a central part in the investigations.

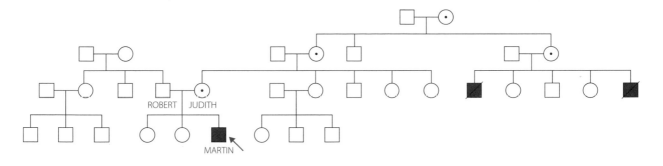

Figure 1.10 – Pedigree of Martin Davies's family.
Assuming this is X-linked muscular dystrophy, the women marked with dots
are **obligate carriers** of the disease gene – that is, they must be carriers
because they have both parents and offspring who are affected or carriers.
Other females (e.g. the sisters of affected boys) may or may not be carriers.

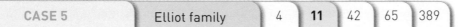

| CASE 5 | Elliot family | 4 | **11** | 42 | 65 | 389 |

- Miscarriage
- Very small dysmorphic baby girl (Elizabeth), parents Elmer and Ellen
- Heart problems
- Blood taken for chromosome analysis
- Pedigree suggests autosomal dominant condition with reduced penetrance

The family history of miscarriages, stillbirth and liveborn infants with malformations in several generations might suggest an autosomal dominant condition with reduced penetrance (see *Section 1.4* for an explanation of penetrance). However, clinical experience suggests the most likely explanation is a balanced chromosome structural abnormality. The next step is to perform chromosome analysis on the parents and the surviving abnormal child (see *Chapter 2*).

After the birth of a child with malformations or other problems parents experience a whole range of emotions including shock, anxiety, denial and confusion. They often also experience a sense of loss for the normal baby they hoped to have. Naturally other family members have their own responses to the difficult situation and tensions are raised further, particularly if one 'side' blames the other. The role of the pediatric team caring for the baby is to keep the family fully informed about their findings in the baby and about tests and consultations that are being arranged. The roles of the clinical geneticist are to help establish a diagnosis as soon as possible and to convey complex results to the parents in a comprehensible way, and also to explain what they mean for the baby's future. Genetic counseling about recurrence risks and implications for the extended family is often arranged later after urgent clinical management issues have been dealt with.

The clinical geneticist and pediatrician agreed that the most likely explanation for Elizabeth's problems is a chromosomal abnormality. Blood was therefore taken from the baby and both parents for chromosome analysis. The results and implications are discussed in *Chapter 2*. Over several sessions the counselor built up the pedigree shown below. The poor reproductive outcomes (miscarriages or abnormal babies) in this family appear to show an autosomal dominant pattern. As explained below, this is not incompatible with the suspicion that the problems are caused by a chromosomal abnormality.

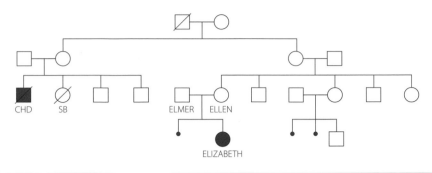

Figure 1.11 – Pedigree of the Elliot family.
This shows the family history of reproductive problems. SB denotes stillbirth and CHD congenital heart disease.

| CASE 6 | Fletcher family | 5 | **12** | 67 | 137 | 156 | 389 |

- Frank, aged 22, with increasingly blurred eyesight
- Family history of visual difficulties
- Pedigree suggests X-linked recessive inheritance but not conclusive
- ? LHON
- Order blood test to check for mutation in mtDNA

Frank attended the genetic clinic with his mother. He was still very shocked after having the diagnosis and poor prognosis explained to him by the ophthalmologist. He hadn't even started to come to terms with the major changes this would bring in his life, including losing his job and not being able to drive. It had, however, begun to occur to him that because of the family history his own children might be at risk. When he came to the clinic he very much wanted to discuss this aspect of things since his girlfriend and he were very worried.

The clinical geneticist first of all drew up a detailed family tree with the help of Frank's mother Freda. Her brother, Derek, was registered blind and had been diagnosed as having optic atrophy. He had first noticed problems like Frank in his 20s; encouragingly he had attended college after his diagnosis and now worked for a large company in their telephone sales department. He had also told Frank about the national organization for people with visual disabilities and about all the help and advice they could offer. Freda's sister Doreen didn't develop any problems until she was in her 40s and her visual deterioration was slower, although still affecting her central vision. At a recent check-up she had been found to have an unusual heart rhythm and had requested Freda to find out in the clinic if that was linked to the eye problems.

The following clues led the geneticist to a hypothesis about the condition in Frank's family:

- the nature of the eye problems
- the rapid progression of symptoms in the affected males
- the later onset and slightly milder disease in Doreen
- Doreen's heart rhythm problems

Based on these observations, the geneticist thought the condition could be Leber hereditary optic neuropathy (LHON). LHON (OMIM 535000) has a wide range of symptoms and ages of onset. It is caused by a mutation in mitochondrial DNA (mtDNA – see *Chapter 3*). The geneticist therefore arranged for blood samples to

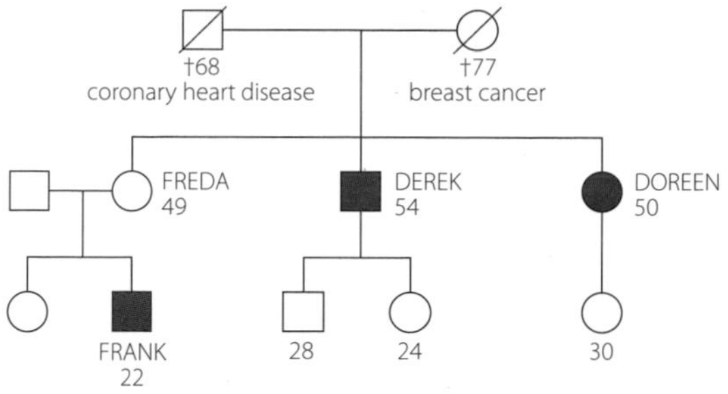

Figure 1.12 – Pedigree of Frank Fletcher.
This pedigree was difficult to interpret. At first sight the geneticist considered X-linked recessive inheritance because of two similarly affected males linked through a normal female. However, Doreen was also affected, which made X-linked inheritance less likely. This nevertheless remained a possibility because sometimes in such families there are 'manifesting female carriers' with milder problems than affected males (see *Chapter 7*). Other types of inheritance such as X-linked dominant and mitochondrial inheritance have to be considered when affected people are linked through the female line.

be taken from Frank and Freda. If this type of inheritance is confirmed then it is good news for any children Frank and his girlfriend may have, since a male does not pass on his mtDNA to his children.

1.4. **Going deeper...**

The art of pedigree interpretation

In laboratory animals like fruit flies or mice, the mode of inheritance of a character can always be established beyond doubt by breeding experiments. With humans we have to take pedigrees as we find them, and they are rarely large enough to define the mode of inheritance unambiguously. For research purposes, collections of pedigrees can be analyzed statistically, using the tools of segregation analysis to work out the most likely mode of inheritance. In the clinic, pedigree interpretation is an art as much as a science. It is more a matter of forming hypotheses for subsequent investigation. The hypothesis might involve any of the following causes:

- a chromosomal abnormality
- an autosomal dominant condition, fully or partially penetrant
- an autosomal recessive condition
- an X-linked condition, dominant or recessive
- a condition caused by a defect in the mitochondrial DNA
- a multifactorial condition
- a non-genetic cause

Case 5 (Elliot family) showed that chromosome abnormalities can give a mendelian pedigree pattern. A mendelian pattern will be seen whenever a phenotype is caused by something at a single fixed chromosomal location – whether that 'something' is a classical gene or a chromosomal abnormality.

Box 1.4 summarizes the features of the main mendelian pedigree patterns. Possible investigations include:

- clinical identification of a syndrome – but bear in mind that some clinically defined syndromes can show more than one mode of inheritance
- karyotyping (see *Chapter 2*)
- analysis of candidate genes for mutations (see *Chapter 5*)
- checking for biochemical abnormalities, including abnormalities of mitochondrial function (see *Chapter 8*)
- checking for skewed X-inactivation (see *Chapter 7*)

Summary of modes of inheritance

Autosomal dominant:

- a vertical pedigree pattern, with multiple generations affected
- each affected person normally has one affected parent
- each child of an affected person has a 1 in 2 chance of being affected
- males and females are equally affected and equally likely to pass the condition on

Autosomal recessive:

- a horizontal pedigree pattern, with one or more sibs affected; often only a single affected case
- parents and children of affected people are normally unaffected
- each subsequent sib of an affected child has a 1 in 4 chance of being affected
- males and females are equally affected
- affected children are sometimes the product of consanguineous marriages. In families with multiple consanguineous marriages, affected individuals may be seen in several generations

X-linked recessive:

- a 'knight's move' pedigree pattern – affected boys may have affected maternal uncles
- parents and children of affected people are normally unaffected. Never transmitted from father to son
- affects mainly males: females can be carriers, and affected males in a pedigree are linked through females, not through unaffected males
- subsequent brothers of affected boys have a 1 in 2 risk of being affected; sisters are not affected but have a 1 in 2 risk of being carriers

X-linked dominant:

- features very similar to autosomal dominant pedigrees, except that all daughters and no sons of an affected father are affected
- condition is often milder and more variable in females than in males

Y-linked:

- a vertical pedigree pattern
- all sons of an affected father are affected
- affects only males

Mitochondrial:

- a vertical pedigree pattern
- children of affected men are never affected
- all children of an affected woman may be affected, but mitochondrial conditions are typically extremely variable even within a family

BOX 1.4

To form a hypothesis, individual pedigrees are checked to see what mode of inheritance gives the best fit. The initial hypothesis is based on two questions:

(1) Does the pedigree show that affected people have at least one affected parent? If the answer is yes, the condition is most likely dominant; if no, it is most likely recessive. A dominant condition is manifest in anybody who carries the relevant gene. Barring new mutations, an affected person must have inherited the gene from one parent, who should therefore also be affected.

(2) Are there any gender effects? For example, does the condition affect both sexes, and can it be passed on by a parent of either sex to a child of either sex? If there are no gender effects, the condition is most likely autosomal. Look especially for male-to-male transmission: this is a powerful pointer against X-linked inheritance because a father should never transmit his X chromosome to a son. If there appear to be gender effects, then it may be X-linked, although as explained below, there can be other reasons for a sex bias. Unless the pedigree is exceptionally large, apparent effects may be just random fluctuations.

Having arrived at an initial hypothesis, the next step is to test it by writing in genotypes, as in *Figure 1.13*. Given sufficient coincidences (new mutations, carriers of the disease happening to marry into the family, etc.) almost

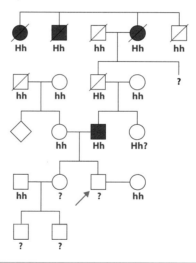

Figure 1.13 – The Huntington disease pedigree of *Figure 1.1* with genotypes written in.
By convention, upper case is used for the allele determining the dominant character and lower case for the allele determining the recessive character. In this example the disease allele is dominant. Note that affected people in this family are heterozygotes. This is the normal situation with human dominant conditions. Homozygotes are usually extremely rare or unknown; when they are recorded, they are often far more seriously affected than heterozygotes. Nevertheless, such a condition is correctly described as dominant (not semi-dominant). Dominance and recessiveness are properties of phenotypes (characters, diseases...) not genes. A character is dominant if it is manifest in the heterozygote, and this is the case for Huntington disease. As it happens, Huntington disease is one of the rare human cases where homozygotes are known to exist and to be phenotypically identical to heterozygotes.

any pedigree can be made to fit almost any mode of inheritance. The most likely mode of inheritance is the one that requires the least number of such coincidences – preferably none. If you require any coincidences to make your initial hypothesis fit, then you should see if an alternative hypothesis gives a better fit. Pedigrees in student examination papers should always have one 'right' answer. Real life is not always so kind: many real pedigrees are ambiguous, or do not fit any of the standard mendelian patterns. The condition may be multifactorial, or other evidence may suggest a chromosomal abnormality or a non-genetic cause.

Penetrance and expressivity – pitfalls in interpretation and counseling

Many human conditions show a mainly autosomal dominant pedigree pattern, but occasionally skip a generation: that is, an unaffected person who has an affected parent produces one or more affected children. Thus occasionally a person can carry the relevant gene but not manifest the condition. Such occurrences are described as non-penetrance. The **penetrance** of a character is defined as the proportion of people with the relevant genotype who show the character.

Penetrance is a property of both the gene and the character. Different syndromes show characteristically different penetrances, but different features of a syndrome can also have different penetrances. Penetrance can also be age-related, as with Huntington disease.

Non-penetrance is a pitfall in both pedigree interpretation and counseling. *Figure 1.14* shows an example. Individual III-11 must carry the disease gene despite being unaffected. Before starting a family he might have requested counseling to find out his risk of having a child with the family disease. The counselor would have had to know the penetrance of that particular condition in order to be able to calculate the risk that, despite being phenotypically normal, he might be a non-penetrant gene carrier. Fortunately in many cases a molecular test would be available that could give a definitive answer.

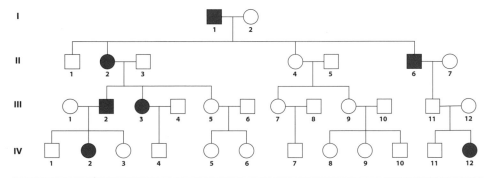

Figure 1.14 – Pedigree of an autosomal dominant condition with reduced penetrance.
The condition is non-penetrant in individual III-11. Other unaffected individuals in generation IV who have an affected parent might also be non-penetrant gene carriers.

Reduced penetrance is a nuisance for counselors, but there is no mystery about why it happens. The surprise is really that some conditions show 100% penetrance. For such a condition, if you have the relevant gene then you will inevitably manifest the condition, absolutely regardless of all your other genes, your environment and your lifestyle. For many conditions, having the gene means that you are highly likely to manifest the condition, but occasionally a lucky combination of other genes and/or environmental factors will save you.

There is a complete spectrum of characters and genes, from 100% penetrance down to very low penetrance (*Figure 1.15*). For example, in cancer research there is much interest in identifying low-penetrance genes that make a person more likely to develop cancer, but do not in any way make that fate inevitable (see *Chapter 12*). Characters at the high-penetrance end of the spectrum are usefully described as mendelian, while those at the low-penetrance end would be called multifactorial (see *Chapter 13*). There is no hard and fast rule where the changeover occurs. Reduced penetrance must occur with characters showing recessive inheritance, but it would be much less obvious from the pedigree, so in practice incomplete penetrance is largely a problem of dominant conditions.

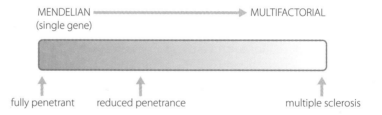

Figure 1.15 – Continuum of penetrance.
There is a continuum of penetrance from fully penetrant conditions, where other genes and environmental factors have no effect, through to low-penetrance genes that simply play a small part, along with other genetic and environmental factors, in determining a person's susceptibility to a disease. Multiple sclerosis is used as an example of a multifactorial condition where genetic factors play a major part in determining susceptibility, but current research suggests that each individual factor has very low penetrance (see *Chapter 13*).

Genetic conditions often show **variable expression**. That is, the full-blown condition involves a number of features, but many affected people show only some of those features, or may show a certain feature to differing degrees. Type 1 neurofibromatosis (NF1; see *Disease box 1*) is an example of a common autosomal dominant condition that is very variable. We could say that each feature of the syndrome has its own characteristic penetrance, or we could say that the syndrome as a whole shows variable expressivity. Either way, this is a reflection of the fact that genes do not act in isolation, but against a background of innumerable other genes and a variable environment. Each child of somebody with NF1 has a 50% chance of inheriting the disease gene, and this might be checked with a DNA test, but the test cannot tell us how severely a child would be affected.

Type 1 Neurofibromatosis (OMIM 162200)

NF1, also known as von Recklinghausen disease, is an autosomal dominant condition caused by mutations in the *NF1* gene on chromosome 17. The disease affects about 1 person in 3500 and is seen in both sexes and all ethnic groups. Penetrance is complete, in that some feature of the condition can be found in every affected person, but the disease can manifest in many ways and varies greatly in severity (see *Box figure 1.1*).

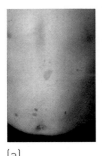

(a)

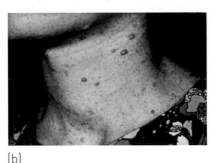

(b)

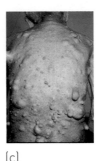

(c)

Box figure 1.1 – NF1. Mildly affected patients show only café-au-lait skin macules (a), Lisch nodules (hamartomas in the iris) and/or axillary freckling. Dermal neurofibromas (b) are frequent, and they can be numerous and grossly disfiguring (c).

NF1 patients are also liable to develop a variety of benign or malignant tumors, including nerve sheath tumors and gliomas and other tumors in the central nervous system. Occasionally NF1 patients have learning difficulties, short stature or seizures.

Counseling in NF1 can be difficult. Approximately half of all cases represent new mutations (a common observation with clinically severe dominant conditions, see *Chapter 10*). Patients with no family history may not understand the genetic risks, and mildly affected people may not appreciate that their children could be severely affected. Although the *NF1* gene has been cloned, molecular testing for mutations is difficult because the gene is large (59 exons covering 350 kb of genomic DNA, see *Chapter 3*). Even if DNA analysis does characterize the mutation in a family, it cannot predict how severely affected a mutation carrier will be.

NF1 is a prime example of the problems of variable expression in an autosomal dominant disease.

Rarer modes of inheritance

X-linked dominant inheritance

For males, X-linked diseases are neither dominant nor recessive, because dominance and recessiveness are properties of heterozygotes, and males have only a single X chromosome. As explained further in *Chapter 7*, the phenomenon of X-inactivation means that even for heterozygous females, dominance and recessiveness are not as clear-cut for X-linked as for autosomal conditions. Most X-linked diseases seldom affect heterozygous females significantly, and so are described as recessive. Occasional X-linked conditions do commonly affect heterozygotes badly, and so are dominant. An example is X-linked hypophosphatemia (OMIM 307800; an inability of the kidneys to retain phosphate, leading to vitamin D-resistant rickets). At first sight the pedigree pattern (*Figure 1.16*) might well be interpreted as autosomal dominant. Consistent with this interpretation, there is a vertical pedigree pattern and on average 50% of the children of an affected person are affected. However, a male passes his X chromosome to all his daughters but none of his sons. Thus all the daughters but none of the sons of an affected father are affected. Because of X-inactivation, X-linked dominant conditions tend to be milder and more variable in females than in males.

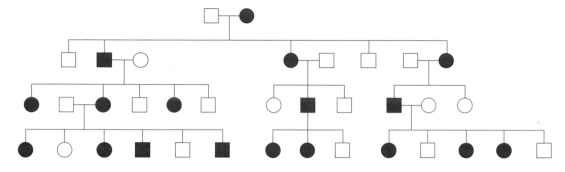

Figure 1.16 – Pedigree of an X-linked dominant condition.
Although heterozygous females are affected, such conditions are usually milder and more variable in females than in males.

X-linked inheritance with cellular interference

The X-linked craniofrontonasal syndrome (CFNS, OMIM 304100) shows a very unusual pattern of inheritance: heterozygous females are more severely affected than hemizygous males. Females have a variety of craniofacial and skeletal problems, while males have no or minimal signs, despite carrying the causative mutation in every cell (*Figure 1.17*).

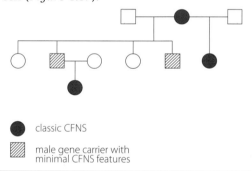

● classic CFNS

▨ male gene carrier with minimal CFNS features

Figure 1.17 – A pedigree of craniofrontonasal syndrome.
Females with filled symbols have typical features of the syndrome; males with hatched symbols are proven gene carriers but have only slight hypertelorism (wide spacing of the eyes). Redrawn from Wieland *et al.* (2004).

CFNS is caused by loss of function mutations in *EFNB1*, a gene that encodes an ephrin cell-signaling molecule. Ephrin on a cell surface causes repulsive interactions with cells that carry a matching ephrin receptor. These interactions are important for establishing boundaries between cell types during development. Because of X-inactivation, females heterozygous for a loss of function mutation in *EFNB1* have clones of cells lacking this ephrin, which therefore fail to establish correct tissue boundaries. The mild phenotype in males, who totally lack the *EFNB1* product, suggests that other members of the ephrin gene family are able to take over, provided there are no *EFNB1*-positive cells to confuse the picture. A similar interference between allelic gene products might occur in other molecular interactions, for example between subunits of a multimeric protein, where homozygotes for either allele are normal but heterozygotes show abnormalities.

Other causes of sex bias

A sex bias is not a reliable indicator of X-linkage. An autosomal condition may affect just one sex for anatomical or physiological reasons. For example, ovarian cancer may be caused by mutations in the *BRCA2* gene on chromosome 13, but obviously affects only females. Such conditions are called **sex-limited**. Sometimes a condition may be lethal in one sex but not the other. If this happens before birth, the result is a condition seen in only one sex. This is most likely with X-linked dominant conditions where heterozygous females survive but affected males die *in utero*. An example is Rett syndrome (OMIM 312750 – see *Disease box 7*). Affected males normally miscarry early in pregnancy, so the classical syndrome is only seen in girls. A few affected males do in fact survive to birth, but their phenotype is so different that its cause was not recognized until molecular tests demonstrated that they had mutations in *MECP2*, which is the gene mutated in most cases of Rett syndrome.

Y-linked inheritance

For a condition determined by a gene on the Y chromosome the inheritance pattern would be simple and striking. It would affect only males, and all the sons of an affected man would be affected. However, the Y chromosome carries only about 50 genes, and since females manage perfectly well without any of them, none of these genes can be essential to life or general health. Y-linked genes are important for male sexual function, and abnormalities of the Y chromosome are a common cause of male infertility. Such abnormalities are clinically important, but because the resulting phenotype is infertility, they do not segregate in multi-generation pedigrees.

Mitochondrial inheritance

The problem in the Fletcher family – Case 6 (*Figure 1.12*) illustrates an unusual mode of inheritance. All the previous cases have involved the chromosomal DNA in the cell nucleus. But, as we shall see in *Chapter 3*, mitochondria also contain DNA. Mutations in the mitochondrial DNA (mtDNA) are responsible for a few diseases, including the Fletcher case. Note four important points:

(1) All the mitochondria of an embryo are derived from the egg, and none from the sperm. This gives rise to a matrilineal pattern of inheritance: mitochondrial mutations are passed on by the mother, but never by the father. Most conditions caused by mutations in mtDNA affect both sexes equally. Leber hereditary optic neuropathy is unusual in that, for unknown reasons, it affects mostly males.

(2) Most of the components and functions of mitochondria are controlled by genes located on the chromosomes in the nucleus (see *Chapter 3*). Most diseases caused by malfunction of mitochondria therefore follow typical mendelian inheritance patterns. Only a very few mitochondrial diseases are caused by mutations in the mtDNA and follow the pattern of inheritance we see in the Fletcher case.

(3) Because each cell contains many mitochondria, people can have a mix of normal and mutant mitochondria in each cell (**heteroplasmy**). The proportion can vary between tissues and in the same tissue over time.

This helps explain why diseases caused by mitochondrial mutations typically have low penetrance and extremely variable expressivity.

(4) Ova contain many mitochondria; therefore a heteroplasmic mother can have heteroplasmic children. This is in stark contrast to mosaicism for nuclear abnormalities (chromosomal or single gene), which cannot be inherited (see below and *Chapter 2*)

Some further problems in pedigree interpretation

A condition is not necessarily genetic just because it is **congenital** (present at birth) or **familial** (tending to run in families). Huntington disease is an example of a condition that is genetic but not congenital, while many birth defects (congenital by definition) are caused by environmental teratogens (rubella or thalidomide, for example). Unless a familial condition shows a clear-cut mendelian pedigree pattern or a demonstrable chromosomal abnormality, it can be very difficult to decide what role genes play in its causation. Innumerable behavioral and occasional physical characters can be the result of shared family environment rather than genes. *Chapter 13* describes how these 'nature – nurture' problems can be approached. The converse is also true: a negative family history does not rule out a genetic cause for a problem. This is especially true of autosomal recessive conditions, as illustrated here by the cystic fibrosis case of the Brown family (Case 2), but it may also be seen with an autosomal dominant or X-linked condition where cases are often the result of new mutations. *Chapter 10* explains why new mutations are frequent with some genetic conditions and rare with others.

Mosaicism

A person whose body contains two or more genetically different cell lines is called a **mosaic**. As explained in *Chapter 2*, the process of mitosis should ensure that every cell in the body carries a complete and identical set of genes. Our discussion so far has tacitly assumed that if a person has a mutation, it is present in every cell of his body. This is true of inherited mutations, but what about freshly arising mutations? Mutations can happen to any cell at any time. Only the descendants of that cell will carry the mutation. Given the number of cells in the human body, and typical mutation rates of genes, it is clear that everybody will have the odd cell or small clone of cells carrying a mutation in almost any gene you care to think of. Normally these odd rogue clones will have absolutely no effect. There are three circumstances in which mosaicism may be clinically important:

(1) if the mutant cells have a tendency to grow and take over – see *Chapter 12*

(2) if the mutation arose sufficiently early in embryonic development that the mutant line makes up a significant part of the whole body. The person may show features of the disease, maybe with a milder phenotype (if the product of the mutated gene is diffusible) or with a patchy distribution reflecting the distribution of mutant cells (if the gene product remains in the cell where it is produced)

(3) if the mutation affects the **germ line** (sperm or egg cells or their progenitors)

Germ-line mosaicism is a major source of uncertainty and confusion in pedigree interpretation and genetic counseling. A person who by all clinical and genetic tests is entirely normal may produce several children with the same dominant or X-linked disease if he or she has a germ-line clone of mutant cells. When a normal couple have a child with a dominant condition, with no previous family history, this is evidently a new mutation. The counselor must remember that one or other parent may be a germ-line mosaic. The risk of recurrence is rarely possible to quantify, because we have no idea what proportion of germ-line cells carry the mutation, but it is not negligible. If a normal couple have two or more affected children, the pedigree pattern (*Figure 1.18*) looks recessive because the parents are unaffected. Misinterpreting the condition as recessive would cause serious errors when the affected children ask about their risk of passing it on. The risk would be very low for a rare recessive condition, but 50% for a dominant condition.

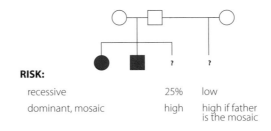

RISK:		
recessive	25%	low
dominant, mosaic	high	high if father is the mosaic

Figure 1.18 – A problem in counseling.
A couple with no previous family history of this condition have two affected children. Is this an autosomal recessive condition, or is it autosomal dominant with one of the parents being a germinal mosaic? The risks are very different depending which theory is correct.

1.5. References

Weiland I *et al*. (2004) Mutations of the Ephrin-B1 gene cause craniofrontonasal syndrome. *Am. J. Hum. Genet.* **74**: 1209–1215.

Useful website

For detailed information on genetic deafness see the Hereditary Hearing Loss Homepage: http://hereditaryhearingloss.org

1.6. Self-assessment questions

Each of the following 10 pedigrees shows a rare disease.

(a) Identify the most likely mode of inheritance, chosen from autosomal dominant (fully penetrant), autosomal dominant with about 90% penetrance, autosomal recessive or X-linked recessive

(b) Define the risk that the next child of the arrowed person or people will be affected.

Hints on pedigrees 1–4 are provided in the *Guidance* section at the back of the book.

SAQ 1

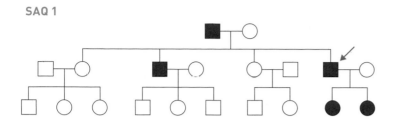

SAQ 2

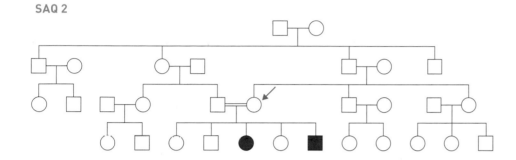

SAQ 3

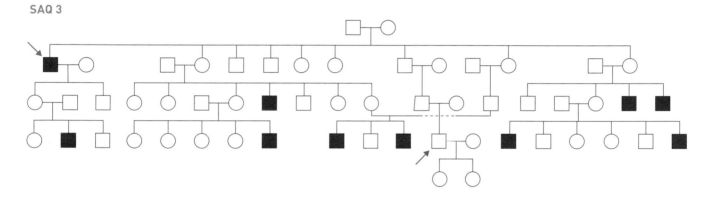

SAQ 4   SAQ 5

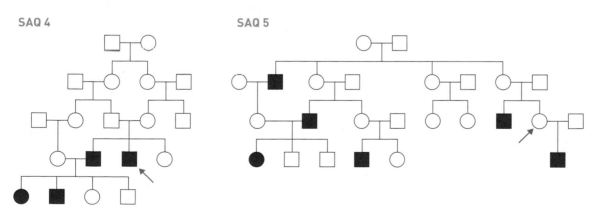

SAQ 6

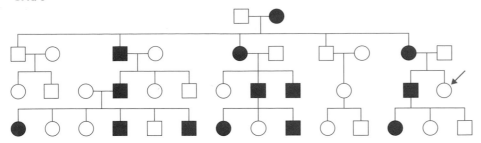

SAQ 7

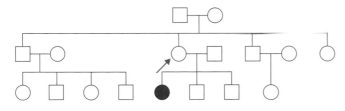

SAQ 8

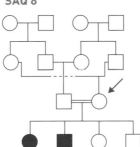

SAQ 9

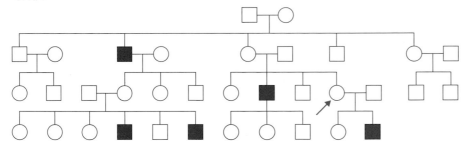

SAQ 10

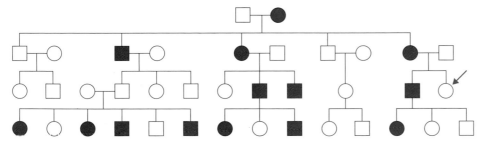

02 | How can a patient's chromosomes be studied?

After working through this chapter you should be able to:

- Describe the results of mitosis and meiosis, and how these are achieved
- Identify normal and simple abnormal karyotypes
- Describe human sex determination and the effects of errors
- Describe triploidy, trisomy, reciprocal translocations, robertsonian translocations, paracentric inversions, pericentric inversions, deletions and copy number variants
- Explain the origins of the main types of numerical and structural chromosome abnormalities
- Work out the main possible reproductive outcomes for carriers of translocations or inversions

2.1. Case studies

| CASE 7 | Green family | **25** | 38 | 68 | 101 | 389 |

- Girl (Gillian) aged 3 years
- Slow to develop
- ? Chromosome abnormality
- Order tests to check for microdeletion at 22q11

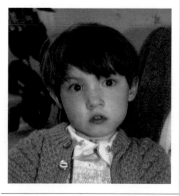

Figure 2.1 – Child with 22q11 deletion. Note small mouth, narrow nose and upward slant of her eyes.

Gillian is the second child born to healthy parents. Everything seemed fine at birth although her birth weight was less than her sister's. At her routine neonatal examination the doctor heard a heart murmur and referred her for an echocardiogram. This showed that she had a small hole between the two lower chambers of her heart (a ventricular septal defect - VSD). It was not considered serious and follow-up was recommended. By 3 years of age the murmur had disappeared and a further echocardiogram showed the VSD had closed. However, Gillian's parents were still worried about her since all her developmental milestones had been slower than her sister's. Her speech development had been particularly slow and she was difficult to understand. The pediatrician referred her for speech studies and she was found to have poor movements of her palate. He then asked the opinion of a clinical geneticist. The geneticist noted that Gillian had a very narrow nose, over-folding of the upper part of her ears, and long fingers. He organized a chromosome test and in addition to the routine karyotype requested a molecular test to see if there was a deletion of part of chromosome 22 (22q11).

| CASE 8 | Howard family | **26** | 38 | 69 | 102 | 277 | 389 |

- Helen – new-born daughter of Henry and Anne (33 years old)
- Down syndrome
- Risk of recurrence if they have more children?

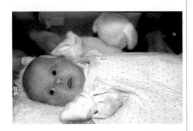

Figure 2.2 – A child with Down syndrome.

Pregnancy was a surprise for Helen's parents Anne and Henry who were both 33 years old. They had had a son and daughter when they were in their early 20s. Nevertheless when they got used to the idea they were pleased. At the antenatal clinic they were offered screening tests for Down syndrome but they decided against these since they had had no tests in their previous pregnancies, and anyway, they both agreed they wouldn't really consider a termination of pregnancy. Everything went well in pregnancy and labor started at full term. When Helen was born, Anne thought she looked like her sister but the midwife was worried because she was very hypotonic (floppy), had loose skin at the back of her neck and single creases across her palms. The pediatrician was called and gently told Anne and Henry that he was concerned that Helen might have Down syndrome. He arranged to send a blood sample to the cytogenetics laboratory and requested that the result be sent as soon as possible since by now the parents and grandparents were extremely anxious. The pediatrician and the midwife saw the family several times over the next two days until the result was available. This confirmed that Helen did indeed have Down syndrome. The parents had lots of questions about Helen's future which the pediatrician answered, but he suggested he refer them to the genetic clinic in a few weeks' time to respond to their questions about how Down syndrome occurs and whether, if they were to have more children, there would be a high risk of recurrence.

| CASE 9 | Ingram family | **26** | 41 | 69 | 104 | 187 | 389 |

- Isabel – first daughter of Irene and Ian
- Small stature despite tall parents

Isabel was the first baby born to Irene and Ian who were both quite tall. She had some swelling of her feet for the first few months, and was quite petite, but in general she was a healthy little baby. She developed normally in childhood but was always the smallest in the class. By 10 years of age, her classmates' growth rate had increased and a couple of her friends had even started puberty. Although Irene and Ian were not really worried, the school nurse suggested that Isabel be referred to a pediatrician since her small stature seemed unusual given her parents' height. As part of her initial investigations the pediatrician requested a chromosome analysis.

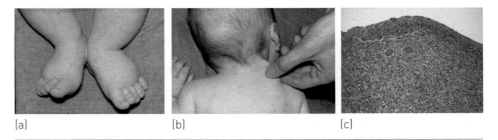

(a)　　　　　　　　　(b)　　　　　　　　　(c)

Figure 2.3 – Turner syndrome.
(a) Puffy feet, (b) redundant skin at back of neck. (c) Histology of gonads: ovarian cortical stroma devoid of germ cell elements. Photo. (c) courtesy of Dr Godfrey Wilson, Manchester Royal Infirmary.

2.2. **Science toolkit**

Why clinicians need to know about chromosomes

Chromosome abnormalities are important in a number of different clinical situations:

- they are a cause of infertility and recurrent miscarriages
- over 50% of embryos that abort spontaneously in the first trimester have a chromosomal abnormality
- about 1 newborn in 200 has multiple congenital abnormalities because of a chromosomal abnormality. Prenatal screening can detect most such abnormalities in time for the pregnancy to be terminated, if the parents so wish
- most chromosomally abnormal babies are born to parents who are entirely normal, but about 1% of people have a subtle chromosomal change that has no effect on their own health, but puts them at high risk of having miscarriages or abnormal babies
- cancer cells typically acquire extensive chromosome abnormalities not present in the normal cells of the patient, and many particular abnormalities have diagnostic and prognostic significance

How are chromosomes studied?

If you want to study chromosomes under the microscope you need dividing cells. As described below, chromosomes are only visible in cells that are in the act of dividing. Taking blood, skin or other samples from a person will yield plenty of cells, but few if any will be dividing. Thus chromosome analysis usually involves taking a sample of non-dividing cells, which are then cultured in the laboratory and persuaded to divide (*Figure 2.4*). Suitable sources are shown in *Box 2.1*. In addition to the methods for studying chromosomes that are described in this chapter, a set of more recent techniques collectively called molecular cytogenetics can be used either to study chromosomes in much finer detail or to check chromosome numbers in non-dividing cells. These are described in *Chapter 4*.

Karyotyping by standard microscopic analysis involves preparing a slide on which a number of dividing cells can be examined, following the protocol of *Figure 2.4*. *Figure 2.10* shows one such cell. The cytogeneticist counts the chromosomes, identifies each one and checks that its structure appears normal. The analysis is typically based on 10 cells, so that if a particular feature is not clear in one cell it can be checked in others. For record-keeping, the chromosomes in one cell are arranged (usually by manipulation of a digital image) into a standard karyogram (often loosely called a karyotype) as in *Figures 2.9* or *2.11*. This is the only method of surveying the entire genome for *any* numerical or structural chromosomal abnormality.

Chromosomes are always prepared from dividing cells, in which the DNA has already been replicated, and therefore under the microscope they are always seen to consist of two identical sister chromatids joined at the centromere. In former times the standard preparation protocols made this structure very clear (see inset

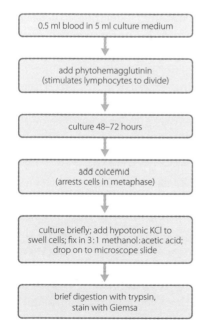

Figure 2.4 – Flowchart for processing a blood sample to obtain a standard G-banded chromosome preparation.

BOX 2.1

Material for chromosome analysis

- **Peripheral blood lymphocytes** are the commonest material used. 0.5–10 ml of blood is treated with phytohemagglutinin, which stimulates lymphocytes to divide. Cultures are harvested after 48 hours. The protocol is summarized in *Figure 2.4*.

- **Chorionic villi** are used for early prenatal diagnosis. They are usually collected at 10–12 weeks' gestation by transvaginal or transabdominal routes. The procedure carries around an additional 2% risk of causing a miscarriage over the background risk. Spontaneously dividing cells are present and can be used for rapid analysis, but results are best confirmed on cultured cells. It is important to dissect out fetal material in order to avoid culturing maternal cells.

- **Amniotic fluid** collected at 14–18 weeks' gestation contains shed fetal cells. These are slow to grow and require around 2 weeks in culture to provide enough dividing cells for analysis. Amniocentesis carries an increased risk of around 0.5–1% over the background risk of causing a miscarriage.

- **Skin biopsies** are used to look for chromosomal abnormalities that may not be present in blood.

- **Testicular biopsies** are the only way to study male meiosis. In females, meiosis takes place in the fetal ovaries before birth, so there is no way of investigating meiosis clinically in a female patient.

to *Figure 2.10*). The centromere and sister chromatids are much less obvious in chromosomes prepared according to current protocols, which leave the sister chromatids pressed tightly together. Cytogeneticists rely more on the banding pattern for identifying each individual chromosome and detecting structural aberrations. Banding makes each chromosome stain in a reproducible and characteristic pattern of dark and light bands. The usual method is G-banding. This involves subjecting the chromosomes, spread out on a microscope slide, to a brief digestion with trypsin, followed by staining with Giemsa stain. Other banding methods are sometimes used for particular analyses. R-banding produces a reversed pattern of dark and light bands, useful for checking chromosome ends. Other specialized procedures stain centromeres (C-banding) or the short arms of the acrocentric chromosomes (silver staining).

Chromosomal locations are named according to the Paris Convention as described in *Box 2.2*. Bands are numbered counting outwards from the centromere. *Figure 2.5* shows the standard ideograms and nomenclature of G-banded chromosomes at a resolution of 550 bands. Higher resolutions can be obtained by harvesting the cells well before the chromosomes become maximally contracted at metaphase of cell division (see *Figure 2.6*). In these highly extended chromosomes, bands split into sub-bands and sub-sub-bands, allowing more precise localizations such as 7q11.23 (pronounced '7q one one point two three'). However, longer chromosomes are more likely to be tangled up, making analysis under the microscope at the highest resolutions (1500–2000 bands) very difficult. Abnormalities too small to be seen by standard 550-band analysis are best detected by switching to molecular methods. We will see this process in action as we follow the case of **Gillian Green (Case 7)**.

BOX 2.2

Chromosomes and their abnormalities: nomenclature and glossary

Karyotypes are described by the number of chromosomes, the sex chromosome constitution, and any abnormality. Locations on chromosomes are described in relation to the Paris Convention of nomenclature shown in *Figure 2.5*. p means the short arm, q the long arm, t signifies a translocation, del a deletion, dup a duplication, inv an inversion, and der a derivative chromosome, whose structure would then be specified.

- 46,XX – a normal female
- 47,XY,+21 – a male with trisomy 21
- 46,XX,t(1;22)(q25;q13) – a female with a translocation between chromosomes 1 and 22 with breakpoints at 1q25 and 22q13 (the abnormality in **Case 5**, *Figure 2.14*)
- 46,XY,del(2)(q34;q36.2) – a male with a deletion on the long arm of chromosome 2 taking out the material between 2q34 and 2q36.2.

This is enough detail for present purposes. For the full nomenclature, covering every possible abnormality, see Shaffer and Tommerup (2005).

Acrocentric – a chromosome that has its centromere close to one end – chromosomes 13, 14, 15, 21, 22 and Y.

Autosome – any chromosome that is not the X or Y sex chromosome.

Centromere – the position on a chromosome where the sister chromatids are joined, and where the spindle fibers attach during cell division to pull the chromatids apart.

Chromatid – in a dividing cell, a chromosome consists of two identical sister chromatids joined at the centromere. After cell division, and until the DNA is next replicated, a chromosome consists of a single chromatid.

Chromatin – a general term for the DNA–protein complex that makes up chromosomes.

Euchromatin – chromatin with a relatively open structure in which genes can be active; the opposite of heterochromatin.

G-banding – a standard procedure in which chromosomes are treated so that they stain in a characteristic and reproducible pattern of dark and pale bands, as shown in *Figure 2.5*.

Heterochromatin – chromatin that is highly condensed and genetically inactive. Found mainly at centromeres.

Homologous chromosomes – the two no.1s or 2s etc. in a person. Note that unlike sister chromatids, homologous chromosomes are not copies of one another, and they may differ in small ways (minor DNA sequence differences) or sometimes in large ways (because of translocations, etc.).

Inversion – a structural abnormality in which part of a chromosome is in the wrong orientation compared to the rest (see *Figure 2.19*).

Karyotype – a person's chromosome constitution – also used loosely to describe a display of a person's chromosomes, as in *Figure 2.9*, etc.

Metacentric – a chromosome that has its centromere in the middle (e.g. chromosomes 3 and 20).

Monosomy – having one copy of one particular chromosome, but two of all the others (i.e. 45 in total for an autosomal monosomy).

Robertsonian translocation – a special type of translocation in which two acrocentric chromosomes are joined close to their centromeres as in *Figure 2.20*.

BOX 2.2 – continued

Sister chromatids – the two chromatids of a chromosome as seen in a dividing cell. Sister chromatids are copies of each other, made during the preceding round of DNA replication.

Submetacentric – a chromosome that has a long arm and a short arm, e.g. most human chromosomes.

Telomere – the special structure at the end of a chromosome arm.

Translocation – a structural abnormality in which two chromosomes swap non-homologous segments.

Triploidy – having three complete sets of chromosomes.

Trisomy – having three copies of one particular chromosome, but two of all the others (i.e. 47 in total).

Chromosome abnormalities

Chromosomal abnormalities can involve having the wrong number of chromosomes, or having one or more structurally abnormal chromosomes. The nature and origin of chromosome abnormalities are discussed in more detail in Section 2.4. Several numerical chromosome abnormalities occur sufficiently frequently to produce syndromes that are recognizable clinically (*Box 2.3*). So, for example, the midwife recognized the characteristic features of Down syndrome in Helen Howard (Case 8). Abnormalities of chromosome structure are usually the result of chromosome breakages. Certain chromosome regions are predisposed to specific breakages which produce recognizable syndromes (*Box 2.4*). An alert clinician would suspect one such syndrome in the case of Gillian Green (Case 7). Most structural abnormalities, however, are one-off events caused by random chromosome breaks. Although these do not produce specific named syndromes, clinicians have learned to suspect a chromosomal abnormality in babies who have multiple congenital abnormalities that are not ascribable to failure of one specific developmental event, or in patients with a combination of mental retardation and dysmorphism. For these reasons it would be appropriate to request chromosome analysis in the case of Elizabeth Elliot (Case 5).

Why do we have chromosomes?

A human cell contains 2 m of DNA. Imagine a typical cell, 10 µm across, expanded to the size of a lecture room 10 m across. The DNA would be represented by 2000 km of string, occupying much of the space in the room. Now replicate the DNA, turning each single strand of string into a double strand like a twin electric flex. And now you must divide the cell. In about an hour a cell succeeds in precisely dividing its replicated DNA, so that each daughter cell gets exactly one copy of every piece of DNA. If you are going to avoid hopeless tangles and confusion in your lecture room full of twin flex, you need to organize it in some very precise way. That is what chromosomes do in a cell.

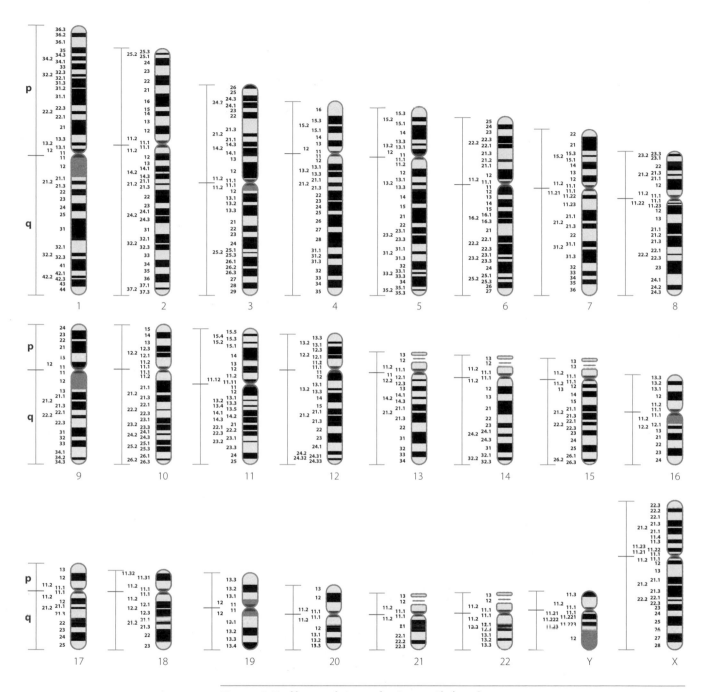

Figure 2.5 – Nomenclature of cytogenetic bands.
The ideograms show ideal G-banding patterns at 550 band resolution. Major bands are labeled 1, 2, 3, etc., going from centromere to telomere. Major band 11q1 (11q means the long arm of chromosome 11, 11p the short arm) is divided into sub-bands 11q11 – 11q14, and at the highest resolution 11q14 splits into 11q14.1 – 11q14.3. Redrawn from Shaffer and Tommerup (2005) with permission from S. Karger AG, Basel.

BOX 2.3

Syndromes due to numerical chromosome abnormalities

Triploidy (69,XXX, XXY or XYY)

Triploidy is common at conception but triploid embryos and fetuses almost never survive to term, and those that do so do not live for long.

Autosomal trisomies

All possible autosomal trisomies can be found among early miscarriages, but only trisomies 13, 18 and 21 generally survive to term. It may be significant that chromosomes 13, 18 and 21 have the lowest density of genes of any chromosomes in our genome. This means that fewer genes are present in abnormal numbers in these trisomies, compared to trisomies of other similar sized chromosomes. How trisomies originate is discussed below.

- +21 Down syndrome – see **Case 8**. The only autosomal trisomy compatible with survival into adult life.

- +18 Edwards syndrome – affected babies normally die in the first year of life. Although they can be externally relatively normal, they have subtle signs, are growth retarded and have many internal malformations. Rare long-term survivors show very little developmental progress.

- +13 Patau syndrome – 50% of affected babies die in the first month, and the rest within the first year. They can have mid-line malformations of the head and face, ranging from mild (closely-spaced eyes, central cleft lip) to very severe (gross malformations of the face with a single central eye and holoprosencephaly – failure of the brain to develop two hemispheres). Polydactyly is another common feature.

Sex chromosome abnormalities

Having wrong numbers of sex chromosomes is much less deleterious than having wrong numbers of autosomes. For the Y chromosome this is because it carries very few genes, and none are essential to life. The X chromosome is different: it carries about 1000 genes including many that are essential to life, but the mechanism of X-inactivation (see *Chapter 7*) greatly reduces the effect of having differing numbers of X chromosomes.

As the examples below show, a person is male if he has a Y chromosome, regardless of the number of X chromosomes. The *SRY* gene on the Y chromosome is believed to be the master switch in sexual differentiation (see *Disease box 6*).

- 45,X   Turner syndrome – females, pubertal failure, infertile, often short stature, normal intelligence. May have neck webbing, heart defects (coarctation) and horseshoe kidneys.

- 47,XXY   Klinefelter syndrome – males, pubertal failure, infertile and often tall with female distribution of body fat. There may be a slightly lowered IQ compared to siblings.

- 47,XXX   females, mostly undiagnosed because they are relatively normal. There may be a slightly lowered IQ compared to siblings.

- 47,XYY   males, tall, possibly mildly reduced intelligence but within the normal range. The great majority of XYY men are living normal lives and are not diagnosed, but there may be a slightly increased risk of behavior problems.

BOX 2.4

Recurrent microdeletion and microduplication syndromes

A number of well-recognized clinical syndromes are caused by **microdeletions** or **microduplications**. These involve a change in a chromosomal segment that is too small to be noticed on a standard chromosome preparation like the one shown in *Figure 2.9*. When an alert clinician suspects such a change on clinical grounds it can be detected and characterized using the molecular cytogenetic techniques described in *Chapter 4*. Some well-defined microdeletion or microduplication syndromes are listed in the table below.

Syndrome	Location of change	Comments
3q29 duplication	Dup at 3q29	Mental retardation, facial dysmorphism
Wolf–Hirschhorn	Del at 4p16	Low birthweight, mental retardation, fits, typical face
Cri-du-chat	Del at 5p15	Mental retardation, typical face, high-pitched cry
Williams–Beuren	Del at 7q11.23	See *Disease box 3*
Angelman	Del at 15q11–q13	See *Chapter 7*
Prader–Willi	Del at 15q11–q13	See *Chapter 7*
Miller–Dieker	Del at 17p13	Lissencephaly, mental retardation, typical face
Smith–Magenis	Del at 17p11.2	Mental retardation, behavioral problems, abnormal sleep patterns
Potocki–Lupski	Dup at 17p11.2	Developmental delay, autistic spectrum disorder
Di George–VCFS	Del at 22q11	See **Case 7, Green family**
22q11.2 duplication	Dup at 22q11	Phenotype very variable, mild mental retardation to multiple defects

Many other one-off or recurrent microdeletions have been described. Of those listed in the table, Wolf–Hirschhorn, cri-du-chat and Miller–Dieker syndromes involve deletion of the end of a chromosome arm. These are usually the result of random breakages and the proximal breakpoint varies between different patients but the deletion always encompasses a critical region specific to the syndrome. The other syndromes in the table normally have exactly the same breakpoints in every patient. These usually arise through recombination between misaligned low-copy DNA repeats, as explained in *Disease box 3*. For each of these microdeletion syndromes, there is a corresponding microduplication syndrome, although the clinical features of the duplication syndrome may be less specific.

Centromeres and telomeres

Chromosomes are not simply passive packages of DNA. They are functional cellular organelles, and parts of their function depend on two special structures, centromeres and telomeres.

- A functional chromosome must have one, and only one, centromere. As mentioned previously, the two sister chromatids are joined at the centromere. Importantly, the centromere (or strictly, the kinetochore, a structure located at the centromere) is the attachment point for the spindle fibers that pull the chromosomes apart during cell division (see below).

- Telomeres are special structures at each end of a chromosome. Telomeres contain long arrays of tandemly repeated DNA sequences, $(TTAGGG)_n$. Because of the detailed enzymology of DNA replication, each chromosome end loses around 10–20 repeat units each time a cell divides (see *Figure 12.3*). If the telomere is totally lost the chromosome becomes unstable, normally leading to cell death. Some theories link this process with ordinary aging, but that is controversial. Telomeres have enough repeats to survive the cell divisions that occur within the lifetime of a person, but between generations they need to be renewed. Germ-line cells, and also cancer cells, produce a special enzyme, **telomerase,** that is able to restore telomeres to full length, helping to make such cells immortal.

The behavior of chromosomes during cell division

Preparing to divide

As discussed above, the primary function of chromosomes is to allow cells to distribute their DNA to daughter cells in an orderly fashion.

(a) *Replicating the DNA.* Each chromosome initially contains a single immensely long DNA double helix. When a cell is preparing to divide, during S phase of the cell cycle, the DNA is replicated, but the two copies remain attached to each other. Each chromosome then consists of two identical sister chromatids, each containing a full copy of the DNA double helix and joined together at the centromere. As seen under the microscope, chromosomes always have this structure (even though, as mentioned above, the two sister chromatids are rarely distinct in standard preparations) – but it is important to remember that the normal state of a chromosome in a non-dividing cell is as a single chromatid.

(b) *Condensing the chromosomes.* During the early part of cell division (**prophase**) the chromosomes become much more compact, until they become visible under the microscope.

What is seen next depends on what daughter cell is to be produced. There are two sorts of cell division:

- **Mitosis** is the normal form of cell division, and the form in which chromosomes are almost always studied for clinical purposes. In mitosis the replicated DNA is divided exactly equally between the two daughter cells, so that they are genetically identical.
- **Meiosis** is a specialized form of cell division that is used only to produce gametes (sperm or eggs). Meiosis has two purposes. First, the number of chromosomes must be reduced from 46 to 23, so that when the sperm and egg fuse, the result is a 46 chromosome zygote. Second, meiosis uses two mechanisms, described below, to ensure that every gamete carries a novel and unique combination of the parental genes. As mentioned in *Box 2.1*, clinically meiosis can be studied in males through a testicular biopsy, and this may be part of investigations of male infertility. Female meiosis is virtually impossible to study in humans because most stages take place in the fetus before birth. However, the consequences of errors in meiosis are central to clinical cytogenetics.

Mitosis

In mitosis (*Figure 2.6*), when each chromosome becomes visible it consists of two highly condensed sister chromatids held together at the centromere. At the end of prophase the nuclear membrane dissolves and the chromosomes move to the center of the cell. The positions of the nuclei of the two daughter cells are already marked by radiating arrays of microtubules. These attach to the centromere of each individual chromosome. Each chromosome is held by microtubules radiating from both ends of the cell. The microtubules contract, pulling the chromosomes to lie on the equatorial plane of the cell (**metaphase**). Eventually the centromere of each chromosome splits, so that as the microtubules continue to contract, one chromatid of each chromosome is pulled to each pole of the cell (**anaphase**). Once all the chromatids have arrived at the poles they decondense, nuclear membranes are formed round them, and the cell divides into two daughter cells.

Note the essential feature of mitosis:

- the sister chromatids are copies of each other, and each daughter cell receives one chromatid of each chromosome
- each chromosome behaves independently. Although there are two copies (homologs) of each chromosome, the two do not interact in any way. Look at *Figure 2.10* and note the random arrangement of the chromosomes in the spread. This is a key difference between mitosis and meiosis.

Meiosis

As mentioned above, meiosis is the highly specialized form of cell division that is used only to produce gametes (*Figure 2.7*). Gametes have 23 chromosomes and each gamete is genetically unique. Meiosis consists of two successive cell divisions; meiosis II is similar to mitosis, but meiosis I has special features.

During prophase I the chromosomes condense and become visible, as in mitosis, but in meiosis I the bodies that appear are not 46 separate chromosomes but 23 bivalents (*Figure 2.8*). Each bivalent is a four-stranded structure, consisting of two homologous chromosomes (the two no. 1s, etc.), each of which consists of two sister chromatids. The two sister chromatids of a chromosome are identical, because they are copies of each other, but the two homologs are not identical. You might think of each as a long line of pigeon-holes. Each will have the same set of pigeon-holes, but the content of corresponding pigeon-holes on the two may be different. For example, near the bottom of the long arm of each copy of chromosome 9 there is a locus (a pigeon-hole) for ABO blood group. But one homolog may carry the A gene and the other the O gene. They are not copies of each other.

The pairing of homologs is extraordinarily accurate. When there is a structural abnormality, so that the homologs do not completely match, matching segments pair (unless this involves tying the chromosomes in impossible knots). *Figure 2.17* shows an example of this effect when there is a translocation, and *Figure 2.21* shows what happens when one homolog has an inversion. In male meiosis the X and Y chromosomes also pair. Although most of their sequence is completely different, there is a short region of homology at the tips of the short arms (the

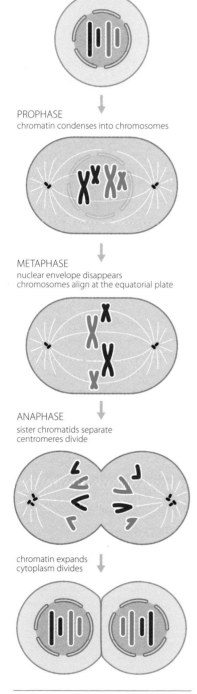

PROPHASE
chromatin condenses into chromosomes

METAPHASE
nuclear envelope disappears
chromosomes align at the equatorial plate

ANAPHASE
sister chromatids separate
centromeres divide

chromatin expands
cytoplasm divides

Figure 2.6 – The stages of mitosis.

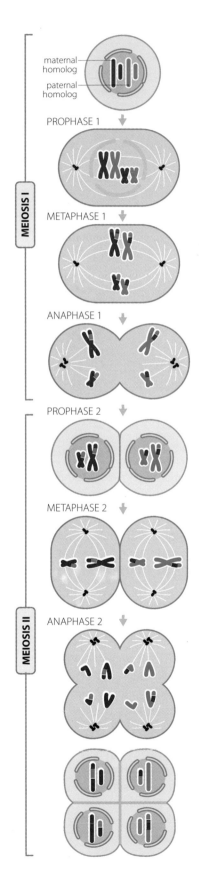

pseudoautosomal region, see *Section 7.2*) and the X and Y use this to pair end-to-end.

At anaphase I the spindle fibers pull the chromosomes apart. In mitosis the centromere of each individual chromosome splits and the two sister chromatids are pulled apart; but in meiosis I the two homologous chromosomes pull apart, each still consisting of two sister chromatids joined at the centromere. Thus at the end of meiosis I each daughter cell has 23 chromosomes, each of which consists of two sister chromatids. In meiosis II the sister chromatids are pulled apart, just as in mitosis, so that the final product of meiosis is four cells, each containing 23 single-chromatid chromosomes. Case 8 (Howard family) and Case 5 (Elliot family) show examples of what can go wrong at this stage.

Whatever its other merits and demerits, sex has one sole purpose in biology: to produce novel combinations of genes. Partly this is achieved simply by involving two different people in the process of sexual reproduction. But there are two additional mechanisms at work generating yet more novelty, and both of these depend on the way chromosomes behave during meiosis (*Figure 2.7*).

(1) When a person forms a gamete, only one of his two no.1 chromosomes will be picked to go into the gamete. It might be the one he got from his mother or it might be the one he got from his father. With each chromosome we have two choices – we could pick the maternal or the paternal one. Over all 23 chromosomes we have $2 \times 2 \times 2 \times 2 \times... = 2^{23}$ different ways of picking the one no. 1, one no. 2, etc. that go into a particular gamete; 2^{23} is 8 388 608.

(2) A second mechanism increases the number of possible variations from 8 million to effectively infinity. As previously mentioned, in the early stages of meiosis homologous chromosomes (the two no. 1s, etc.) pair up. But they don't simply stick together (synapse); they exchange segments. This is genetic recombination. The DNA of one homolog is physically cut and joined to the DNA of the homologous chromosome. Not surprisingly, the mechanism of recombination is complicated. It appears to involve cutting the DNA of the two chromosomes at precisely the same position to the nearest single nucleotide, and joining the ends the other way round. Actually that is not exactly how it is done – in reality, after the first cut, the second is made somewhere in the right vicinity, and then DNA is resynthesized around the position of the crossover to get the correct matching sequences. This complicated process requires many enzymes and is still not very well understood.

Regardless of the precise molecular mechanism, the effect is that homologous chromosomes swap segments. Normally there is at least one crossover (point of recombination between synapsed chromosomes) in each arm of each chromosome

Figure 2.7 – The stages of meiosis.
Meiosis is used only for the production of sperm and eggs. It consists of two successive cell divisions, producing four daughter cells (although in oogenesis only one of these develops into a mature oocyte; the others form the polar bodies). Meiosis has two main functions: to reduce the chromosome number in the gamete to 23, and to ensure that every gamete is genetically unique.

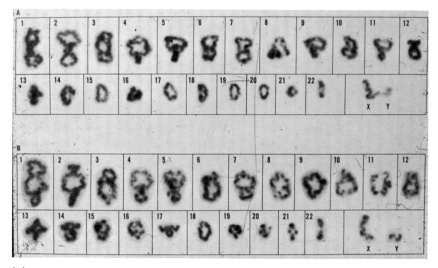

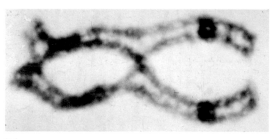

(a)

(b)

Figure 2.8 – Examples of chromosomes during meiosis.
(a) Two cells from a testicular biopsy showing chromosomes during prophase I of male meiosis. Each of the 23 structures is a bivalent, consisting of two homologous chromosomes, each having two chromatids. Note the end-to-end pairing of the X and Y chromosomes. (b) A bivalent seen in meiosis in an amphibian, which has large chromosomes that make the four-stranded structure clear.

pair. On average there are about 60 crossovers in each cell in spermatogenesis, and about 90 in oogenesis, though the actual number varies considerably between people and between cells. To a first approximation, crossovers are distributed at random along each of the 23 pairs of chromosomes (although closer investigation reveals some interesting non-random features). Thus each chromosome in every sperm or egg that a person produces carries a unique combination of genes that came from his or her father and mother. This topic is discussed further in *Chapter 9* where we consider how disease genes can be mapped to a particular chromosomal location, because recombination is the key to genetic mapping.

As a result of these mechanisms, every conceptus is a unique combination of a unique sperm with a unique egg. The only people who are not genetically unique are monozygotic twins, whose cells are all derived by mitosis from a single original conceptus. The fact that monozygotic twins are unique individuals despite being clones reminds us that genetics is not everything in life.

2.3. **Investigations of patients**

CASE 7	Green family	25	**38**	68	101	389

- Girl (Gillian) aged 3 years
- Slow to develop
- ? Chromosome abnormality
- Order tests to check for microdeletion at 22q11

The combination of slow development, a heart defect, palatal problems and mildly dysmorphic features in Gillian suggested a chromosomal abnormality. Blood was taken for cytogenetic analysis, but the result (*Figure 2.9*) was a normal female karyotype, 46,XX. Because of her particular combination of clinical features the geneticist suspected that Gillian might have the Di George – velo-cardio-facial syndrome (VCFS) which is caused by a microdeletion at chromosome 22q11. As described in *Box 2.4*, the Di George–VCFS deletion is too small to be visible under the microscope. He therefore requested a molecular test. The test and its result are described in *Chapter 4*.

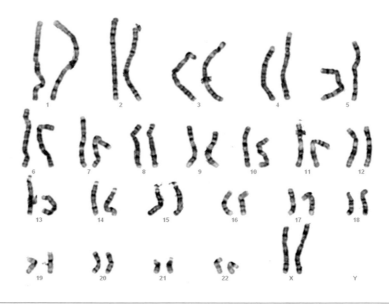

Figure 2.9 – Gillian Green's karyotype.
The result (at this resolution) shows a normal female karyotype, 46,XX.

CASE 8	Howard family	26	**38**	69	102	277	389

- Helen – new-born daughter of Henry and Anne (33 years old)
- Down syndrome
- Risk of recurrence if they have more children?

The clinical diagnosis of Down syndrome in Helen was confirmed by karyotyping. A 2 ml blood sample was taken and, as shown in *Figure 2.4*, the cells were cultured, harvested after 48 hours, spread on a microscope slide and stained by G-banding. The cytogeneticist analysed 10 cells by eye down the microscope (one of the cells is shown in *Figure 2.10*), and for record purposes she used an image analyzer program to arrange chromosomes from one cell into a standard karyotype (*Figure 2.11*). Her report gave the karyotype as 47,XX,+21, confirming that Helen had typical Down syndrome, trisomy 21. An additional reason for checking Helen's karyotype is discussed below in *Section 2.4*.

As expected, the pedigree showed nothing noteworthy (no previous abnormal babies or recurrent miscarriages) in either Anne's or Henry's family, and it is

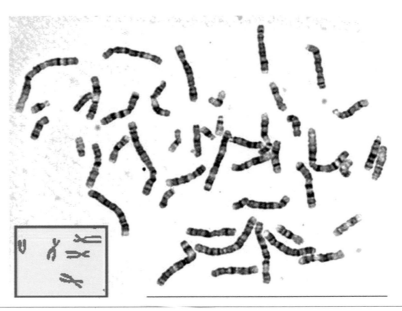

Figure 2.10 – 47,XX,+21 spread.
There are three copies of chromosome 21. Note that homologous chromosomes (the two no. 1s etc.) behave entirely independently in mitosis. The preparation method used here leaves the two sister chromatids of each chromosome tightly pressed together, so that the position of the centromere is not obvious to the eye. This makes the banding pattern easier for the cytogeneticist to recognize. The inset shows some chromosomes that have been handled differently, to make the structure of sister chromatids joined at the centromere more obvious.

not illustrated here. Their first question was why it had happened, and why to them? The counselor explained that it was a one-off accident in meiosis (see *Figure 2.12*). Either the two paired chromosomes 21 (in the first meiotic division), or the two sister chromatids of the one copy of 21 in the second division, had

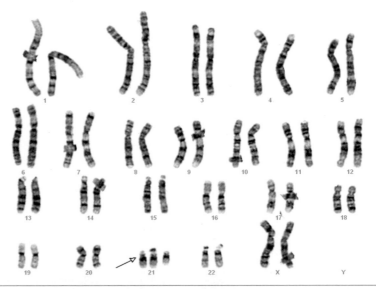

Figure 2.11 – Karyotype showing trisomy 21 (47,XX,+21).

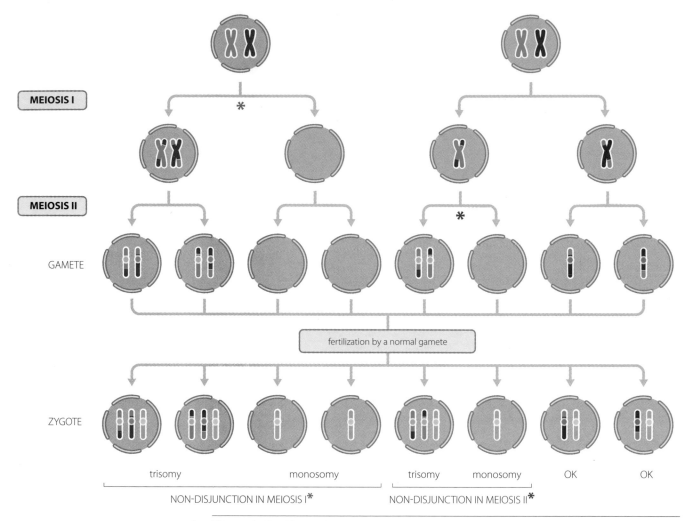

Figure 2.12 – The effects of non-disjunction in meiosis.
The non-disjunction involves only the single pair of chromosomes (meiosis I) or the single chromosome (meiosis II) shown; all the other chromosomes (not shown) disjoin and segregate normally.

failed to disjoin at anaphase and segregate into separate daughter cells. They had both ended up in the same daughter cell, producing an egg or sperm with 24 chromosomes, including two copies of no. 21.

Anne asked if it was always the woman's fault, as she had heard that said. No; in the first place these things are nobody's fault, and secondly, in principle the non-disjunction could happen at either division of meiosis in either parent, though DNA marker studies showed that 70% of cases were due to non-disjunction in the first meiotic division in the mother. This might possibly be a reflection of the extremely long duration of that stage in women, from before birth until whenever the relevant egg ovulated. In men, meiosis goes on continuously in the testes from puberty to old age. The individual risk rises sharply with the age of the mother (*Table 2.1*) but because most babies are born to younger women, most Down syndrome babies are also born to younger mothers. This led to the discussion of population screening that is summarized in *Chapter 11*.

Table 2.1 – Risk of Down syndrome vs. maternal age

Age (years)	20	30	34	36	38	40	42	45
Risk	1 in 1500	1 in 900	1 in 500	1 in 300	1 in 200	1 in 100	1 in 60	1 in 30

With the exception of Turner syndrome (45,X), all the numerical abnormalities listed in *Box 2.3* show a similar age dependence.

Later, Anne and Henry requested an appointment to discuss options for prenatal diagnosis in any subsequent pregnancy. This led to the discussion and intervention described in *Chapter 4*.

| CASE 9 | Ingram family | 26 | **41** | 69 | 104 | 187 | 389 |

- Isabel – first daughter of Irene and Ian
- Small stature despite tall parents
- ? Turner syndrome

As described earlier, although Isabel had a few mildly abnormal features at birth, she only came to medical attention because she was small compared to her parents' heights and her peer group. Her phenotype and history of swollen hands and feet were strongly suggestive of Turner syndrome. Chromosome analysis confirmed this (*Figure 2.13*). This is the only human monosomy that is not lethal early in development. Because males survive with only one X chromosome, maybe it is not surprising that Turner syndrome is not always lethal. But in fact it is lethal in over 90% of cases. Fetuses with Turner syndrome can be grossly distended with fluid and the great majority abort spontaneously. The survivors are often born with puffy (edematous) hands and feet and with redundant skin on the neck, which represent the remains of presumably milder fetal edema.

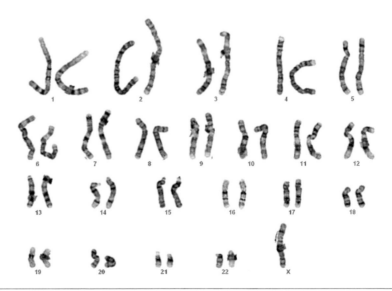

Figure 2.13 – Karyotype of Isabel Ingram.
Although Isabel will never be able to have children normally, treatment with estrogens can allow her to develop normal secondary sex characteristics and greatly assist her personal and social life. Modern reproductive technology has allowed some Turner syndrome patients to bear children using donor eggs. Treatment with growth hormone can result in improved growth and final height.

Unlike all the trisomies, the risk of Turner syndrome does not increase with maternal age. The mechanism is different. Rather than non-disjunction, Turner syndrome is the result of anaphase lag, in which one of the sex chromosomes moves too slowly to the pole of a daughter cell during cell division, and ends up outside the nucleus, whereupon it is broken down. It can arise during gametogenesis or after conception during an early mitotic division. Many Turner women are mosaics (see *Section 1.4*, and below), and they can be either 45,X / 46,XX or 45,X / 46,XY mosaics. Where there is XY tissue in the gonad, it has a propensity to become malignant, and therefore the gonads are best surgically removed.

| CASE 5 | Elliot family | 4 | 11 | **42** | 65 | 389 |

- Miscarriage
- Very small dysmorphic baby girl (Elizabeth), parents Elmer and Ellen
- Heart problems
- Blood taken for chromosome analysis
- Pedigree suggests autosomal dominant condition with reduced penetrance

Previously it had been found that baby Elizabeth suffered from multiple congenital abnormalities (*Figure 1.5*). This suggested she had a chromosomal imbalance, but did not allow the geneticist to guess which chromosomes might be involved. Ellen had had one previous miscarriage, not in itself remarkable, but it was noted that her sister had also had two miscarriages. Further enquiries revealed a family history of reproductive problems – the pedigree is shown in *Figure 1.11*. Blood was taken from the baby and both parents for chromosome analysis. The results showed:

- Elmer – normal male karyotype, 46,XY
- Ellen – a balanced translocation between chromosomes 1 and 22 (*Figure 2.14*)
- Elizabeth – an unbalanced segregation product (*Figure 2.15*)

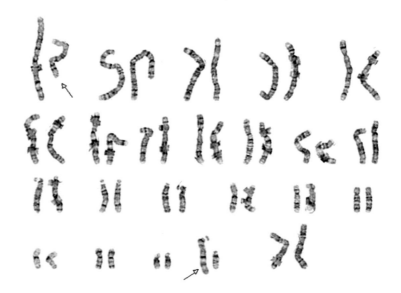

Figure 2.14 – **G-banded karyotype of Ellen's chromosomes.**
There is a balanced translocation. Chromosomes 1 and 22 have exchanged segments (arrows). The translocation is described as 46,XX,t(1:22)(q25:q13).

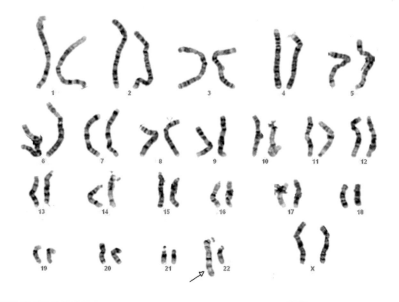

Figure 2.15 – G-banded karyotype of baby Elizabeth.
She has inherited Ellen's normal chromosome 1 but her translocated chromosome 22 (arrow). She is trisomic for the portion of chromosome 1 distal to 1q25, the translocation breakpoint, and monosomic for chromosome 22 distal to 22q13.

When they learned these results, the parents, as well as being very distressed and wanting to know the implications for Elizabeth, were keen to understand exactly what had happened and why. An explanation of the cytogenetics was given using language familiar to the family and explaining technical terms.

Ellen was a constitutional carrier of a balanced translocation – that is, it was present in every cell of her body (see below for a discussion of balanced vs. unbalanced abnormalities). The translocation had been present in the fertilized egg from which Ellen developed, and the pedigree suggested it was already present in one of Ellen's maternal grandparents. At some time in that person or a more distant ancestor, chromosomes 1 and 22 had undergone breakages. Chromosome breaks are common events, but cells have machinery to repair them so that most go unnoticed. In this case, two simultaneous breaks had generated four broken ends, and by bad luck the repair machinery had joined those up the wrong way round (*Figure 2.16*). Alternatively, maybe the translocation had been produced by the machinery responsible for genetic recombination during meiosis activating inappropriately and cutting and joining non-matching chromosomes in a germ-line cell. Because each derivative chromosome nevertheless had a single centromere, mitosis proceeded with no problems, and because no genetic material was extra or missing, there was no phenotypic effect.

Although Ellen's cells could go through mitosis with no problems, meiosis was a different matter. In the first division of meiosis, homologous (matching) chromosomal segments pair (*Figure 2.7*). In this case, pairing would produce a cross-shaped structure containing four whole chromosomes – a tetravalent. When spindle fibers attached to the four centromeres and pulled them

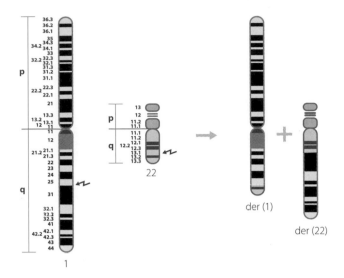

Figure 2.16 – How the 1;22 translocation in Ellen Elliot originated.
Chromosomes 1 and 22 broke at the positions indicated by the arrows, and the cell's DNA repair machinery rejoined the ends to form the two derivative chromosomes as shown. The derivative chromosomes are labeled der(1) and der(22).

apart, they could segregate in various ways (*Figure 2.17*). She could produce entirely normal gametes, gametes carrying the balanced translocation, or various unbalanced forms, one of which had produced Elizabeth. The baby had partial trisomy of chromosome 1 and simultaneously partial monosomy of chromosome 22. The resulting genetic imbalance was the cause of her abnormalities.

There was a risk of problems in future pregnancies, which could take various forms depending on the way the translocated chromosomes segregated. The result could be another child with the same problems as baby Elizabeth, or a different segregation pattern could result in a child with a different set of multiple abnormalities; maybe the result would be severe enough to cause a miscarriage; or of course they could hope to be lucky and have a normal baby. All these various outcomes could be seen in other family members on the pedigree (*Figure 1.11*). The risk was substantial, but it was not easily quantifiable for several reasons:

- we can't predict the exact probability that the translocated chromosomes would segregate in each of the various possible ways
- with some possible unbalanced outcomes a conceptus might abort so early that it would not be recognized as a problem
- it is uncertain whether other less fatally unbalanced karyotypes would result in a miscarriage or a live-born abnormal baby

If it had been Elmer who carried the translocation the risk would be lower, because abnormal sperm are less likely to win the race to fertilize the egg. If Elmer and Ellen wished, it would be possible in future pregnancies to check prenatally and offer termination where the fetus had one of the unbalanced karyotypes. The ways this might be done are discussed in *Chapter 14*.

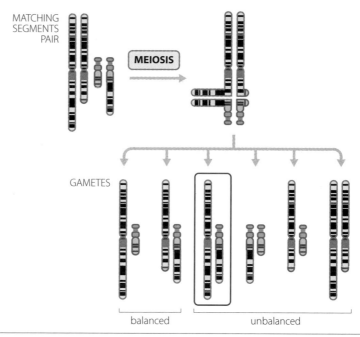

Figure 2.17 – Possible ways the chromosomes in Ellen could segregate in the first meiotic division.
During prophase I matching chromosome segments pair, resulting in a cross-shaped tetravalent containing the normal and translocated copies of chromosomes 1 and 22. At anaphase I they pull apart, and the diagram shows various ways this could happen. The gamete that gave rise to Baby Elliot is circled. Other more complex segregation patterns (3:1 segregation) are also possible.

Months later, once Elmer and Ellen had begun to cope with Elizabeth's health problems, and had absorbed the information about the translocation and their own risks for future children, the question of family risk was discussed. The family history suggested that Ellen's aunt and sister could well be carrying the same balanced translocation, as might her younger sister, who was not yet married. The counselor explained that they needed to be made aware of the risk, preferably by Elmer and Ellen having a word with them to raise the subject. The counselor offered to see the relatives to explain the situation and the options available, including genetic testing. In the genetic clinic it is important to deal with each branch of a family separately, unless family members indicate otherwise. Confidentiality should be maintained and information about one family member only given to another with permission.

2.4. **Going deeper...**

What are chromosomes?

Chromosomes are packages of DNA. Each chromosome contains a single immensely long DNA double helix, packaged by a diverse set of proteins. Chief among these are four types of histones H2A, H2B, H3 and H4, but there are also many other proteins. Chromatin is the generic name for the resulting DNA–protein complex. The basic structure of chromatin is a string of beads

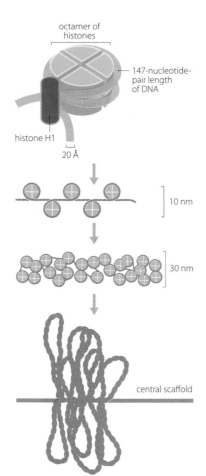

octamer of
histones

147-nucleotide-
pair length
of DNA

histone H1

20 Å

10 nm

30 nm

central scaffold

Figure 2.18 – Packaging DNA into a chromosome.
If you stretched out the DNA in one of the chromosomes in *Figure 2.9*, it would be 10 000 times the length of the chromosome. The DNA in chromosomes exists as a DNA–protein complex called chromatin. The most basic component of chromatin is the nucleosome, consisting of approximately 147 bp of double–stranded DNA wrapped round an octamer of histone proteins. This 'string of beads' is coiled up into a 30 nm fiber then hung in loops from the protein scaffold of the chromosome.

(*Figure 2.18*). The string is DNA and the beads are called nucleosomes. A nucleosome has a roughly spherical core made up of eight histone molecules, with 147 bp of DNA wrapped round it, and a ninth histone molecule on the outside. The chromatin forms large loops, anchored at their bases to a protein scaffold that forms the backbone of a chromosome.

Above this basic structure, chromatin exists in several alternative configurations, depending on what that particular stretch of DNA and that particular cell are doing. Most of the time the string of beads is coiled into an extended 30 nm fiber. The nucleosomes can be loosely or tightly packed, depending whether or not the genes in that stretch of DNA are being expressed (see *Chapter 3* for a description of transcription). When cells are dividing the chromatin is much more tightly packaged. At this time the chromosomes can be seen under the light microscope (*Figures 2.10* and *2.11*). Chromosomes are equally present in non-dividing cells but cannot be seen under the microscope because the 30 nm chromatin fibers are so thin.

Numerical and structural chromosome abnormalities

Chromosome abnormalities can be **numerical** (wrong number of chromosomes, e.g. Helen Howard (*Figure 2.11*), Isabel Ingram (*Figure 2.13*) and the examples in *Box 2.3*) or **structural**, when one or more chromosomes contain the wrong DNA, as with Ellen Elliot (*Figure 2.14*).

Numerical abnormalities
These are of two types:

- **Errors of ploidy** are errors where there are the wrong number of complete sets of chromosomes. Normal cells are **diploid** ($2n$ = 46 chromosomes). Gametes are **haploid** (n = 23). Occasionally two sperm fertilize one egg, producing a triploid ($3n$ = 69). Triploids can also be produced if the whole meiotic process fails, resulting in a diploid gamete that then fertilizes a normal haploid gamete. As mentioned in *Box 2.3*, triploidy in humans is a common error at conception, but triploids virtually never survive to term. Tetraploidy results when a cell replicates its DNA but then does not divide. Tetraploidy and higher degrees of ploidy (polyploidy) may be seen in individual cells, but not in a whole person.
- **Aneuploidy.** All the above abnormalities involve cells with complete sets of chromosomes, which are called **euploid**. **Aneuploid** cells have just one or more single chromosomes extra or missing. Cells or people with one chromosome extra or missing are trisomic or monosomic for that chromosome. Tetrasomy and nullisomy are also possible. The reasons why aneuploidy causes clinical problems are discussed in *Chapter 7*.

Structural abnormalities
These include:

- **Reciprocal translocations.** These arise when any two chromosomes swap non-homologous segments (see *Figure 2.16*). A carrier of a balanced reciprocal translocation is at risk of producing offspring with trisomy of one of the translocated segments and, at the same time, monosomy of the other (*Figure 2.17*). This was the problem in Case 5 (Elliot family).

- **Robertsonian translocations.** These involve a translocation between two acrocentric chromosomes (13, 14, 15, 21, 22 or Y) with the breakpoints in the proximal short arm, just above the centromere (*Figure 2.20*). A carrier of a Robertsonian translocation is at risk of producing a conceptus with either complete trisomy or complete monosomy for one of the chromosomes involved. For example, somebody carrying a Robertsonian translocation involving chromosome 21 is at risk of producing a child with trisomy 21. About 3–4% of Down syndrome cases are due to such translocations. Phenotypically such a child will be indistinguishable from any other child with Down syndrome, but the recurrence risk is much higher. That is an additional reason why Helen Howard (Case 8) was karyotyped, even though there was little doubt about the diagnosis of Down syndrome.
- **Deletions** can be interstitial or terminal, though a chromosome must always have telomeres, so any stable terminal deletion must have somehow acquired a telomere. Ring chromosomes (see *Figure 2.19*) are a special type of terminal deletion. Deletions generally have severe effects, and large deletions are lethal.
- **Duplications** normally have less severe effects than the corresponding deletions.
- **Inversions** can be of any size. If they involve the centromere (pericentric inversions) they change the overall chromosome shape; if not (paracentric inversions) they can only be detected by careful examination of the banding pattern.

Copy number variants

Duplications or deletions of chromosomal segments large enough to be visible under the microscope have severe, often lethal, effects. For many years it was therefore assumed that most of the genetic variation between normal healthy people would consist of changes of single nucleotides in the DNA. The new technique of comparative genomic hybridization (described in *Section 4.2*) showed that this view was wrong. Deletions and duplications ranging from a few nucleotides up to one megabase (1 million nucleotides) are common in normal healthy people. One survey of 40 healthy individuals of European or African ancestry identified over 10 000 copy number variants (CNVs) involving sequences of 450 bp or greater. Only some parts of the genome can vary in this way without causing problems. Databases are being built up to catalog common non-pathogenic CNVs, to assist clinical geneticists to interpret the significance of a variant found in a patient.

Balanced and unbalanced abnormalities

A chromosomal abnormality is described as **balanced** if there is no material extra or missing: the DNA is just divided into packages incorrectly. Provided each chromosome has a single centromere and proper telomeres, a cell can proceed normally through mitosis. Thus a fertilized egg with a balanced abnormality

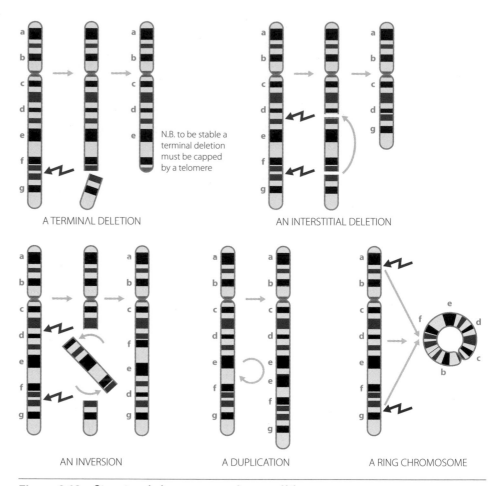

N.B. to be stable a terminal deletion must be capped by a telomere

A TERMINAL DELETION

AN INTERSTITIAL DELETION

AN INVERSION

A DUPLICATION

A RING CHROMOSOME

Figure 2.19 – Structural chromosome abnormalities.
These can arise either through mis-repair of chromosome breaks or through inappropriate function of the genetic recombination machinery. See *Figures 2.16* and *2.20* for translocations.

should be able to develop into a normal adult. **Ellen Elliot** (*Figure 2.14*) is an example of a person who has a balanced chromosomal abnormality but is phenotypically normal. However, if there is pathogenic extra or missing material the abnormality is described as **unbalanced**.

The distinction between balanced and unbalanced abnormalities is a useful tool for thinking about the consequences of chromosomal variants, but it becomes fuzzy when pushed too far. Robertsonian translocations are regarded as balanced even though two acrocentric short arms have been lost (*Figure 2.20*). The short arms of all the acrocentric chromosomes carry similar genes (sequences encoding ribosomal RNA), and losing two of the ten short arms has no phenotypic effect. The many CNVs that can be found in normal healthy people stretch the concept of balance still further. One would not describe these variants as unbalanced. Nevertheless, much of our DNA does have to be present in the correct quantity and **Helen Howard** (*Figure 2.11*) and **Elizabeth Elliot** (*Figure 2.15*) exemplify the problems of unbalanced chromosomal abnormalities.

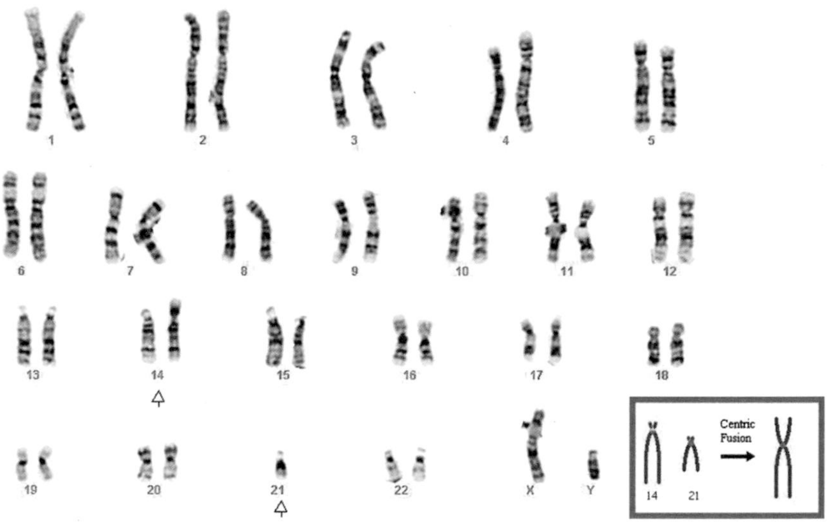

Figure 2.20 – A Robertsonian translocation.
The inset shows how this common type of chromosome abnormality arises. The short arms of all the acrocentric chromosomes (13, 14, 15, 21, 22) contain similar DNA. Inappropriate recombination between two non-homologous chromosomes produces the fusion chromosome, which functions as a normal single chromosome in mitosis. The small acentric fragment comprising the two distal short arms is lost.

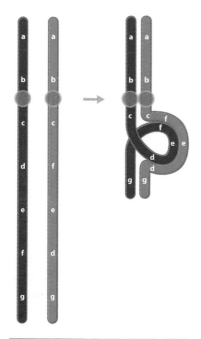

Figure 2.21 – During meiosis I matching chromosome segments pair. If one chromosome has an inversion compared to its homolog, they usually form a looped structure.

Balanced abnormalities become important in meiosis when homologous chromosomes pair up. Things can go wrong in two ways.

- Translocated chromosomes have segments derived from more than one original chromosome. During prophase of meiosis I they will pair with multiple partners, forming trivalents or quadrivalents (associations of three or four chromosomes) instead of bivalents (associations of two homologs). These are liable to segregate incorrectly at anaphase (*Figure 2.17*)
- Chromosomes with inversions pair with a single partner forming a looped structure (*Figure 2.21*), but if a crossover occurs within the loop the recombinant chromosomes are abnormal (see also *SAQ 4*).

Although balanced abnormalities do not normally affect a person's phenotype, there are exceptions.

- One or more of the breakpoints may slice through a gene. This will prevent that gene from working, which may or may not matter to the individual. *Figure 4.20* shows an example where it did matter: an inversion that disrupts the clotting factor VIII gene causes hemophilia.
- Sometimes, as described in *Chapter 3*, a breakpoint does not disrupt a gene itself, but separates a gene from a control element located some way away on the same DNA strand. Again, this may prevent the gene from working.
- Occasionally, when a misplaced recombination or DNA repair joins together segments from different chromosomes, the join creates a novel gene out of parts of two genes that were located near the breakpoints on the different chromosomes. Such chimeric genes are important in cancer (*Chapter 12*).

- Finally, balanced X–autosome translocations cause special problems because of X-inactivation. This is discussed in *Chapter 7*.

Constitutional and mosaic abnormalities

Any genetic variant can be present either in constitutional form (that is, present in every cell of a person) or in mosaic form (present only in some cells). Mosaicism has already been discussed in *Chapter 1* and in connection with Case 9 (Ingram family, Turner syndrome). It is always the result of post-zygotic events: one cell undergoes some change in a person or embryo consisting of more than one cell. Any chromosomal abnormality (except triploidy) that can arise in constitutional form through a meiotic error can also arise in mosaic form through a mitotic error. Many abnormalities that would be lethal if present in constitutional form can survive in mosaics. For example, a patient may have mosaic trisomy 8, but is unlikely to have full constitutional trisomy 8.

Sometimes mosaicism is present only in some tissues, for example mosaic 12p tetrasomy (four copies of the short arm of chromosome 12; the two extra copies are in the form of a small additional metacentric chromosome) causes Pallister–Killian syndrome, where affected individuals have a characteristic appearance and pattern of malformations. But the abnormal cells are seen only in skin and not in the standard blood samples – it is likely that in blood, which has a rapid cell turnover, abnormal cells are at a disadvantage and the normal cell lines come to predominate. Tissue-limited mosaicism can be a particular problem in prenatal diagnosis. The procedure of chorion villus biopsy (*Chapter 14*) provides the cytogeneticist with a sample of the placenta for analysis. Although the placenta is a fetal tissue, if it shows mosaicism there is great uncertainty whether this might be confined to the placenta or whether the fetus itself might also be mosaic. If the fetus is mosaic, predicting the phenotype is difficult. It will lie somewhere along the spectrum between normal and the full constitutional phenotype, but exactly where along the spectrum is unpredictable, because it depends on the proportion of abnormal cells in different tissues and organs.

Although the focus here has been on chromosomal mosaicism, smaller DNA changes may also occur in mosaic form and cause problems in counseling, as described in *Chapter 1*. However, mosaicism is most easily detected by techniques that look individually at each of a large number of cells. Thus cytogeneticists, scanning a spread of dividing cells on a microscope slide, have long been familiar with chromosomal mosaicism. DNA-based techniques normally use the pooled DNA from thousands of cells; in these techniques mosaicism shows as a faint extra band on a gel, or a small extra peak on a sequencer trace, and is easily overlooked. Proving DNA-level mosaicism usually requires a specific test for the abnormal sequence.

Chromatin diseases

As explained above, DNA is packaged by being wrapped round an octamer of histone proteins to form nucleosomes. The string of nucleosomes is then subject to further levels of packaging, under the control of numerous other proteins. There are two basic configurations of chromatin (*Box figure 2.1*). Heterochromatin is tightly packed and genes in heterochromatin are not expressed. Euchromatin is more open and variable; genes in euchromatic regions of chromosomes may or may not be expressed. The local chromatin conformation is a major factor regulating whether or not a gene is expressed.

Chromatin conformation is the result of an interplay between several factors.

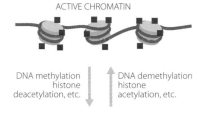

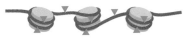

ACTIVE CHROMATIN

DNA methylation
histone
deacetylation, etc.

DNA demethylation
histone
acetylation, etc.

INACTIVE CHROMATIN

■ acetyl groups
▲ methyl groups

Box figure 2.1 – Euchromatin and heterochromatin.

- Modification of histones – the N-terminal parts of histone molecules protrude from the body of the nucleosome, and chemical modifications of amino acids in these 'histone tails' are major determinants of the chromatin conformation. A whole panoply of specific enzymes control the process. Histone acetyltransferases add acetyl ($COCH_3$) groups to the free amino groups of lysines or arginines (see the formulae in *Box 3.6*); histone deacetylases remove them. Histone methyltransferases and histone demethylases add or remove methyl (CH_3) groups. Histone kinases and histone phosphatases add or remove phosphates (PO_3H_2). The spectrum of histone modifications constitute a 'histone code' – but the overall conformation depends also on the chromatin remodeling factors.

- DNA methylation – as described in *Chapter 7*, methyl groups can be attached to certain nucleotides in the DNA.

- Nucleosome positioning – chromatin remodeling factors are multiprotein complexes that can move nucleosomes so as to protect or expose parts of the DNA chain.

These factors can be seen as 'writers', altering the local chemical nature of the chromatin. Their effects are interpreted by 'readers', proteins that attach to differently modified chromatin so as to switch genes on or off. A large number of different proteins are involved in writing and reading the chromatin signals. Mutations in the genes that encode these proteins can cause generalized disorders of gene expression that manifest themselves as a very diverse group of clinical syndromes. One such condition is Rubinstein–Taybi syndrome (RSTS; OMIM 180849). Patients are mentally retarded, have a characteristic facial appearance, and broad thumbs and big toes (*Box figure 2.2*).

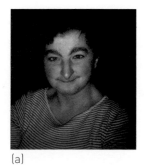
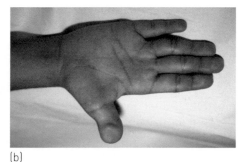
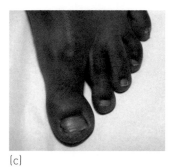

(a) (b) (c)

Box figure 2.2 – Clinical features of Rubinstein–Taybi syndrome.
(a) The typical face; arched eyebrows and long nose with low columella, (b) broad laterally deviated thumb, and (c) broad great toe.

RSTS is caused by mutations in the *CREBBP* or *EP300* genes, both of which encode histone acetyltransferases. Other chromatin diseases include:

- an X-linked syndrome of mental retardation with variable neurologic, behavioral and dysmorphic features (OMIM 300154) that is caused by mutations in the *JARID1C* gene. The gene encodes a histone lysine demethylase that specifically removes methyl groups from lysine 4 of histone H3.

- ICF syndrome (immunodeficiency, centromeric instability, facial anomalies; OMIM 242860) which results from a defect in the *DNMT3B* DNA methyltransferase gene. Patients with this autosomal recessive disease show variable degrees of immunodeficiency and mental retardation, and there is a characteristic facial appearance. When lymphocytes of ICF patients are cultured a proportion of cells show abnormalities of the heterochromatin surrounding the centromeres of chromosomes 1, 9 and 16, including sometimes forming bizarre multiradial structures (*Box figure 2.3a*).

- α-thalassemia / mental retardation syndrome (ATRX; OMIM 301040) which is caused by a defect in an X-chromosome gene encoding a chromatin remodelling factor. Affected males are mentally retarded, have a characteristic facial appearance, sometimes show male-to-female sex reversal and, unexpectedly, have a mild form of α-thalassemia (*Box figure 2.3b and c*). Alpha-thalassemia is normally caused by deletion or inactivation of the α-globin genes on chromosome 16. Lack of the *ATRX* gene product must affect the chromatin structure, and hence the expression, of several genes, including the α-globin genes.

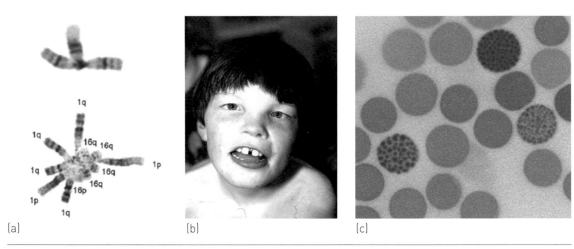

(a) (b) (c)

Box figure 2.3 – Chromatin disease.
(a) Unusual chromosome configurations in lymphocytes of a patient with ICF syndrome. (b and c) ATRX syndrome – facial appearance and lymphocytes showing characteristic inclusions. Photo (a) reproduced from *Am. J. Med. Genet.* 2007; **143A**: 2052–2057 with permission from John Wiley and Sons, (b) reproduced from *J. Med. Genet.* 1991; **28**: 742–745 with permission from the BMJ Publishing Group, (c) courtesy of Dr Richard Gibbon, Oxford.

The clinical features of chromatin diseases are not readily predictable from knowledge of the molecular defect. The chromatin conformation at individual gene loci is governed by subtle interactions between many different factors, so that in the current state of knowledge we are unable to predict which genes will be most affected by a defect in any one player.

2.5. **References**

Conrad DF, Pinto D, Redon R, *et al*. (2010) Origins and functional impact of copy number variation in the human genome. *Nature,* **464**: 704–712. *Reports the large-scale screen for copy number variants described in* Section 2.4.

Gardner RJM and Sutherland GR (2004) *Chromosome Abnormalities and Genetic Counseling,* 3rd edition. Oxford University Press, Oxford. *Gives an in-depth treatment of the material covered in this chapter.*

Hendrich B and Bickmore W (2001) Human diseases with underlying defects in chromatin structure and modification. *Hum. Molec. Genet.* **10**: 2233–2242.

Shaffer LG and Tommerup N, eds (2005) *ISCN 2005, An International System for Human Cytogenetic Nomenclature.* S. Karger AG, Basel.

More detail on mitosis and meiosis can be found in any cell biology textbook.

Useful websites

A useful web resource is the Online Biology Book by MJ Farabee (see the chapters on mitosis and meiosis): www.emc.maricopa.edu/faculty/farabee/BIOBK/BioBookTOC.html

The website of Hironao Numabe at Tokyo Medical University contains many (English language) graphics and animations relevant to this chapter: www.tokyo-med.ac.jp/genet/index-e.htm

2.6. **Self-assessment questions**

(1) Which meiotic divisions in which parent could, by non-disjunction, potentially produce a child with:
(a) 45,X [*guidance provided for this one*]
(b) 47,XXY
(c) 47,XYY

(2) Draw the tetravalent and possible gametes and conceptuses from the following translocations.
(a) t(2;4)(q22;q32) [*guidance provided for this one*]
(b) t(5;10)(p14;p13)
(c) t(7;9)(q32;p21)

(3) Using the diagrams of tetravalents that you drew for the previous question, put in a crossover between the translocated and normal chromosomes in each of the paired segments. Work out the consequences. (*This is not done just to give you a headache – there is normally at least one crossover per chromosome arm during meiosis.*)

(4) Consider the carrier of a balanced Robertsonian 14:21 translocation whose karyotype is shown in *Figure 2.20*. During meiosis the translocation chromosome will form a trivalent with the normal chromosomes 14 and 21. Draw the possible ways this can segregate when

a gamete is formed, and describe the consequences of each of these for any conceptus.

(5) Work out the possible gametes, conceptuses and live-born babies that a carrier of a balanced Robertsonian 21:21 translocation married to a chromosomally normal person could have.

(6) Considering the inversion heterozygote shown in *Figure 2.21*, work out the consequences of a crossover occurring either within the inversion loop or outside it. Is it different if the centromere lies within the inverted segment (a pericentric inversion) rather than outside it as in the figure (a paracentric inversion)?

03 How do genes work?

After working through this chapter you should be able to:

- Name the bases, sugars and nucleosides that form normal DNA and RNA, and sketch a DNA double helix, marking in base pairs and the 5′ and 3′ ends
- Draw diagrams showing the principles (but not the detailed enzymology) of DNA replication, of transcription, of splicing of the transcript and of the way an mRNA sequence specifies the amino acid sequence of a polypeptide
- Describe the general features of the nuclear and mitochondrial genomes
- Sketch a typical human gene structure, showing exons, introns, the promoter, the start and stop codons, the 5′ and 3′ untranslated regions and splice sites
- Describe in outline the role of the promoter, transcription factors and chromatin structure in determining gene expression

3.1. Case studies

| CASE 10 | Johnson family | **55** | 65 | 389 |

- Marfan syndrome

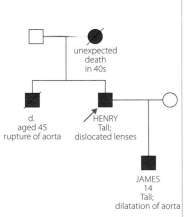

d.
aged 45
rupture of aorta

HENRY
Tall;
dislocated lenses

JAMES
14
Tall;
dilatation of aorta

Figure 3.1 – Pedigree of James Johnson.

James first came to the genetic clinic when he was 14 years old. His father, Henry, and several other relatives had been known to the genetics department for many years. They were originally referred by an eye specialist who had noted that Henry had dislocated lenses and was rather tall. The ophthalmologist was alarmed to find out that Henry's brother had died suddenly at the age of 45 with an aortic rupture and that his mother had died unexpectedly at a similar age. The diagnosis of Marfan syndrome (OMIM 154700) was made and Henry was counseled that his own offspring would have a 50% risk of inheriting this dominant genetic condition. At that time the gene responsible for the syndrome had not been identified, and diagnosis rested on well-defined clinical criteria. These included a positive family history and involvement of the systems that are typically affected in Marfan syndrome (mainly the skeletal, ocular and cardiovascular systems). Years later, when James came to the clinic, the doctor carefully checked for the clinical features of Marfan syndrome using the Ghent criteria (Loeys *et al.*, 2010). An echocardiogram showed early dilatation of the ascending aorta, and James was very tall for his age. The doctor concluded that these features and the positive family history left no room for doubt. By this time the gene involved in Marfan syndrome had been identified, but on clinical criteria alone it was obvious that James was affected.

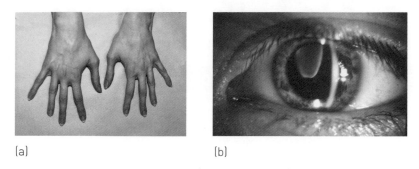

(a)   (b)

Figure 3.2 – Marfan syndrome.
(a) Arachnodactyly (long fingers). (b) Dislocated lens.

3.2. **Science toolkit**

How genes work is the subject of two famous hypotheses. Neither of them is wholly true, but both are nevertheless useful tools for thinking about genes.

- In the 1940s Beadle and Tatum proposed that the job of each gene was to specify one particular enzyme (the **one gene – one enzyme hypothesis**). It is not completely true because many genes specify non-enzymic proteins, and some specify functional RNA molecules rather than proteins – but in the form of 'one gene – one polypeptide' it remains a useful first tool for thinking about what genes do.
- Some years later, Francis Crick defined the essential function of DNA in the 'Central Dogma' of molecular biology (*Figure 3.3*). Genes are functional units of the DNA, and the usual function of a gene is to specify the structure of a protein. There are thought to be about 23 500 such protein-coding genes in the human genome. The Central Dogma is useful but not absolutely true. Occasionally the flow of information from DNA to RNA is reversed, when a special enzyme (reverse transcriptase) makes a DNA copy of an RNA molecule. This is a critical part of the life cycle of RNA viruses, but is not part of the mainstream metabolism of a human cell. More importantly, RNA has many functions apart from

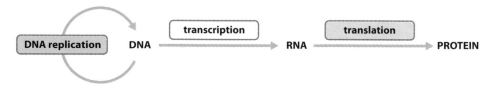

Figure 3.3 – The Central Dogma of molecular biology.
The arrows don't mean that DNA is turned into RNA, etc; they mean the information contained in DNA is transferred to an RNA molecule, which in turn transmits its information to a protein. In other words, genes consist of DNA, but exert their effects through proteins. DNA also specifies the information in other DNA molecules (DNA replication).

specifying the amino acid sequence of proteins and, as mentioned above, some genes specify a functional RNA rather than a protein. Ribosomal RNA and transfer RNA are the best-known examples of such functional RNAs, but there are many others.

A full account of the structure and function of genes would take a whole book. All the processes involved are vastly complicated and involve innumerable proteins and other molecules to affect and control them. Fortunately most of the detail is irrelevant to clinical practice. For clinicians, while there is no limit to the level of detail that it would be desirable to understand, the amount that is essential is much more manageable. The basic essential topics are explained below and in *Boxes 3.2* and *3.3* and are:

- the general structure of nucleic acids as chains of A, G, C and T (or U) units
- the double helix
- 3′ and 5′ ends of DNA
- the exon–intron structure of genes
- splicing of the primary transcript
- the genetic code

If you are interested in finding out more, many excellent textbooks cover these topics in more detail. Additionally there are several websites that provide freely accessible course material (see *Section 3.5*).

Structure of nucleic acids

Nucleic acids (DNA and RNA) are made of subunits called **nucleotides** linked together into long chains. Each nucleotide comprises three modules: a base, a sugar and a phosphate. DNA chains are made of only four types of nucleotide. The sugar is always deoxyribose and the base can be adenine (A), guanine (G), cytosine (C) or thymine (T). The chemical formulae are given in the last section of this chapter, but it is not necessary to know them in order to use this book. RNA is also made up of four types of nucleotide. Here the sugar is always ribose, the bases are A, G and C as in DNA but instead of T, RNA has uracil (U).

DNA, as famously described by Watson and Crick in 1953, normally exists as two polynucleotide chains wrapped round each other – the double helix. Its crucial feature is that the two chains will only fit together correctly if opposite every A in one chain is a T in the other, and opposite every G is a C. Base-pairing, A with T and G with C, explains how DNA is able to be replicated (*Figure 3.4*). This mechanism enables the genetic information in the mother cell to be copied and passed during mitosis to both daughter cells, as described in Chapter 2. RNA does not normally exist as double helices. This is not because of any feature intrinsic to the chemical structure of RNA, but because normal cells do not contain complementary strands of most RNA molecules, nor any enzyme that would construct an RNA strand using an RNA template. Cells use DNA and RNA to do different jobs, and they use the chemical differences between them as recognition signals for targeting enzymes to DNA or RNA as appropriate.

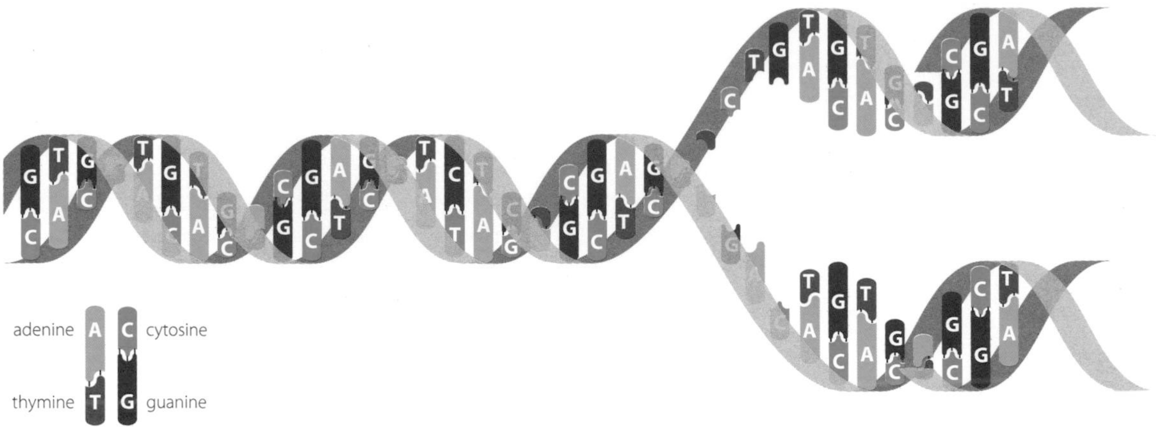

adenine A C cytosine

thymine T G guanine

Figure 3.4 – Principle of DNA replication.
Each strand of the double helix serves as a template for synthesis of an exact replica of the other strand. A similar mechanism is used to make an RNA copy of one strand of the double helix when a gene is transcribed (U in RNA pairs with A in DNA). This diagram shows the principle and the result of DNA replication; the actual molecular events are much more complicated. In particular, this diagram ignores the fact that nucleic acid chains can only grow in the 5′ → 3′ direction (see *Box 3.2* and *Chapter 4*).

The human genome comprises around 3×10^9 bp of DNA (see *Box 3.1* for an explanation of the units). A normal diploid cell contains two copies of the genome (two copies of chromosome 1, two copies of chromosome 2, etc.). As described in *Chapter 2*, each chromosome contains a single immensely long double helix of DNA, packaged by histones and other proteins into chromatin. Chromosome 21, the smallest, contains 47 Mb of DNA, chromosome 1, the largest, 245 Mb. In addition to this nuclear genome, mitochondria have their own little genome, comprising a single circular DNA molecule 16 569 bp long.

A note on units

The size of a piece of DNA is measured in nucleotides (nt), base pairs (bp), kilobases (kb or kbp = 1000 bp) or megabases (Mb or Mbp = 1 000 000 bp). Because DNA is virtually always double-stranded, the distinction between bases and base pairs is often ignored when talking about the size of a piece of DNA. Thus a DNA double helix comprising one million base pairs can be described as either 1 Mbp or 1 Mb – it is not 2 Mb.

BOX 3.1

The structure of genes: exons and introns

Most genes of humans and other higher organisms are organized in a strange and unexpected way. The DNA sequence that will ultimately specify the amino acid sequence of a protein is split into segments (**exons**) interrupted by non-coding sequences (**introns** or intervening sequences). The number and size of introns varies without any evident logic. The average human gene has nine exons averaging 145 bp each and the introns average 3365 bp each, but the range is very wide – see *Table 3.1*.

Table 3.1 – **Structures of some human genes**

Gene	Size in genome (kb)	No. of exons	Average exon size (bp)	Average intron size (bp)	Exons as % of primary transcript
Interferon A6 (*IFNA6*)	0.57	1	570	–	100%
Insulin (*INS*)	1.4	3	154	483	32%
Class 1 HLA (*HLA-A*)	2.7	7	160	269	41%
Collagen VII (*COL7A1*)	51	118	78	358	18%
Phenylalanine hydroxylase (*PAH*)	78	13	206	6264	3.4%
CFTR (cystic fibrosis)	188	27	227	7022	3.2%
Dystrophin (*DMD*)	2090	79	178	26615	0.7%

The number and size of introns varies very widely between genes. You can look at the size and exon–intron structure of any gene using the ENSEMBL genome browser as explained in *Box 3.7*.

BOX 3.2

5′ and 3′ ends

To understand clinical genetics it is not crucial to know a lot about the chemical structure of DNA, but there is one non-obvious feature that does matter. Writing a DNA sequence as a string of letters like AGTTGCACG obscures one important point: the two ends are not chemically identical. Looking at the chemical formula of the sugar–phosphate backbone (see *Box figure 3.1*), successive deoxyribose units are linked through the carbon atoms labeled 5′ ("5 prime") and 3′. The uppermost deoxyribose has its 5′ carbon free, while the lowermost has its 3′ carbon free. Biochemically this difference is crucial. Enzymes that act on the 5′ end of DNA will not act on the 3′ end, and vice versa. This has several important consequences.

- The two chains in a DNA double helix are anti-parallel. If a double helix is drawn vertically one chain will have its 5′ end at the top, and the other will have its 3′ end at the top. The same is true of the DNA–RNA double helices that are temporary intermediates when a gene is transcribed.

- All DNA replication proceeds in the 5′→3′ direction. That is, all the enzymes that string nucleotides together (DNA polymerases) can only add nucleotides to the 3′ end of a polynucleotide. This will turn out to be crucial when we consider the polymerase chain reaction in *Chapter 4*. The same is true of the RNA polymerases that synthesize RNA.

- It is a universal convention that DNA or RNA sequences are written in the 5′ to 3′ direction. The sequence AGTTGCACG means 5′–AGTTGCACG–3′. It is just as wrong to write a

Box figure 3.1 – DNA. A single strand of DNA showing the 5′ and 3′ ends. The carbon atoms of the deoxyribose sugars are numbered 1′, 2′ etc. The prime (′) is to distinguish them from the carbon atoms of the bases, which have their own numbering scheme (not shown here). The phosphate groups carry a negative charge – this is the basis for separating nucleic acids by electrophoresis (see *Box 4.4*).

BOX 3.2 – continued

sequence 3′ to 5′ as it is to write English from right to left. If for any reason you need to write a sequence in the 3′ to 5′ direction, it is essential to label the ends to make this clear.

- Only one strand of the DNA of a gene is transcribed. This is called the **template strand**. Suppose part of this sequence reads 5′–AGTTGCACG–3′. The RNA transcript is complementary to this, with A wherever the template strand has T, G where the template has C, etc. (see *Figure 3.5a*). Writing it in the conventional 5′→3′ direction, its sequence would be CGUGCAACU (remember the strands are anti-parallel and RNA uses U in place of T). Even with very short sequences like these, their relationship is not immediately obvious. To avoid this problem, by convention we write the DNA sequence of a gene not as the template strand but as its complementary strand – CGTGCAACT in this case. This strand is called the **sense strand**. The RNA sequence is just the same as the sense strand, except for replacing T with U.

- Sequences lying 5′ of a gene or sequence of interest (on the sense strand) are often referred to as **upstream**; those 3′ are **downstream**.

Splicing of the primary transcript

When a cell needs to make a particular protein it first makes an RNA copy of one strand of the DNA of just the relevant gene (*Figure 3.5a*). Transcription is a very dynamic process, involving only small segments of a chromosome at any one time, but varying according to the needs of the cell. The way this works is described in a little more detail in the final section of this chapter. The entire sequence of exons and introns is transcribed to make the **primary transcript**. Within the cell nucleus this is then processed by physically cutting out the introns and splicing together the exons (*Figure 3.5b*). The RNA of the introns is broken down and appears to have no useful purpose. Splicing is accomplished within the cell nucleus by a large multimolecular machine called the spliceosome, which is a complex of proteins and small RNA molecules. We can safely ignore most of the complicated molecular details, but we do need to consider how introns are recognized.

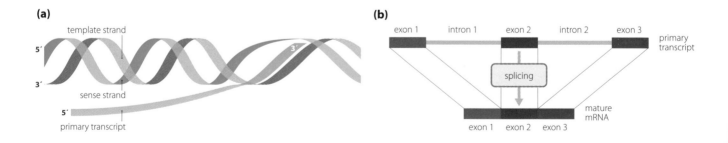

Figure 3.5 – Summary of transcription.
(a) The DNA double helix unwinds locally to allow RNA polymerase to assemble the primary transcript, and rewinds after the polymerase has moved on along the chain. The transcript is made using the template strand; its sequence is complementary to the template strand and identical to the sense strand. (b) The primary transcript is processed by cutting out introns and splicing exons together to form the mature messenger RNA (mRNA).

Almost all human introns start with GU (GT in the DNA of the sense strand – this is called the donor splice site) and end with AG (the acceptor splice site). By themselves these signals would not be sufficient to define splice sites – there are innumerable GU and AG dinucleotides within exons or introns that are not used as splice sites. To be recognized as a splice site the GU or AG must be embedded in a broader **consensus sequence**. A functional splice site has a suitable combination of short sequence motifs that bind proteins or small RNA molecules in the spliceosome. These individual motifs are only loosely defined, making splice sites hard to predict by analysis of DNA or RNA sequences. This is frustrating for clinical geneticists because, as we will see later, sequence variants affecting the efficiency of splice sites are major causes of diseases.

Translation and the genetic code

The mature mRNAs, now comprising just exon sequences, are exported to the cytoplasm where they engage with a ribosome. Ribosomes are yet another large multimolecular machine including many different proteins and several species of non-coding RNA. Again, more details of the mechanism of protein synthesis can be found in textbooks or the recommended websites; for present purposes we need note only the following (see also *Figure 3.6*):

- Amino acids are specified by successive triplets of nucleotides (codons) in the mRNA. The details of the genetic code can be found in *Table 6.1*.
- Ribosomes attach to the 5′ end of the mRNA, and move down it in a 5′→3′ direction.
- The coding sequence starts some way downstream of the 5′ end of the mRNA. It is inaugurated by an invariant AUG embedded in a broader consensus sequence (the Kozak sequence). The parts of the mRNA between the 5′ end and the start codon are called the 5′ untranslated sequence (5′UT).
- The initiating AUG sets the reading frame. The concept of the reading frame is best explained by an example (see *Box 3.3*).

BOX 3.3

The reading frame

Consider the following string of letters:

ISAWTHEBIGBADDOGEATTHECAT

We can read successive triplets of letters in three alternative reading frames:

ISA WTH EBI GBA DDO GEA TTH ECA T ... or:

I SAW THE BIG BAD DOG EAT THE CAT ... or:

IS AWT HEB IGB ADD OGE ATT HEC AT

Similarly the string of nucleotides in an mRNA molecule can be translated by a ribosome in three different reading frames, only one of which gives a sensible message (i.e. encodes the desired protein). The reading frame of an mRNA is defined by the AUG start codon. Mutations that change the reading frame have catastrophic effects on gene function (see *Chapter 6*).

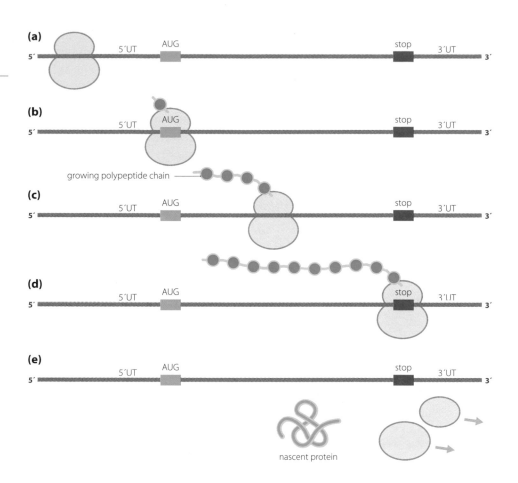

Figure 3.6 – Summary diagram of translation.
(a) A ribosome attaches at the 5′ end of the mRNA.
(b) It moves along the 5′ untranslated sequence until it encounters the AUG initiation codon. At this point it picks up the first amino acid. (c) The ribosome moves along the mRNA, picking up amino acids according to the codons of the mRNA and incorporating them into the growing polypeptide chain.
(d) When it reaches a stop codon, translation of the message is complete. (e) At this point the ribosome falls off the mRNA and dissociates into its two subunits, and the polypeptide is released. The mature functional protein must be correctly folded, perhaps chemically modified, and transported to the appropriate intracellular or extracellular location.

- The ribosome slides along the mRNA, adding the appropriate amino acid to the growing polypeptide chain in accordance with the genetic code. Amino acids are ferried to the ribosome by a family of small RNA molecules, the **transfer RNAs** (tRNA).
- The ribosome works its way along the mRNA until it encounters a **stop codon**. There are three stop codons, UAG, UAA and UGA. When the ribosome meets a stop codon it releases the polypeptide it has made and falls off the mRNA. The parts of the mRNA downstream of the stop signal comprise the **3′ untranslated sequence** (3′UT). They are important for regulating the stability of the mRNA.

Translation is not the end of the story

Translation finishes with the release of the newly synthesized polypeptide chain from the ribosome. However, several more processes are needed to convert the nascent polypeptide into a fully functional protein (see also *Box 3.4*).

- Folding the chain into the correct three-dimensional structure requires no additional information – the amino acid sequence potentially dictates the folding. However, until they are correctly folded, proteins are unstable and vulnerable. It has also recently become apparent that partially folded or incorrectly folded proteins can be toxic to the cell. A number of 'chaperone' molecules assist the folding process and protect the polypeptide during folding, while misfolded proteins are detected and degraded.

- Many proteins incorporate chemical modifications to the basic polypeptide. Often sugars are attached (glycosylation) or a variety of other small molecules. The chain may be cleaved; cysteines may be cross-linked to form S–S (disulfide) bridges that lock the structure in place; other amino acid residues may be chemically modified, for example, prolines may be hydroxylated. All polypeptides initially have an N-terminal methionine, incorporated in response to the AUG initiation codon, but very often this is cleaved off.

- Proteins must be transported to an appropriate location. The destination is often specified by a short N-terminal **signal peptide** that is removed during the process of protein sorting. In other cases the signal is a sequence of amino acids located somewhere within the chain, and is not removed. In the case of **Joanne Brown (Case 2)**, it will turn out that one of her two *CFTR* genes carries a mutation that prevents the protein being correctly located in the cell membrane (her other copy of the gene carries a different mutation – that is, she is a **compound heterozygote**).

- Structural proteins may be further modified in their final location.

Some further examples of the importance of post-translational modification are described in *Section 8.4*.

Biosynthesis of collagens

BOX 3.4

Collagens provide good examples of the way post-translational processing can be required to convert a nascent polypeptide into the functional protein. Almost one-third of the total protein mass of the human body consists of collagens. They are major proteins of the extracellular matrix, the connective and supporting tissue that holds cells together. They form cartilage, tendons, the matrix of bones, and the basic support of many membranes. Humans have 30 or so collagen genes, distributed around the genome. These encode at least 27 forms of collagen, different types being found in different tissues.

The basic collagen structure is a triple helix of three polypeptide chains wound tightly round one another. Collagens may be homotrimers (all three chains the same) or heterotrimers. For example, Type I collagen, the major collagen of skin, tendon and bone, is made of two α-1 chains, encoded by the *COL1A1* gene on chromosome 17, and one α-2 chain encoded by the *COL1A2* gene on chromosome 7. The initial product of these genes is a preprocollagen. The future triple helical region has a repetitive structure, Gly-X-Y where X and Y can be any amino acid, but are often proline or lysine. This preprocollagen undergoes extensive post-translational modification:

- in the rough endoplasmic reticulum (see *Figure 3.10a*) a proportion of the lysines and prolines are hydroxylated by special enzymes that use oxygen, Fe^{2+} and ascorbic acid as cofactors

BOX 3.4 – continued

- sugar residues are attached to some of the hydroxyl groups
- three chains are then wound together, starting at their C-terminal ends, to form the triple helix; see *Box 3.6* for an explanation of N- and C-termini
- this procollagen is secreted, after which special enzymes cleave off the C-terminal and N-terminal propeptides
- finally, the triple helical molecules are assembled into large multimers and crosslinked through lysine residues

Some collagens (I, II, III, V, XI, XXIV, XXVII) form fibrils; collagen VI associates with fibrillin in the microfibrils that are involved in Marfan syndrome (see **Case 10, Johnson family**). Collagens IV, VIII and X form meshworks that support membranes, and the other collagens have various specialized functions.

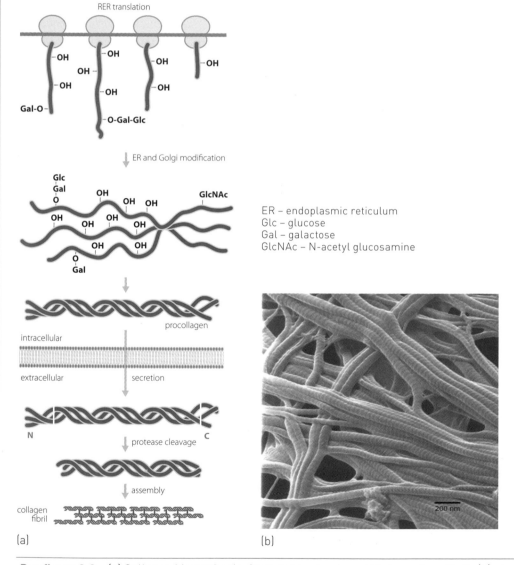

ER – endoplasmic reticulum
Glc – glucose
Gal – galactose
GlcNAc – N-acetyl glucosamine

Box figure 3.2 – (a) Collagen biosynthesis, from nascent polypeptide to mature fibril; (b) electron micrograph of collagen fibers (reproduced courtesy of Zeiss).

3.3. **Investigations of patients**

Many of the cases described so far in the book will require DNA investigations. Here we describe how each case fits into the picture of gene structure developed in the previous section. First, however, we will note two cases where no DNA tests will be used.

| CASE 5 | Elliot family | 4 | 11 | 42 | **65** | 389 |

- Reciprocal translocation

The chromosome analysis tells us all we need to know in this family. DNA testing is not relevant.

| CASE 10 | Johnson family | 55 | **65** | 389 |

- Marfan syndrome

James didn't have a gene test when he first attended the clinic because his diagnosis was obvious on clinical grounds. For most genetic disorders molecular tests were only introduced into clinical practice in the 1990s. For many years diagnoses for most disorders relied on family history, clinical signs and symptoms and on investigations such as X-rays. There is a great deal of information available about Marfan syndrome because it is a relatively common genetic condition, and formal diagnostic guidelines have been assembled as knowledge increases (Ghent criteria, see Loeys *et al.*, 2010). However, even for disorders where a diagnosis is usually possible on clinical grounds alone, there may be a need for molecular testing. This might be for use in prenatal testing, or where a person does not quite fulfil the diagnostic criteria but there remains considerable suspicion.

For the remaining cases, DNA tests are required.

| CASE 1 | Ashton family | 1 | 7 | **65** | 106 | 154 | 389 |

- John – 28-year-old son of Alfred Ashton
- ? Huntington disease
- Other family members with similar symptoms
- Autosomal dominant inheritance shown in pedigree
- Diagnostic test ordered

Huntington disease is caused by a change to the coding sequence of a gene on chromosome 4, position 4p16. The Huntington disease gene *HTT* has 67 exons, covers 169 kb of genomic DNA (*Figure 3.7*) and encodes a 3141 amino acid protein called huntingtin. Huntington disease patients always have a sequence change in exactly the same place in the gene. Part of exon 1 encodes a run of glutamines in the huntingtin protein. Every patient with Huntington disease has an expansion of this sequence, so that the encoded protein contains a much longer run of glutamines. How this makes the patient ill is discussed in *Disease box 4*. The DNA test needs to check the size of the sequence encoding this polyglutamine run.

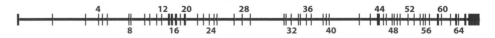

Figure 3.7 – Structure of the Huntington disease gene.
Short vertical bars represent the exons. Human Genome Project data as displayed by GenAtlas (www.dsi.univ-paris5.fr/genatlas/).

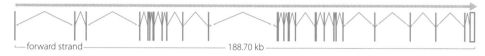

CASE 2   Brown family   2   8   **66**   132   154   281   389

- Girl (Joanne) aged 6 months, parents David and Pauline
- ? Cystic fibrosis
- Order molecular test?

As mentioned previously, cystic fibrosis is always caused by mutations in the *CFTR* gene on chromosome 7. The disease is recessive, so if Joanne has cystic fibrosis both copies of her *CFTR* gene must be mutated. *CFTR* is quite a large gene, with 27 exons spread over 188 kb of chromosome 7 at position 7q31.2 (*Figure 3.8*). Unlike in Huntington disease, mutations may be anywhere in the gene. Different patients with cystic fibrosis may have different mutations – over 1000 different mutations are described in the Human Gene Mutation Database. Joanne's two mutations might be the same or different. All the mutations are changes to a single nucleotide or a small number of adjacent nucleotides. Scanning both copies of the gene for any such change will be a challenge.

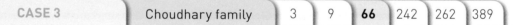

forward strand ———————————————————————— 188.70 kb ————————

Figure 3.8 – Structure of the *CFTR* gene.
An alternative graphical display of Human Genome Project data, as displayed by the Ensembl genome browser. Some closely spaced exons appear as a single bar. The arrow shows the 5'→3' direction of the sense strand.

CASE 3   Choudhary family   3   9   **66**   242   262   389

- Girl (Nasreen) aged 8 months, parents Aadnan and Mumtaz
- Deaf
- Parents are first cousins
- Pedigree suggests autosomal recessive deafness

The problem with deafness is that, even when the cause is genetic, mutations in any one of over 50 different genes can cause it. The reason for this diversity is not hard to understand. Our sense of hearing uses a wonderfully complex and subtle mechanism to convert air pressure waves reaching the ear into nerve impulses. Naturally the mechanism involves many components, encoded by many different genes. If any one of these fails, the whole mechanism may fail. It would be very expensive to check every one of them although the new high throughput sequencing technologies (see *Section 5.2*) make this technically feasible. As described in *Chapter 9*, the usual approach is to check for one particular mutation in one particular gene, *GJB2*, that is a relatively common cause of the problem. If this test is negative a normal diagnostic DNA laboratory would not be able to justify the expense of looking through a whole long list of genes. However, Nasreen's unusually large family and affected uncles means that it might be possible to narrow down the list of candidate genes using linkage analysis. This investigation is pursued in *Chapter 9*.

| CASE 4 | | Davies family | 4 | 10 | **67** | 104 | 155 | 186 | 281 | 389 |

- Boy (Martin) aged 24 months, parents Judith and Robert
- Clumsy and slow to walk
- Family history of muscular dystrophy
- Pedigree shows X-linked recessive inheritance
- Order diagnostic DNA test

Duchenne muscular dystrophy is X-linked, so the causative gene must be located on the X chromosome. It is in the proximal short arm, at Xp21, and encodes a protein, dystrophin, that is essential for making muscle cells robust enough to withstand mechanical stresses over many years. The dystrophin gene (*DMD*) is one of the most remarkable in the human genome. It is huge, covering over 2 million base pairs of DNA – 99.3% of this comprises introns; after they are spliced out of the primary transcript the 79 exons make a 13 kb mature mRNA. Two-thirds of cases are caused by partial deletions of the gene. Because almost all the genomic sequence is intronic, the deletion breakpoints almost always fall in introns, so their effect on the mature mRNA is to remove one or more contiguous exons (*Figure 3.9*). Searching for mutations anywhere in this vast gene would be a major challenge. The initial test is therefore to check the genomic DNA for missing exons, concentrating on those exons that are most commonly deleted. Missing exons are obvious in DNA from an affected boy; in a carrier woman they are masked by her normal X chromosome, which of course has all exons intact.

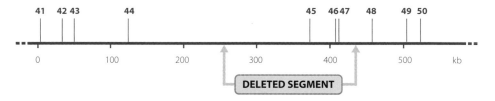

Figure 3.9 – A deletion of part of the dystrophin gene.
This figure shows a 500 kb region containing exons 41–50. These exons are all 100–200 bp long, and so if drawn to scale each exon would be represented by a line occupying less than 0.05% of the width of the figure. Random deletion breakpoints therefore almost always fall in introns. Their effect is to remove one or more complete exons from the mature mRNA. The deletion shown removes exons 45–47 from the mature mRNA, while leaving all the other exons intact.

| CASE 6 | | Fletcher family | 5 | 12 | **67** | 137 | 156 | 389 |

- Frank, aged 22, with increasingly blurred eyesight
- Family history of visual difficulties
- Pedigree suggests X-linked recessive inheritance but not conclusive
- ? LHON
- Order blood test to check for mutation in mtDNA

The pedigree and clinical phenotype suggested a diagnosis of Leber hereditary optic neuropathy (LHON). This is caused by mutations in the DNA of the mitochondria, rather than the DNA of the chromosomes in the cell nucleus.

The small mitochondrial genome (*Figure 3.10b*) is markedly different from the nuclear genome. In many ways it is much more similar to bacterial genomes – an observation consistent with the belief that mitochondria evolved from bacteria that lived in a symbiotic relationship inside some ancestral cell. The mitochondrial genome is circular and compact. Though only 16 569 bp long, it contains 37 genes. Like bacterial genomes, the genes are tightly packed together with very little intergenic DNA – a marked contrast to the nuclear genome which averages only eight genes per megabase. Mitochondrial genes have no introns – another point of resemblance to bacterial genes. However, mitochondria are very far from being independent micro-organisms. Most mitochondrial functions depend on proteins encoded by nuclear genes that are transported to the mitochondrion after being

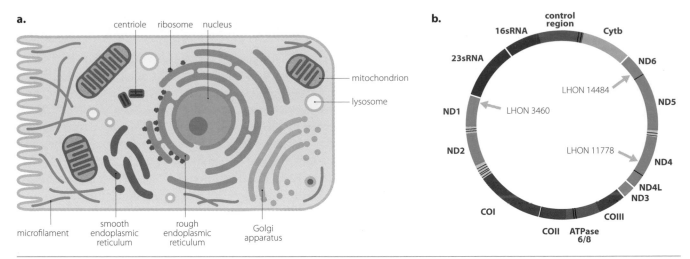

Figure 3.10 – (a) A cell showing the nucleus and mitochondria. (b) The mitochondrial genome. The 13 protein-coding genes are labeled and the locations of the three common LHON mutations shown. The other 24 mitochondrial genes encode functional RNAs: the two ribosomal RNAs (red segments) and 22 transfer RNAs (small genes indicated by unlabeled thin lines).

synthesized. Importantly, this means that diseases caused by mitochondrial dysfunction are not necessarily caused by mutations in the mitochondrial DNA. For example, mtDNA is replicated by DNA polymerase gamma, the gene for which (*POLG1*) is located on chromosome 15q25. Mutation in *POLG1* can cause Alpers syndrome (OMIM 203700), with neurodegeneration and liver failure, or progressive external ophthalmoplegia (OMIM 157640 and 258450). LHON is one of the few diseases caused by mutations in the mitochondrial DNA.

The DNA extracted from a clinical sample includes the mitochondrial as well as the nuclear DNA. The diagnosis in Frank Fletcher will be confirmed if his DNA sample can be shown to have one of the mitochondrial DNA mutations characteristic of LHON (see *Chapter 5*).

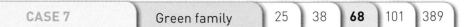

| CASE 7 | Green family | 25 | 38 | **68** | 101 | 389 |

- Girl (Gillian) aged 3 years
- Slow to develop
- ? Chromosome abnormality
- Order tests to check for microdeletion at 22q11

Gillian's combination of learning difficulties and mild dysmorphism suggested a chromosomal abnormality, and her clinical features resembled those of patients with an interstitial deletion of chromosome 22 at position 22q11. Under the microscope her karyotype appeared normal (*Figure 2.9*) but a deletion of less than 3–5 Mbp of DNA would not have been visible. Given an average density of genes across the whole human genome of about eight per Mb of DNA (23 500 genes spread over 3000 Mbp of genomic DNA), a deletion that is too small to see under the microscope can still affect a dozen or more genes. Checking the diagnosis requires a test able to see deletion of a region of DNA that is small in cytogenetic terms but still very large in molecular terms. This will require a different technique from the previous cases.

| CASE 8 | | Howard family | 26 | 38 | **69** | 102 | 277 | 389 |

- Helen – new-born daughter of Henry and Anne (33 years old)
- Down syndrome
- Risk of recurrence if they have more children?

The clinical features and chromosome analysis (*Figures 2.2* and *2.11*) establish the diagnosis. Many couples request prenatal testing for Down syndrome, either because, like Helen's mother, they have had an affected child, or because of the increased risk when the woman is older. As we will see in *Chapter 14*, it takes 2 weeks from obtaining fetal cells to get them dividing well enough for conventional cytogenetic analysis. The waiting can be very stressful for the patient. To avoid this, a DNA test is increasingly used that can give an immediate indication of the number of copies of chromosome 21 that are present, without the need for cell culture.

| CASE 9 | | Ingram family | 26 | 41 | **69** | 104 | 187 | 389 |

- Isabel – first daughter of Irene and Ian
- Small stature despite tall parents
- ? Turner syndrome

Clinical features and chromosome analysis (*Figures 2.3* and *2.13*) establish the diagnosis. As explained in *Chapter 2*, Isabel may have started life as a 46,XY conceptus and lost the Y chromosome in one of the early mitotic divisions. If any of the cells in her streak gonads retains a Y, these cells can give rise to a malignant gonadoblastoma. Therefore it is important to check for the presence of Y-chromosome DNA sequences. If any are found, then gonadectomy is usually recommended.

3.4. **Going deeper ...**

Some chemistry

For reference, *Box 3.5* shows the chemical structures of the bases A, G, C, T and U, and *Box 3.6* shows the 20 amino acids that are used to make proteins.

Chemical formulae of A, G, C, T and U.

The formulae and names show the bases, and indicate how each base is attached to a sugar (ribose in RNA, deoxyribose in DNA). Bases are classified into purines (A, G) and pyrimidines (C, T, U). See *Figure 5.2* for a formula of a complete nucleotide.

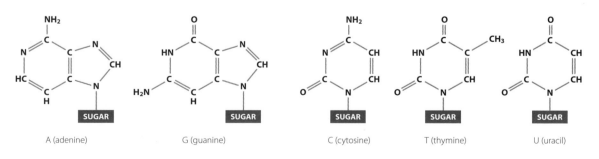

A (adenine)   G (guanine)   C (cytosine)   T (thymine)   U (uracil)

One gene often encodes more than one protein

Contrary to the one gene – one enzyme hypothesis, very often a single gene can encode several different proteins (*Figure 3.11*). The main mechanism for this is alternative splicing. Often there is more than one way of splicing the primary transcript. Certain exons may be variably incorporated or skipped in the mature mRNA, giving rise to **splice isoforms**. Sometimes there are two alternative splice sites marking the beginning or end of an exon. A gene may also have several alternative promoters and first exons (the dystrophin gene has seven). All these variables mean that most genes can encode more than one protein. Some can potentially encode more than 1000 different proteins. The average number of transcripts per locus in one set of intensively investigated genes (from the ENCODE project, see *Section 6.2*) is 5.4. Some of this variability may be just noise in the system, where the cell is bad at recognizing the one correct signal – but in many cases it is functional, with isoforms having distinct functions. Mutations that affect the balance of splice isoforms can be clinically significant, but hard to recognize in the DNA sequence.

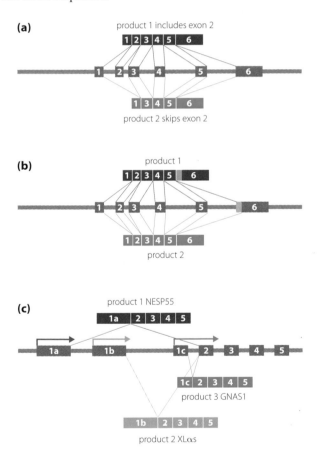

Figure 3.11 – How one gene can encode more than one protein.
(a) Exons may be variably incorporated into the mature mRNA or skipped. (b) An exon may have two alternative splice sites. (c) A gene may have two or more alternative promoters and first exons (this example shows the *GNAS1* gene, which encodes three differently named proteins). The majority of all human genes use one or more of these mechanisms to encode more than one protein.

BOX 3.6

Structure of proteins

(a) Chemical formula of a polypeptide. The amino acids differ according to the nature of the side chain, labeled R_1, R_2, R_3, here. A real protein would probably contain several hundred amino acid residues. (b) Chemical formulae of the side chains (R groups) of the 20 amino acids used to make up proteins. The three letter and single letter abbreviated names of each amino acid are shown.

(a)

N-terminus $H_2N-CH-C-N-CH-C-N-CH-C-OH$ C-terminus

AN AMINO ACID RESIDUE

(b)

GLYCINE (Gly, G)
ALANINE (Ala, A)
VALINE (Val, V)
LEUCINE (Leu, L)
ISOLEUCINE (Ile, I)
SERINE (Ser, S)
THREONINE (Thr, T)

ASPARTIC ACID (Asp, D)
GLUTAMIC ACID (Glu, E)
ASPARAGINE (Asn, N)
GLUTAMINE (Gln, Q)
LYSINE (Lys, K)
ARGININE (Arg, R)
HISTIDINE (His, H)

CYSTEINE (Cys, C)
METHIONINE (Met, M)
PHENYLALANINE (Phe, F)
TYROSINE (Tyr, Y)
TRYPTOPHAN (Trp, W)
PROLINE (Pro, P)

Switching genes on and off – transcription and its controls

All the cells of our body contain the identical set of genes – that is the purpose of mitosis. So how do they come to be so very different from each other – brain cells, liver cells, skin cells, muscle cells, etc? The answer is that they express different subsets of their repertoire of genes. Differential switching of genes is crucial to development. Additionally, an individual cell will switch genes on or off depending on its current needs. Switching can operate at the level of transcription or translation. The major on–off controls operate at the level of transcription. Translational controls operate mainly to fine-tune gene expression.

Selectivity is the key to transcription. Although the DNA of a chromosome is a single huge molecule, the RNAs produced by transcription are a diverse collection of much smaller molecules, made by transcribing selected small segments of the DNA. Choosing appropriate segments to transcribe is crucial to the life of the cell. Partly this is controlled by the way the DNA is packaged by histones and other proteins into chromatin. As explained in *Chapter 2* (*Section 2.4* and *Disease box 2*), the local chromatin structure is determined by an interplay between modification of histones, methylation of DNA and the action of chromatin remodeling complexes. This provides an environment that allows or represses transcription.

Transcription starts when a large multiprotein initiation complex has been assembled at an appropriate place on the DNA, defined by an 'open' chromatin structure and specific sequence motifs. The promoter of a gene contains a number of different short (typically 4–8 nt) sequence motifs that each bind specific proteins. These DNA-binding proteins are called **transcription factors**. They in turn bind other proteins, and so build up a complex including the RNA polymerase that does the actual transcription. Each individual DNA–protein interaction is weak, but once several different transcription factors are loosely bound, protein–protein interactions between them glue the complex together. Proteins bound to distant regulatory sequences, up to a megabase away, can help regulate transcription if the DNA is looped so as to bring them adjacent to the promoter – remember, the 2 m of DNA in each cell has to be intricately folded to fit into the nucleus. Some of the proteins of the initiation complex are present all the time in every cell, but others (themselves the products of genes that are highly regulated) occur only in certain cells, or only when the cell responds to certain signals. By acting in different combinations, a limited (though large) number of transcription factors can achieve flexible control over the expression of a much greater number of genes.

Once started, transcription proceeds until some loosely defined stop signal is reached. The end result (the primary transcript) is a single-stranded RNA molecule, typically 1–100 kb long, corresponding precisely in sequence to the sense strand of the DNA (*Figure 3.5*).

From gene to genome

The Human Genome Project was launched in 1990 and culminated triumphantly with the publication of the 'finished' human genome sequence in 2004. The key publications (International Human Genome Sequencing Consortium, 2001, 2004) do not of course print out all 3 000 000 000 As, Gs, Cs and Ts, but they describe the methods used and key features of the genome. The 2004 paper is quite brief, but the blockbuster 2001 paper ranks with *On the Origin of Species* and Watson and Crick's 1953 paper describing the double helix, as one of the seminal milestones in biology.

The raw sequence is held in freely accessible public databases. To access it you use a genome browser program. Several of these are freely available on the internet as a public service. Widely used ones include the SANTA CRUZ and ENSEMBL browsers. *Box 3.7* shows how to use ENSEMBL to view the intron–exon structure, DNA sequence and chromosomal environment of any gene.

How to use the ENSEMBL genome browser

One of the most frequent uses of a genome browser is to find information about the intron–exon structure and sequence of a gene. Here is how the ENSEMBL browser does this for the *CFTR* gene. The SANTA CRUZ browser (www.genome.ucsc.edu) offers similar tools.

1. Go to www.ensembl.org/Homo_sapiens/index.html

2. Fill in the search boxes to get ENSEMBL to look for a gene with the appropriate name – in this case, *CFTR* (you could also enter 'cystic fibrosis').

3. If you have got the name right, this will produce a screen inviting you to search 'by species' or 'by feature type'. In the latter window, the 'Gene' line in the Feature box listed 31 entries when consulted on 30th January 2010; the number may change.

4. Click on the '31'. This brings up a list of genes, each with a long list of data items. Check carefully to get the right one (for *CFTR* this is ENSEMBL Gene: ENSG00000001626)

5. Having selected the correct gene, you will see one or more transcripts listed, (6 when consulted on 30th January 2010), each with links to Transcript ID and Protein ID. Clicking on a transcript brings a display of the exon structure of that transcript, like *Box figure 3.3*.

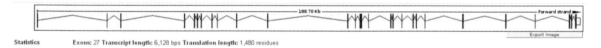

Statistics   **Exons:** 27 **Transcript length:** 6,128 bps **Translation length:** 1,480 residues

Box figure 3.3 – Screenshot of the *CFTR* gene transcript ENST00000003084 as shown by ENSEMBL.

A menu at the left hand side of the screen allows you to bring up details of exons, cDNA or the protein. Clicking on 'Exons' gives a display containing the size of each exon and intron, and the sequence of each exon and a user-specifiable number of nucleotides in the flanking introns.

An alternative common use of the browser is to view genes and other features in a particular chromosomal region. Staying with the example of the *CFTR* gene, when the list of genes has been produced (stage 4 above), clicking on 'Region in detail' produces a display like *Box figure 3.4*.

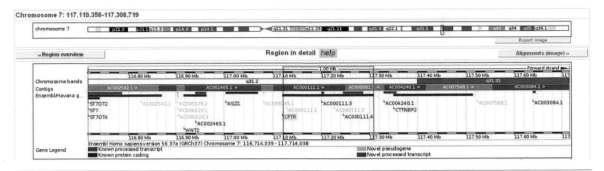

Box figure 3.4 – **Screenshot of the chromosomal region around the *CFTR* gene (red box), as shown by** Ensembl.

The display, currently of 1 Mb, can be zoomed in or out, and many more user-selectable tracks of information can be displayed. Clicking on items in the display brings up further information and links.

The finished sequence was obtained by piecing together literally millions of short runs of sequence, derived from several different anonymous donors. Thus it does not represent the sequence of any one person. Indeed, probably nobody has exactly this sequence. But just as we are all recognizably human despite our individual differences in appearance, so we all have recognizably human genomes despite individual variants. A major interest now is in cataloging those variants. The rapid progress in DNA sequencing technology has now made it feasible – indeed, almost routine – to sequence the genomes of specific individuals. Several major collaborative projects, such as the HapMap and 1000 Genomes projects, are generating a comprehensive view of how the genomes of normal healthy individuals vary. For clinicians, this information provides an essential background for interpreting the likely effect of variants found in patients.

The human genome sequence is a stunning achievement, but it is important to understand its limitations. In fact, by itself, the raw sequence does not tell us very much. It needs to be annotated to identify the genes and other functional elements contained in the sequence. Annotation is based on a combination of laboratory experiments to identify transcripts and computer analysis of the sequence to identify features such as protein-coding exons, RNA genes and regulatory elements. Genome browsers like Ensembl use huge amounts of annotation data to turn the raw sequence into useful information.

Even when we have a full catalog of genes, this will not in itself tell us what any gene does. **Functional genomics** tries to provide this information. Again, the analysis uses both laboratory data and computer analysis of gene sequences. The human **proteome** (the complete set of all proteins) includes maybe 100 000 different proteins (many more than the number of genes because most genes encode several proteins – see *Figure 3.11*). However, proteins obtain much of their function through combinations of a much more limited number (maybe 1000) of functional modules (*Figure 3.12*). Thus one protein might have a DNA binding module, a protein–protein interaction module and a steroid hormone receptor. Recognizing the modules encoded by a gene can help identify the function of its protein product.

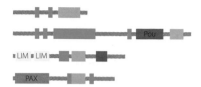

Figure 3.12 – Domain architecture of proteins. Each line represents one family of proteins and each colored shape represents a structural and functional protein domain. The homeodomain (green) is found in all the proteins shown here, together with a variety of other functional domains. These in turn can be found in different combinations in other proteins.

When the focus moves from individual protein-coding genes to the whole genome, a number of puzzling features emerge. The human genome contains around 23 500 protein-coding genes. The number of exons in a gene varies widely: some genes consist of a single exon with no introns, while the gene encoding the muscle protein titin has over 300 exons (*Table 3.1* gave a few examples); the average number is about 9. Exons average around 145 bp in size (compared to 3365 bp for introns). Considering all these numbers leads to two surprising conclusions. First, if you add up the sizes of every exon of every protein-coding gene, the total comes to only around 30 Mb – hardly more than 1% of the total amount of DNA in our genome. This raises the question, what does the other 99% of our DNA do? Secondly, it appears that we have scarcely any more genes than the 1 mm long nematode worm *Caenorhabditis elegans*. It takes 20 158 protein-coding genes to build this worm, a creature much studied as an example of an extremely simple animal. Surely it is not just anthropocentric arrogance to think that we are far more complex creatures than these worms? If we don't have more genes than worms, maybe we use the same number of genes in a smarter way? Maybe the fact that we have so much noncoding DNA is at least partly because much of it is involved in regulating the expression of genes? We need to take a closer look at the noncoding DNA.

Looking at our noncoding DNA

Figure 3.13 gives an overall picture of our genome. A small portion of our DNA has known functions. Apart from the protein-coding sequence, some noncoding DNA is required to make the centromeres and telomeres of chromosomes, or is present in the heterochromatin. For the rest, we can ask several questions:

- **Is it conserved?** If you compare the human genome with genomes of distantly related mammals like mice, a few percent of our non-coding sequence is identical or very similar, while the rest shows no relationship. Presumably chance variants arose in these sequences, as elsewhere in

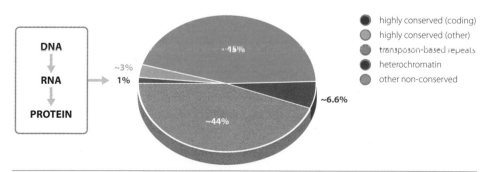

Figure 3.13 – What does all our DNA do? About 1% does what the Central Dogma says DNA does. A further ~3% is conserved between humans and mice, implying that it has some sequence-dependent function. Some of the heterochromatin functions as the centromeres of chromosomes. About half of the rest of our DNA is made up of many copies of transposable elements that have spread within the genome like an infection. Data from the Draft Human Genome Sequence (2001).

the genome, but have been eliminated by natural selection. This implies that these **conserved sequences** have some important function, most likely connected with gene regulation. The functions may be specific to mammals, since very little non-coding sequence is conserved between humans and more distantly related organisms like the nematode worm.

- **Is it unique?** Almost half of our DNA consists of short sequences present in huge numbers of copies scattered across the genome. There are 1.5 million copies of 100–300 bp sequences called SINEs (Short Interspersed Nuclear Elements) and 850 000 copies of LINEs (Long Interspersed Nuclear Elements). These comprise about 13% and 21% of our genome, respectively. Complete LINE elements are 6–8 kb long, but the majority are incomplete. Other large families of repeats make up a further 11% of our genome. All these repetitive elements are believed to have multiplied within our genome like an infection. They can be seen as a sort of genomic parasite. Originally they had the ability to jump from one chromosomal location to another, hence their name, **transposons**. Most have lost this ability, but a few retain it. Whether they have any function useful to us, their hosts, is controversial. At least they are for the most part harmless.

  In addition to these high copy-number repeats, there are many low copy-number repeats that have arisen by recent duplication events. There are many traces of sequences, including gene sequences, being duplicated and then the copies diverging by accumulation of mutations. Often when genes are duplicated only one copy stays functional, the other becoming a non-functional **pseudogene**. Some 12 500 pseudogenes have been identified in the human genome – see **Case 19** (*Chapter 8*) for an example.

- **Is it transcribed?** In addition to transcription of the protein-coding genes, it has long been known that some of our DNA is transcribed to make functional noncoding RNAs such as the ribosomal and transfer RNAs. In recent years there has been an explosion in the number of functional noncoding RNAs that have been identified. In addition to our 23 500 protein-coding genes there are at least 6500 genes for noncoding RNAs. A major class are the **microRNAs (miRNAs)**. These 21–22 nt single-stranded RNAs modulate the translation of many mRNAs by binding to sequences in the 3′ untranslated region. Around 1000 miRNAs have been identified in the human genome, and they have widespread and overlapping effects on gene expression. A single miRNA can affect the expression of hundreds of genes.

  As well as miRNAs, many other noncoding RNAs have been identified. Some of these have known regulatory functions. The *XIST* gene encodes a large spliced RNA that has a vital role in X-inactivation (see *Section 7.2*). Several other examples are known where the expression of a gene is regulated by an antisense RNA that is transcribed from the opposite strand of the gene sequence. A major surprise in recent years has been the discovery of pervasive transcription: the great majority of all the DNA in our genome gets transcribed, at least in some cells and at some time.

Williams–Beuren syndrome (OMIM 194050)

Children with Williams–Beuren syndrome (WBS) are recognized by their combination of learning difficulties, small size and characteristic face with full lips and cheeks and short nose (*Box figure 3.5*). Many have a heart problem, supravalvular aortic stenosis (SVAS), which may require surgery, and some suffer from infantile hypercalcemia, which worsens their failure to thrive and may lead to kidney damage, but which tends to resolve spontaneously. WBS occurs sporadically; there is almost never any family history. About 1 in 20 000 births is affected in both sexes and all ethnic groups.

WBS is interesting both for its mechanism of origin and for its cognitive and behavioral phenotype. The mechanism of origin relates directly to the presence of low copy number repeats, as described above. All WBS patients have a microdeletion that takes out 1.4 Mb of DNA at position 7q11.23. The WBS deletion is a recurrent one, almost always arising *de novo* in each new case. The reason why the same pathogenic deletion occurs over and over again is that the deleted region is flanked by low copy repeats. Over a 300–500 kb region the DNA either side of the WBS-critical region shows greater than 98% sequence homology. When the two copies of chromosome 7 pair during meiosis, occasionally these repeats mispair. If there is then a crossover within the mispaired repeats, the result is to generate one chromosome carrying the WBS deletion and another carrying a duplication of the region (*Box figure 3.6*).

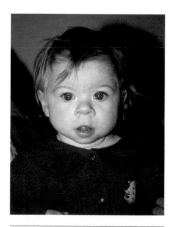

Box figure 3.5 – **Williams–Beuren syndrome.**

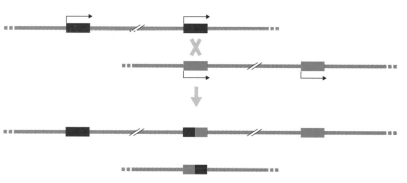

Box figure 3.6 – **Generation of a deletion and the reciprocal duplication by recombination between mispaired repeats flanking the WBS-critical region.** Low copy repeats are a common feature of the human genome, and recombination between mispaired repeats (non-allelic homologous recombination) is a frequent cause of recurrent duplications or deletions of various sizes that cause a number of different human syndromes.

A particular fascination of WBS comes from the cognitive and behavioral phenotype that affected individuals display. Although WBS children have a global IQ similar to children with Down syndrome (usually in the range 40–85), their pattern of abilities and deficiencies is strikingly different. They have relatively good verbal skills which contrast with their poor spatial skills. Asked to draw an object or copy a diagram, a WBS child will crudely reproduce the details but fail to integrate them into any overall picture (*Box figure 3.7*). On the other hand, they can be very eloquent verbally. They also have characteristic behavior and personality traits. They manifest anxiety in unfamiliar situations but may be inappropriately friendly to strangers.

Although the WBS deletion is too small to be seen by conventional cytogenetics, this WBS-critical region contains around 29 genes. There is great interest in trying to relate individual features of the syndrome to the deletion of individual genes. Deficiency of one gene, the elastigene, is known to be responsible for the heart problem. Many researchers hope that this syndrome will give us clues to the more general genetic determinants of normal speech acquisition, cognition and behavior.

DISEASE BOX 3 – continued

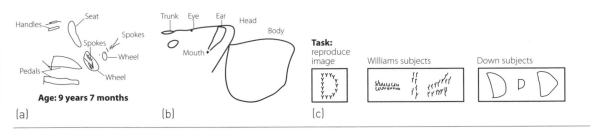

Box figure 3.7 – Drawings by people with WBS.
(a) A bicycle and (b) an elephant. In each case the drawing consists of disconnected parts (labeled by the tester), not integrated into a whole. (c) Children with WBS and children with Down syndrome matched for age and IQ were asked to copy the diagram on the left. Again, note how the WBS children see the details but not the overall design. Illustrations reproduced with permission from Dr Ursula Bellugi, The Salk Institute for Biological Studies.

Overall, the human genome appears chaotic. Evidently there has been no selective pressure for a tidy genome. The contrast with the elegance and efficiency of most of our anatomy and physiology is very striking. It is fascinating to speculate on how and why all this has evolved. The discovery of pervasive transcription has caused a reappraisal of the traditional view of the genome as containing thinly scattered genes separated by long stretches of 'junk DNA'. It raises many unanswered questions. Does most of this activity represent noise in the system, accidental transcription of non-functional sequences because the cell is not very good at recognizing genes? Is there some reason why much of the DNA should be transcribed even if the transcripts have no function? Or is there a whole world of functional RNA species waiting to be discovered? We don't know.

3.5. References

International Human Genome Sequencing Consortium (2001). Initial sequencing and analysis of the human genome. *Nature*, **409**: 860–921.

International Human Genome Sequencing Consortium (2004). Finishing the euchromatic sequence of the human genome. *Nature*, **431**: 931–945.

Loeys BL, Dietz HC, Brauerman AC, *et al*. (2010) The revised Ghent nosology for the Marfan syndrome. *J. Med. Genet.* 47: 476–485.

General background

NCBI Science primer – www.ncbi.nlm.nih.gov/About/primer/

The Online Biology Book produced by MJ Farabee – www.emc.maricopa.edu/faculty/farabee/BIOBK/BioBookTOC.html Chapters 14–19 are good background reading for *Chapters 3–6* of this book

More detail of DNA structure and function can be found in any reasonably recent genetics or cell biology textbook, such as:

- Strachan T and Read AP (2010) *Human Molecular Genetics, 4th edn.* Garland, New York.

- Alberts B, *et al* (2007) *Molecular Biology of the Cell, 5th edn.* Garland, New York.

Earlier editions of both these books are freely available as searchable text on the NCBI Bookshelf – www.ncbi.nlm.nih.gov/entrez/query.fcgi?db=Books

Useful websites

ENSEMBL genome browser: www.ensembl.org/Homo_sapiens/

Human Gene Mutation Database: www.hgmd.org/

SANTA CRUZ genome browser: http://genome.ucsc.edu

3.6. **Self-assessment questions**

(1) Consider the DNA sequence:

CCAGCTTCGCAAGTC

Which base is immediately downstream of a CpG dinucleotide (a) in the strand shown (b) in the complementary strand?

(2) A partial gene sequence from the database reads:

CAGCTGGAGGAACTGGAGCGTGCTTTTGAG

Write out the sequence of the template strand and the mRNA.

(3) The sequence of a 150-nucleotide section of chromosome 7 is shown. It is written in groups of 10 to make counting easier. The sequence in upper case is exon 1 of a gene. Flanking nucleotides shown in lower case are not part of the exon. The initiation codon is double-underlined.

```
  1   gcagccaatg gagggtggtg ttgcgcggggg ctgggattag ggccggggcg
                                    a
 51   aaatgGGATC CTCCAAGGCG ACCATGGCCT TGCTGGGTAA GCGCTGTGAC
                   b                  c
101   GTCCCCACCA ACGGCgttag acctcagtac tgaatcagga cctcactcct
                        d                      e
```

a) What number nucleotide in the sequence is the first one to be transcribed into mRNA?
b) Name the parts of the sequence underlined and labeled a–e, choosing from the following list:
   3′ untranslated region
   3rd codon
   5′ untranslated region
   9th codon
   acceptor splice site (the 3′ end of an intron)
   donor splice site (the 5′ end of an intron)

part of exon 2

part of intron 1

part of intron 2

part of promoter

(4) Here are two nucleic acid sequences. Sequence (A) is a genomic sequence and (B) is the corresponding mRNA.

(A)

```
ATGACCACGCTGGCCGGCGCTGTGCCCAGGATGATGCGGCCGGGCCCGGGGCAGAACTACCCGCGTAGC
GGGTTCCCGCTGGAAGGTAAGGGAGGGCCTCAGCGCGCCGCGCTTCTCTTTTTCACCTTCCCACAGTGT
CCACTCCCCTCGGCCAGGGCCGCGTCAACCAGCTCGGCGGTGTTTTTATCAACGGCAGGTACCAGGAGA
CTGGCTCCATACGTCCTGGTGCCATCGGCGGCAGCAAGCCCAAGGTGAGCGGGCGGGCCTTGCCCTCCT
CGCCTGCCCGCCTGTTCTCTTAAAGCAGGTGACAACGCCTGACGTGGAGAAGAAAATTGAGGAATACAA
AAGAGAGAACCCGGGCGTGCCGTCAGGTACTAGGCCCATTAACCTCTCCCCGCTTCCTTCCTCCTCCCG
CCCCCAGTGAGTTCCATCAGCCGCATCCTGAGAAGTAAATTCGGGAAAGGTGAAGAGGAGGAGGCCGTC
CTGAGCGAGCGAGGTAAGCGGTGGCGCCTTGGGCGGCGGTTGAAGTAGCTTTTATGCCCTCAGGAAAGG
CCCTGGTCTCCGGAGTTTCCTCGCATTAAAGGAGAGAGAGAGAGTACTCTTTTGACTGGT
```

(B)

```
AUGACCACGCUGGCCGGCGCUGUGCCCAGGAUGAUGCGGCCGGGCCCGGGGCAGAACUACCCGCGUAGC
GGGUUCCCGCUGGAAGUGUCCACUCCCCUCGGCCAGGGCCGCGUCAACCAGCUCGGCGGUGUUUUUAUC
AACGGCAGGUACCAGGAGACUGGCUCCAUACGUCCUGGUGCCAUCGGCGGCAGCAAGCCCAAGCAGGUG
ACAACGCCUGACGUGGAGAAGAAAAUUGAGGAAUACAAAAGAGAGAACCCGGGCGUGCCGUCAGUGAGU
UCCAUCAGCCGCAUCCUGAGAAGUAAAUUCGGGAAAGGUGAAGAGGAGGAGGCCGUCCUGAGCGAGCGA
GGAAAGGCCCUGGUCUCCGGAGUUUCCUCGCAUUAAAGGAGAGAGAGAGAGAGUACUCUUUUGACUGGU
```

How many exons does this gene have? Make a little table, showing the nucleotide number (in the genomic sequence) of the start and end of each exon, and the length of each exon and intron. Note that in real genes the introns are likely to be much longer than here.

(5) Look up the following genes using a genome browser such as the ENSEMBL or SANTA CRUZ browser: *BRCA1*, *GJB2*, *DYS*.

(a) How many transcripts are recorded for each?

(b) Choosing one transcript for each gene, note its ID number and report how many exons it has.

(c) What is the relationship between the different transcripts?

(d) What is the size of the gene, from the 5′ end of exon 1 to the 3′ end of the last exon? Note that nucleotides are counted from the tip of the short arm of the chromosome. Because the two strands of the double helix are antiparallel, genes on one strand are transcribed from the short arm tip towards the long arm tip, while those on the other strand are transcribed in the opposite direction. Therefore for genes on one strand the numbering of the nucleotides goes up as you move 5′→3′ through the sense strand, for those on the other strand the numbering goes down.

04 | How can a patient's DNA be studied?

4.1. Case studies

| CASE 11 | Kavanagh family | **81** | 97 | 156 | 389 |

- Healthy first baby boy
- Second child, Celia, pale with low hemoglobin levels
- Sickle cell disease

Ken and Carol are a healthy couple whose first child Keith was born when they were living in their native Kenya. He thrived and soon after Carol became pregnant again. This coincided with the family moving to England for Ken to undertake postgraduate studies and, soon after they arrived, baby Celia was born. Things didn't go so well for her; at three months of age she developed swelling of her fingers which seemed painful and she was referred to a pediatrician who noticed that she seemed pale and found she had an enlarged spleen. Her hemoglobin levels were low, only 7 g/dl, and the reticulocyte count was 12%, indicating she had a hemolytic anemia. The diagnosis of sickle cell disease was made on examination of a blood film which revealed sickled erythrocytes. Carol had trained as a nurse in Kenya and knew a lot about sickle cell disease and was devastated about the implications for Celia. She knew she would be likely to have crises leading to serious bone and abdominal pain necessitating hospital admissions, and that she may need transfusions as well as lifelong penicillin. The next few months were very difficult for the family trying to settle in a new country and adjust to the news about Celia. Although they hadn't planned any more children yet, Carol found that she was pregnant again. Ken and Carol were very upset; they had always wanted three children but were really concerned about the risk of sickle cell disease in the new baby. They thought that their only option would be an abortion. However, when they went to see the gynecologist he explained that it would be possible to have tests early in pregnancy to see if a child was affected or not. They knew the risk of an affected child was 1 in 4 and of a child who was unaffected or a carrier 3 in 4, so they began to feel more optimistic.

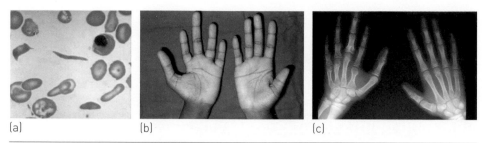

Figure 4.1 – Sickle cell disease.
(a) Blood film showing a sickled cell, marked poikilocytosis (abnormally shaped red cells) and a nucleated rell cell. (b and c) Bony infarctions in the phalanges and metacarpals can result in unequal finger length. Photos courtesy of Dr Andrew Will, Royal Manchester Children's Hospital.

| CASE 12 | Lipton family | **82** | 98 | 389 |

- Family history of learning difficulties
- Baby boy, Luke, with poor head control
- ? Fragile X syndrome
- Blood taken for DNA extraction

Linda and Laurence Lipton were delighted when their son Luke was born and appeared healthy. He weighed 3.6 kg, fed well and seemed a 'good' baby who didn't cry much and lay still when his diaper was changed. Linda had a friend with a baby of the same age and as time went on Linda became concerned about Luke's head control and how slow he was compared to her friend's baby. Linda's anxieties were made worse by the fact that she had an older brother, Len, who had learning difficulties and lived in a group home. She hadn't been worried about risks to her children because she had been told that her brother had been 'starved of oxygen' during birth. Linda told the doctor at the baby clinic about her worries, but an examination didn't reveal any problems other than that Luke was a little hypotonic; in fact the doctor said he had a very good head size for his age. The doctor also asked about family history, particularly in the female line.

Linda had always known that she had two male half-cousins who had learning difficulties. As a biology teacher, she knew about X-linked inheritance and, having drawn up a pedigree (*Figure 4.2b*), she suddenly realized that the pattern in the family might indicate an X-linked condition. But subsequently she dismissed the idea because her mother and her two aunts were the products of three separate marriages of her maternal grandfather Luigi. X-linked inheritance would either require Luigi's three unrelated wives all coincidentally to be carriers of the condition, or else would require Luigi himself to be the source of the mutant allele in all three of his daughters. Three independent mutations would be too much of a coincidence, while Luigi himself was clearly unaffected, having founded a very successful business. Also, there was the question of her cousin Lydia. Lydia was strikingly slow, had left school without any qualifications and worked as an unskilled care assistant. If there were an X-linked condition segregating in the family, Lydia could be a heterozygote – but all the other women in the family who, on this hypothesis, would also be heterozygotes were graduates following professional careers. Linda asked to be referred to the genetic clinic because she wanted to go through all her reasoning and to see whether an expert agreed the pedigree was incompatible with X-linked inheritance. The doctor in the genetic clinic, however, thought the pedigree and phenotypes to be very suggestive of

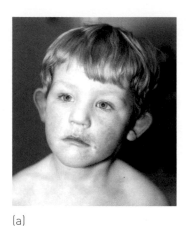

(a)

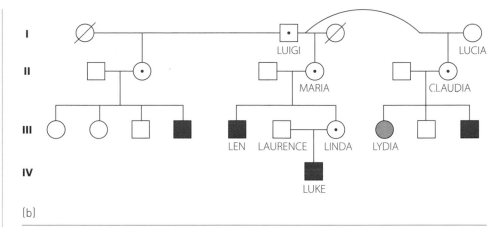

(b)

Figure 4.2
(a) Typical facial appearance of a boy with Fragile X syndrome. (b) Pedigree of the Lipton family. Affected males are shown in black; III-8 (gray) is a mildly affected female. Obligate carriers are indicated. Note that the normal male I-2 is the source of the Fragile X chromosome in his daughters. He is an example of a normal transmitting male (see *Section 4.3*).

Fragile X syndrome. She explained why she thought this to Linda and gave her some literature about the syndrome and arranged to take blood for DNA extraction.

| CASE 13 | Meinhardt family | **83** | 102 | 389 |

- Baby girl, Madelena, with small head, large ears and needing to be tube fed
- Normal 46,XX karyotype
- ? Underlying chromosome problem

Madelena was the second child born to Manfred and Margareta. Their older son was healthy and developing normally. Madelena was born at term weighing 2.7 kg but there were problems from the beginning, even though scans in pregnancy had been reassuring. Madelena was hypotonic; she wouldn't suck from a bottle and needed to be tube fed. She was also noted to have a relatively small head, a ridged metopic suture and large ears. In view of these problems the pediatrician arranged for a routine chromosome test which showed a normal 46,XX karyotype. Although her mother managed to get her onto bottle feeds and the family was able to go home, this progress did not last long and Madelena was readmitted to hospital 2 weeks later with constant crying. In spite of tube feeding being restarted she did not settle and so the specialist undertook another detailed examination. He was worried to find that Madelena's corneas appeared cloudy and asked for an urgent ophthalmic check, which confirmed that she had severe congenital glaucoma known as buphthalmos. Surgery was performed immediately to save her sight. Madelena's further development was slow; she didn't smile until she was 5 months old, she was only able to sit at 16 months, and the decision was made to feed her directly into her stomach through a gastrostomy tube because of recurrent chest infections due to inhalation of milk. Manfred and Margareta didn't think matters could get much worse but the next problem they faced was the onset of seizures in Madelena at 2 years of age, leading to more hospital admissions and tests. The family was desperate to know what might be the underlying cause of

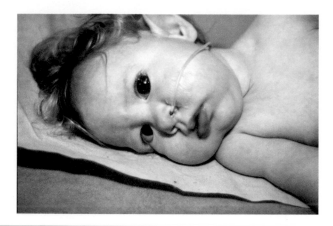

Figure 4.3 – A child with multiple congenital abnormalities suggestive of a chromosomal abnormality.
Note small head, prominent metopic region (above bridge of nose) and large ear.
Note also buphthalmos (large eyes) due to congenital glaucoma.

all their daughter's problems and they were referred to a geneticist who strongly suspected an underlying chromosome problem. However, it was several years before a test became available that could scan the whole genome for small copy number changes (duplications or deletions).

4.2. Science toolkit

A diploid human cell contains 6×10^9 bp of DNA, all chemically identical, all consisting of A, G, C and T nucleotides. Progressing the analysis of most of our cases will require us to examine specific genes or chromosomal regions in DNA samples provided by the patients. How can we achieve this, against a background of so much chemically identical but irrelevant DNA?

All the many laboratory methods boil down to one of two essential approaches:

a) hybridize the sequence to a labeled matching sequence (a **probe**).
b) amplify the sequence of interest; it is repeatedly copied to generate a large excess of just that sequence.

The principles and the applications that will be used in this chapter's investigations are described below. Some further applications that are important in clinical genetics are described in the final section of the chapter.

Nucleic acid hybridization

The two strands of a double helical DNA molecule are held together by relatively weak chemical bonds (hydrogen bonds) between paired bases. The bonds can be broken by boiling the solution containing the DNA, or by exposing it to a high pH. This is called **denaturing** the DNA. The process is reversible. Complementary single-stranded nucleic acids will **hybridize** or **anneal** (stick together to form a double helix) if they are mixed in solution at a moderate (typically below 50–60°C) temperature and pH (*Figure 4.4*). The ability of matching strands to hybridize is the basis of much of DNA technology.

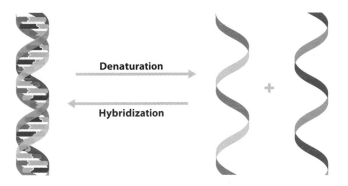

Figure 4.4 – Denaturation of double-stranded DNA; hybridization of two complementary single strands.

Hybridization does not necessarily require a perfect match between the strands. Two strands will hybridize if there are enough correctly matching base pairs that can form hydrogen bonds, even if some bases are mismatched. Strands with mismatches will denature at a lower temperature than perfectly matched strands, and equally will require a lower temperature to hybridize successfully. Short strands will denature more easily than long strands because there are fewer hydrogen bonds holding them together. They need a lower temperature for hybridization, and hybridization is more sensitive to mismatches. By manipulating these variables, hybridization can be used in various different ways for DNA testing.

Using hybridization as the basis for DNA testing

Hybridization tests used in clinical genetics fall into two general types:

- Sometimes a test is used to check for a point mutation or very small sequence change in the test DNA. In the Kavanagh family (Case 11; sickle cell), if we are to check their fetus for the sickle cell mutation by a DNA test, we need to look for a substitution of one specific nucleotide out of the 3 000 000 000 in its genome. One way to do this is to use a short synthetic oligonucleotide (a piece of DNA typically 15–30 nucleotides long) as the hybridization probe. For such a short probe, the hybridization conditions can be such as to require a perfect match. Even a mismatch of a single nucleotide will be enough to prevent hybridization. Highly specific hybridization is also a prerequisite for the polymerase chain reaction (PCR, see below), which therefore also depends on using oligonucleotides. Although PCR is not primarily a test for hybridization, it does depend on specific hybridization for its ability to amplify just one specific sequence.

- At other times we want a hybridization test that will work on anybody's DNA, regardless of any minor differences between the DNA of different people. When we use a hybridization test to check for chromosomal microdeletions in Gillian Green (Case 7; ?22q11 deletion), we don't want hybridization to fail just because the corresponding sequence in the

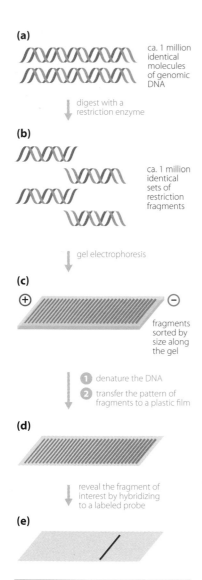

(a)

ca. 1 million
identical
molecules
of genomic
DNA

↓ digest with a
restriction enzyme

(b)

ca. 1 million
identical
sets of
restriction
fragments

↓ gel electrophoresis

(c)

⊕ ⊖

fragments
sorted by
size along
the gel

↓ 1 denature the DNA
2 transfer the pattern of
fragments to a plastic film

(d)

↓ reveal the fragment of
interest by hybridizing
to a labeled probe

(e)

**Figure 4.5 – Southern blot
analysis of DNA**
The test DNA (a) is digested with
a restriction endonuclease (b).
The fragments are separated
by size by gel electrophoresis
(c), denatured by immersing
the gel in alkali, and then
transferred to a nitrocellulose
film (d). The nitrocellulose sheet
is then immersed in a solution
containing the labeled probe,
revealing any fragments that
hybridize (e). See *Box 4.1* for
more details.

patient has a few variant nucleotides. Lack of hybridization should mean that the whole sequence is deleted. For these tests we use a much longer hybridization probe, typically a cloned piece of natural DNA. A probe 1 kb long will hybridize to its cognate sequence even if this varies a bit between individuals.

Whichever procedure we use for a hybridization test, we need to be able to tell whether or not the probe has hybridized to the test DNA. Most commonly this is achieved by labeling one of the two hybridizing partners, then separating out the other partner and seeing whether or not the label has accompanied it. In former times DNA was usually labeled by incorporation of radioactive ^{32}P; nowadays it is more usual to tag it with a fluorescent dye. Usually the separation is achieved by fixing one partner to a solid support – a piece of nitrocellulose film or a microscope slide, for example. This is immersed in a solution containing the labeled partner, left to hybridize, then taken out and washed. The label will then mark any areas of the solid support where hybridization has taken place. The investigations in this chapter use the following procedures.

- **Dot blotting** – for the Kavanagh family (Case 11; sickle cell) fetal DNA is spotted onto a nitrocellulose film that is immersed in a solution containing labeled oligonucleotide probes specific for the normal and sickle cell sequences. This is illustrated in *Figure 4.11*.
- **Southern blotting** – for the Lipton family (Case 12) the diagnosis of Fragile X syndrome is made by demonstrating a large expansion of a $(CGG)_n$ trinucleotide repeat in the 5′ untranslated region of the *FMR1* gene, as described below. A Southern blot (summarized in *Box 4.1* and *Figure 4.5*) is used rather than PCR to check for large expansions because long highly CG-rich sequences are difficult to amplify by PCR. As shown in *Figure 7.8*, G–C base pairs are held together by three hydrogen bonds, compared to only two for A–T base pairs, and so these sequences do not denature readily.
- **Fluorescence *in situ* hybridization (FISH)** is used to check the presence or absence, copy number and chromosomal location of a particular DNA sequence in chromosomes of a patient. For Gillian Green (Case 7; ?22q11 deletion) we want to check for a megabase-sized deletion at a specific chromosomal location. If a deletion is present it will affect only one of the two homologous chromosomes. To retain the information about the chromosomal location the hybridization target is a spread of her chromosomes on a microscope slide, rather than extracted DNA. By very careful treatment the DNA in the spread-out chromosomes can be denatured without destroying the recognizable form of the chromosomes. Although each sequence has its partner nearby, because they are stuck down on the glass slide, the partners cannot move to find each other, so the chromosomal DNA remains single-stranded. The slide is exposed to a solution containing the labeled probe. A cloned piece of the relevant DNA, tens of kilobases long, is used as the probe so that, as mentioned above, minor sequence variations do not affect the hybridization. The probe is labeled with a fluorescent dye. After hybridization the slide is washed and examined under the microscope. Where the probe has hybridized, a pair

BOX 4.1

Principle of Southern blotting

The test DNA is first cut into specific fragments using a special enzyme (a restriction endonuclease – see *Box 4.2* and *Figure 4.5b*). These enzymes cut the DNA in a reproducible way, so that every molecule gives the same set of fragments. The mixture of fragments is subjected to gel electrophoresis (*Box 4.3*) so that fragments of different sizes are located at different positions in the gel (*Figure 4.5c*). The fragments, still in their size-dependent pattern, are denatured in alkali to make them single-stranded. We want to see which fragments will hybridize to our probe, but the hybridization reaction will not work efficiently on DNA immobilized in a gel. The molecules cannot move about to find partners. The next step is therefore to transfer the fragments on to nitrocellulose paper, while retaining their spread-out pattern. This is the actual Southern blotting procedure. It is usually done by laying the sheet of nitrocellulose paper on top of the gel, putting a stack of dry paper towels on top of that, and very carefully pressing so that the liquid in the gel is sucked through the nitrocellulose paper into the towels. The denatured DNA sticks to the nitrocellulose (*Figure 4.5d*). As before, this is immersed in a solution containing a labeled probe that will stick to just the fragment of interest and reveal its position (*Figure 4.5e*). Depending on the label used, the location of the probe is detected by autoradiography or by fluorescence. The technique provides information on whether a sequence matching the probe is present and, if so, on what size restriction fragment it is located.

of fluorescent spots is seen over the relevant chromosome (a pair of spots because at this stage in the cell cycle each chromosome consists of two sister chromatids, see *Chapter 2*). *Figure 4.6* shows the principle, *Figure 4.14* an actual example.

- **Interphase FISH** – Anne Howard (Case 8, Down syndrome) has been offered a prenatal test to see if her fetus has Down syndrome. Fetal cells have been obtained by amniocentesis (see *Chapter 14*). Interphase FISH allows specific chromosomes to be counted without waiting for the cells to divide in culture. As with the standard FISH protocol (above), the cells

BOX 4.2

Restriction endonucleases

These bacterial enzymes cut double-stranded DNA whenever they encounter some specific short sequence, usually 4, 6 or 8 bp long. Bacteria use them as part of a defense mechanism against foreign DNA. Many different restriction enzymes have been isolated from a wide range of bacterial species. Each has its own recognition sequence – for example, the enzyme *Eco*RI cuts GAATTC.

For molecular biologists, restriction enzymes are very valuable tools. They provide a means to cut a DNA molecule reproducibly into large fragments. It is easy to forget that virtually everything one does with DNA involves a large collection of identical molecules. For example, a Southern blot would typically use 5 µg of DNA extracted from blood. One human cell contains 6.4 pg of DNA, so 6.4 µg of DNA would be the DNA content of 1 million cells. Thus the starting material is a very large collection of identical molecules. Unless the restriction enzyme cuts each molecule in exactly the same places, the fragments would be a complete jumble and would not run as sharp bands on a gel. The average size of fragment depends on the choice of restriction enzyme. On average, a 4-bp restriction site will occur by chance once every $4^4 = 256$ bp, while a 6-bp site will occur on average every 4096 bp. Restriction sites are randomly distributed in human DNA so there will be a wide spread of fragment sizes around these averages.

BOX 4.3

Gel electrophoresis

Along with PCR, gel electrophoresis is a central tool of molecular genetics. DNA molecules carry a negative charge because of the phosphate groups (see *Box 3.2*). In an electric field a DNA molecule will move towards the positive pole. If the DNA is contained in an agarose or polyacrylamide gel, the DNA molecules have to fight their way through a jungle of long polymer molecules. How fast a double-stranded DNA molecule moves depends almost entirely on its size, and hardly at all on its sequence. Small molecules move quickly, large ones

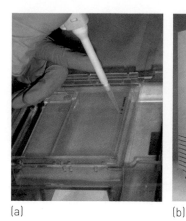
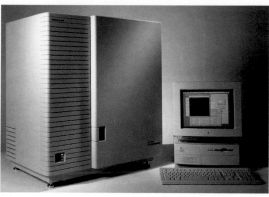

(a)   (b)

Box figure 4.1 – Gel electrophoresis.
(a) Loading an electrophoretic gel. The DNA samples, mixed with blue dye to make them visible, are pipeted into wells formed in the agarose gel. The gel is submerged in a buffer solution to cool it and make electrical contact. (b) An automated gene analyzer. The machine electrophoreses 96 fluorescently labeled DNA samples in parallel through very thin capillaries. For each sample it records the time it takes for each fragment to emerge from the capillary, and the intensity of the fluorescence.

move slowly. Molecules of a given size will form a sharp band. The position of a fragment, revealed by hybridization or staining, is a measure of its size. As mentioned later, single-stranded DNA, or double helices containing mismatched bases show anomalous migration rates, which is the basis of some methods for detecting mutations. Electrophoresis is most simply carried out manually through a slab gel, as illustrated in *Box figure 4.1a*, but for diagnostic purposes it is usual to use an automated gene analyzer (*Box figure 4.1b*). The software displays the result as a trace with peaks (an electropherogram; see *Figure 4.18*). The position of a peak determines the size of a fragment, and the area under the peak measures the quantity.

are immobilized on a microscope slide, the DNA carefully denatured and a fluorescently labeled probe applied. The probe consists of a sequence specific for the chromosome in question. The number of fluorescent spots in the cell nucleus is counted. Spots are counted in 50 cells, and if more than 60% of them show three spots for the chromosome in question, this is taken to indicate trisomy (the hybridization never works in 100% of cells).

- **Comparative genomic hybridization (CGH)** is a general method of looking for copy-number variants. That is, it checks for any sequence that is present in a greater or smaller number of copies per genome in the test DNA compared to a normal control DNA. It can detect variants that are too small to be seen under the microscope and, unlike FISH, it does not require prior knowledge of the chromosomal location of any variant.

  The probes are in the form of a **microarray**. Microarrays use the dot blot principle on a massively parallel scale. In this case it is the probe rather than the test DNA that is anchored to a solid support, and the

(a)

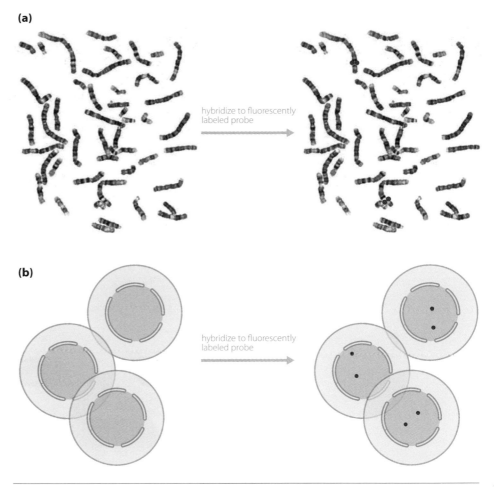

hybridize to fluorescently
labeled probe

(b)

hybridize to fluorescently
labeled probe

Figure 4.6 – Fluorescence *in situ* hybridization (FISH).
FISH can be used on either a chromosome spread (a) or on non-dividing cells (b). In either case the material, on a microscope slide, is very carefully denatured and then hybridized to a fluorescently labeled probe. See *Figures 4.14* and *4.15* for examples.

test DNA rather than the probe that is labeled with a fluorescent dye. Thousands of different probes are anchored in a grid pattern to a glass slide, which is then immersed in a solution containing the labeled test DNA. The slide is divided into thousands of cells, like the pixels of a digital image, each of which contains many thousands of molecules of one particular probe. CGH uses competitive hybridization. DNA from the patient and DNA from a normal control are labeled with two different fluorescent dyes, for example, the patient green and the control red. The two labeled DNAs are mixed in equal proportions and allowed to hybridize to the microarray (*Figure 4.7*). Green DNA fragments from the patient compete with red fragments from the control for hybridization to the molecules of the probe in each cell of the array. After hybridization and washing, the slide is examined under a microscope to determine the relative amounts of red and green fluorescence bound to each cell. Where the two are present in equal amounts the cell fluoresces yellow. Sequences where one or both copies are deleted in the patient give cells

Figure 4.7 – Principle of CGH using a microarray of genomic clones (array-CGH). Adapted with permission from an original by Dr Joris Veltman, Nijmegen.

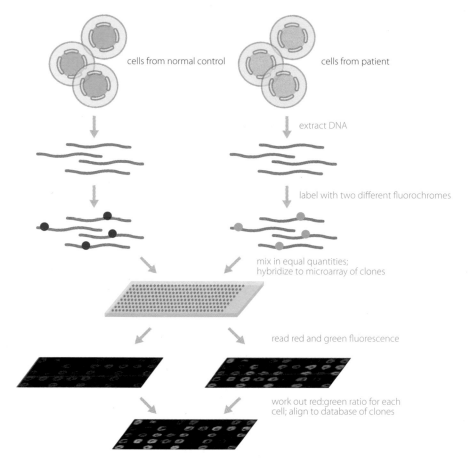

cells from normal control

cells from patient

extract DNA

label with two different fluorochromes

mix in equal quantities; hybridize to microarray of clones

read red and green fluorescence

work out red:green ratio for each cell; align to database of clones

with more red fluorescence, because for that sequence there is relatively more control DNA. Duplications give green cells (*Figure 4.8*).

Array-CGH has many powerful features. The availability, through the Human Genome Project, of huge numbers of precisely mapped and characterized clones allows total control over the specificity and resolution of a CGH array. Arrays can be constructed that are specific for one particular chromosome, or that cover the entire genome. The resolution depends on the number and size of probes used and their distribution across the genome. Because each probe is precisely mapped on the human genome sequence, any deletion or duplication detected can be immediately linked to a list of the genes involved. An earlier version of CGH used a spread of normal chromosomes on a microscope slide in place of the microarray. This has now been superseded by array-CGH. CGH is a very powerful tool but it has two main limitations in clinical testing. It cannot detect balanced chromosomal rearrangements such as translocations or inversions, only copy number changes, and it is quite expensive.

- **SNP chips** offer an alternative application of microarray technology to detect copy number changes. These microarrays use allele-specific oligonucleotides to genotype a DNA sample for a large number of common single nucleotide polymorphisms (SNPs). Around 1 nucleotide in 300 across the human genome is polymorphic – that is, at a certain

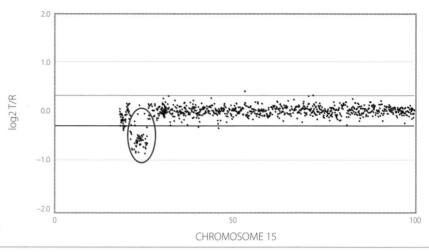

Figure 4.8 – Example of array-CGH output.
The test DNA (labeled green) and control DNA (labeled red) were mixed and hybridized to a microarray containing over 30 000 Bacterial Artificial Chromosome (BAC) probes, each from a known chromosomal location. The ratio of green to red signal for each cell of the array is plotted on the vertical axis. Ratios above the upper normal limit (green line) indicate a duplication in the test DNA; ratios below the lower normal limit (red line) indicate a deletion. The results are arranged along the horizontal axis according to the chromosomal location of the probe. Here only results from probes from chromosome 15 are shown. The circle shows a set of contiguous clones from 15q11–q13 that are present in only a single copy in the test DNA, indicating heterozygosity for a deletion. Courtesy of Dr Joris Veltman, Nijmegen.

position in the genome, two (or occasionally more) alternative nucleotides are each quite frequent in the population. The great majority of SNPs are in noncoding DNA and have no phenotypic effect. SNP chips are versatile tools: they are used in linkage analysis as described in *Chapter 9*, and in the search for genetic susceptibility factors for non-mendelian diseases as described in *Chapter 13*. They are also increasingly replacing array-CGH as the method of choice for identifying copy number variants, as the case of Madelena Meinhardt (Case 13) will illustrate (*Figure 4.16*).

A typical SNP chip would carry oligonucleotides specific for each allele of maybe 500 000 SNPs spaced across the genome. Unlike array-CGH, the test does not use competitive hybridization. Only the DNA of the patient is used. Both the hybridization intensity and the SNP genotypes (homozygous or heterozygous) can provide useful information. If there is a microdeletion, this would show as a series of contiguous SNPs where the DNA only hybridized to the probe for one allele, but with a hybridization intensity only half what one would see with DNA from somebody who was homozygous for that allele. A duplication would show as an increased intensity of hybridization, compared to the probes mapping either side of the duplicated region. Comparing genotypes and intensities in the patient and his parents can shed light on the origin and nature of any variants detected.

Amplifying the sequence of interest

When the sequence of interest forms only a very small fraction of a DNA sample, it may be made visible and followed by means of specific hybridization, as described above. Alternatively, it can be studied after selective amplification. Traditionally this was done by cloning the sequence in a living cell, usually in *E. coli* bacteria. This enabled the researcher to obtain many copies of the sequence in pure form, uncontaminated by all the other DNA originally present. This method is described in *Box 4.4*. For most clinical purposes cloning in living cells has been superseded by PCR. This is a form of *in vitro* cloning. Like conventional cloning, it works by making many copies of just the sequence of interest, but in a much quicker and

---

BOX 4.4

Amplifying a sequence by cloning

Until the mid 1980s, cloning was the only way to isolate a DNA fragment for study. It exploited the idea that if a DNA fragment was put into a cell in the right way, and then the cell was allowed to grow to form a colony of daughter cells, each of the daughter cells would contain a copy of the inserted fragment. The cells used are usually *E.coli* bacteria, but can be yeast, mammalian cells, or other types.

Cloning requires a **vector**. Getting a DNA fragment into a cell is surprisingly easy, but a loose DNA fragment inserted into a cell will normally be rapidly degraded and will certainly not be replicated when the cell divides. Vectors are pieces of DNA containing features that cause the host cell to tolerate their presence and replicate them. They are derived from naturally occurring viruses or plasmids. The fragment to be amplified is ligated into the vector so that together they form a single recombinant DNA molecule. A vast amount of ingenuity has gone into engineering vectors optimized for specific tasks. Engineered vectors incorporate various ingenious arrangements for identifying host cells that contain the recombinant vector, and for isolating the cloned DNA after the host cells have been grown up. For present purposes the only important point to note is that each type of vector has a maximum size of inserted fragment that it can accommodate (see *Box table 4.1* below). This maximum size is always very much smaller than a chromosome, and smaller than many individual human genes:

Box table 4.1 – **Some vectors used for cloning DNA fragments.**

Vector	Host cell	Maximum cloning capacity	Comments
Plasmid	*E. coli*	5–10 kb	Simple vectors for cloning small fragments
Cosmid	*E. coli*	45 kb	Mainly historical importance
Bacterial artificial chromosome (BAC)	*E. coli*	150 kb	Workhorse of the Human Genome Project
Yeast artificial chromosome (YAC)	Yeast	1000 kb	Technically tricky; special purposes only

The ability to cut and patch DNA, so central to genetic engineering, depends on the restriction endonucleases, described above, and on another enzyme, DNA ligase. Many restriction enzymes make a staggered cut when they cut a double helix, leaving short single strands ('sticky ends') protruding. Fragments with complementary sticky ends can hybridize end-to-end (see *Box figure 4.2*). DNA ligase then joins the abutting strands permanently with a standard (covalent) chemical bond.

BOX 4.4 – *continued*

Cloning is an essentially random process. A large collection of molecules of the test DNA is broken into random fragments. These are incorporated *en masse* into millions of vector molecules which in turn are used to infect millions of host cells. Vectors are engineered so that host cells containing a recombinant vector can be selected, usually through a particular pattern of antibiotic resistance. Next, single cells are picked and used to grow colonies. Each colony is an inexhaustible source of one specific human DNA fragment. The resulting collection of clones is called a **library** and ideally would contain cloned examples of every sequence in the test DNA. 'Library' is a very misleading name – in a real library the books are ordered on shelves and there is a catalog that enables you to go straight to any book you want. Recombinant DNA libraries might better be called haystacks, that may or may not contain the needle you want.

During the period 1970–1990, the rate of progress of human molecular genetics was largely determined by the rate at which interesting clones could be found by screening libraries. For a view of this heroic phase of human genetics, flip through any human genetics or molecular biology textbook from the 1980s. Nowadays the Human Genome Project has made available a complete collection of fully characterized and mapped BAC clones covering the entire genome. We also have a much easier way of amplifying selected DNA fragments from the genome of a patient, by PCR. As a result, making and screening recombinant DNA libraries is no longer part of mainstream clinical investigation, though it is still an important research activity.

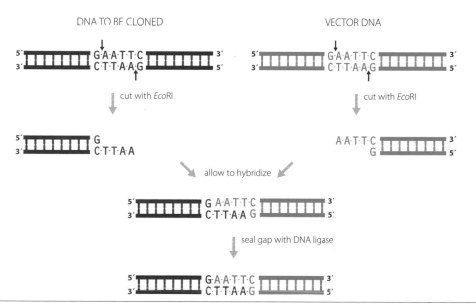

Box figure 4.2 – Creating a recombinant DNA molecule.
Two different molecules are digested with the same restriction enzyme to create complementary sticky ends. They hybridize, and are permanently joined by DNA ligase.

easier way. Unlike conventional cloning, the PCR process does not separate the amplified sequence from the original mixture. If necessary this can be done in a separate step, but for many purposes this is not required. The amplified sequence is present in such large excess that the whole product can be treated as a slightly impure preparation of just the sequence of interest. PCR has several advantages over *in vivo* cloning – it is easier and quicker, but crucially, it is selective. With PCR you choose which bit of the DNA you want to amplify. With *in vivo* cloning you clone everything, then have to search through thousands or millions of clones to find the one you want.

The polymerase chain reaction

PCR revolutionized molecular genetics. Before PCR, only skilled researchers could amplify and characterize DNA. From around 1990, improved PCR methods allowed selective amplification of sequences from patient samples to become a routine tool in diagnostic laboratories.

PCR depends on three features of DNA replication.

(1) A new chain requires a **primer**. DNA polymerase (the enzyme that replicates DNA by synthesizing a strand complementary to a single-stranded template) cannot simply start assembling isolated nucleotides; it can only work by extending an existing chain. The primers used in PCR are chemically synthesized single-strand oligonucleotides, normally around 20 nt long.

(2) Chain extension can only proceed in the 5'→3' direction (see *Box 3.2*)

(3) The two strands of a DNA double helix are anti-parallel, as shown in *Figure 3.5a.*

The requirement for a primer makes it possible to force DNA polymerase to copy just a selected sequence in a complex DNA sample. A chemical oligonucleotide synthesizer is used to make a large number of molecules of a specific single-stranded oligonucleotide, whose sequence is such that it will hybridize to only one particular sequence in the human DNA. A large excess of this primer is added to the DNA. The whole sample is denatured by brief heating to 95°C, then cooled to a temperature at which hybridization can take place (typically 55–60°C). Some of the original double helices in the complex DNA will re-form, but because there are so many more molecules of the primer, the sequence that matches the primer will most likely end up hybridized to the primer, rather than to its original partner. If the starting material consists of DNA from many cells, as is usually the case, some copies of the relevant sequence may re-hybridize to their original partner, but most will end up hybridized to a molecule of the primer. If DNA polymerase is then allowed to act on the mixture, most of the action will consist of adding nucleotides on to the 3' end of the primer, building up a strand complementary to that bit of the genomic DNA. *Figure 4.9* summarizes this process.

The PCR uses this principle, but converts the linear reaction of *Figure 4.9* into an exponential chain reaction by using two primers and multiple cycles of denaturation, hybridization and synthesis. *Figure 4.10* shows how it works. The primers hybridize specifically to opposite strands of the DNA either side of the sequence to be amplified, and are oriented so that 5'→3' chain extension from each primer runs towards the other primer. Thus each strand being synthesized by extending the forward primer comes to include the sequence to which the reverse primer can hybridize, and each strand made by extending the reverse primer comes to include the sequence to which the forward primer can bind. *Box 4.5* explains the process in more detail.

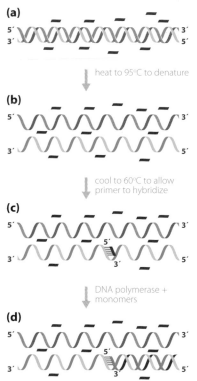

(a)

5' 3'
3' 5'

heat to 95°C to denature

(b)

5' 3'
3' 5'

cool to 60°C to allow primer to hybridize

(c)

5' 3'
5'
3'
3' 5'

DNA polymerase + monomers

(d)

5' 3'
5'
3'
3' 5'

Figure 4.9 – Using a synthetic primer to force DNA polymerase to synthesize just a strand complementary to a specified part of a large DNA molecule.
(a) The primer (red) is present in a large molecular excess. (c) It hybridizes only to one specific sequence. (d) Only sequence downstream of the primer is copied.

BOX 4.5

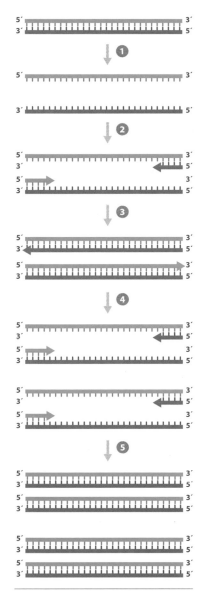

Figure 4.10 – Principle of PCR.
The PCR reaction contains the target DNA, the DNA polymerase enzyme, large amounts of both primers and a supply of mononucleotides. (1) The starting DNA is denatured by heating to 95°C. (2) At 55–60°C the primers anneal to their target sequences. Note the 5′ and 3′ directions. (3) At 72°C the polymerase extends the primers in the 5′→ 3′ direction. (4) Another round of denaturing and annealing primers. (5) Another round of polymerization. After two rounds of PCR we have four strands where originally we had one.

Understanding PCR

In each round of denaturation, hybridization and synthesis, not only the original template but also all the copies made in previous rounds are replicated. Thus the amount of target DNA is doubled in each round – 20 rounds of PCR should suffice to amplify the target sequence one million-fold. Cycles of PCR are controlled by varying the temperature. A few seconds at 95°C denatures everything. Then a few seconds at around 55–60°C allows the primers to anneal to every possible template. Finally a few seconds at 72°C, the optimum temperature for the special polymerase used, sees each primer extended by adding nucleotides to the 3′ end. A typical amplification of 20–25 cycles with each stage lasting 30–60 seconds can be set up and completed in under 2 hours. A programmable heating and cooling block is used that will hold 20 or more individual reaction tubes, so that a number of samples can be PCR-amplified in parallel (*Box figure 4.3*).

The selectivity of PCR depends on having primers that will anneal only to the desired target and not to any other sequence in the whole genome. The necessary specificity is achieved by using short primers (usually 18–22 nt) and fine-tuning the temperature. If the annealing temperature is too low, the primers may be able to hybridize to mismatched targets, while if it is too high they will not hybridize at all. Usually a temperature in the 55–60°C range allows specific hybridization. Possible primers are checked against the complete genome sequence database to make sure that no other sequence matches the primer. The length and nucleotide composition of the

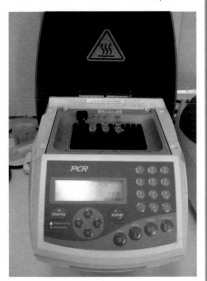

Box figure 4.3 – A typical thermocycler, used to carry out PCR amplification.
When in use an insulating lid covers the tubes.

primer can affect the efficiency of the PCR process, and there are computer programs to assist with primer design.

When working out what goes on in PCR it is useful to think of two classes of PCR product:

- Product A is synthesized using the original DNA as the template. Molecules of Product A have a defined 5′ end (the 5′ end of the primer) but are of indeterminate length.

- Product B is synthesized using Product A as template. Both ends of Product B are defined. The 5′ end is the 5′ end of the primer used to make it, and the 3′ end is defined by the end of its template (the 5′ end of Product A). All molecules of Product B are exactly the same size.

BOX 4.5 – continued

In later cycles of the PCR reaction, Product B is also used as the template for the next round of synthesis (see *Box table 4.2*). The end of a strand made by extending primer 1 is complementary to primer 2, and so in the next cycle primer 2 can hybridize to it and prime synthesis of a complementary strand. The end of this strand, in turn, is complementary to primer 1. The newly synthesized strand is exactly the same length as its template. After the first few cycles, virtually all the product is made in this way, using Product B as the template.

The best way to understand how PCR works is to take a large sheet of paper and draw out what happens in the first three or four cycles of the reaction. Check your effort against *Figure 4.10*. Take care to mark 3′ and 5′ ends. Make sure that hybridized strands are always anti-parallel and that strand extension is always 5′→3′.

Box table 4.2 – **Progress of the PCR reaction.**

	Starting DNA	Product A template is starting DNA; 1 defined end		Product B template can be Product A or Product B; 2 defined ends		
	Single strands	Made in this cycle	Cumulative total	Made in this cycle using Product A as template	Made in this cycle using Product B as template	Cumulative total
After 1 cycle	2	2	2			
After 2 cycles	2	2	4	2	–	2
After 3 cycles	2	2	6	4	2	8
After 4 cycles	2	2	8	6	8	22
After 5 cycles	2	2	10	8	22	52

We imagine starting with one molecule of double-stranded DNA. After the first few rounds, almost all the product consists of just the sequence between the outside ends of the two primers. The numbers are numbers of single strands that are present when all the DNA is denatured.

PCR has certain limitations:

- you need to know enough about the sequence to be amplified to be able to design specific primers
- PCR works best for amplifying sequences of 100–400 bp. Sequences longer than 1–2 kb are difficult, and sequences above 20 kb almost impossible to amplify

At the end of the PCR reaction, although all the original irrelevant DNA is still present, the amplified sequence is present in such excess that the product can be treated as a slightly impure preparation of just the target sequence.

Similarly to Southern blotting, PCR can be used to detect the presence or absence of a sequence or to measure its size. Examples of both those applications are shown below. Additionally, PCR products are suitable for sequencing and testing for point mutations, as we shall see in *Chapter 5*.

4.3. **Investigations of patients**

We will first consider cases that were investigated by hybridization. The DNA regions involved range from a single nucleotide in the first case through successively larger parts of the genome until in the fourth case the entire genome was surveyed. The final three cases use PCR to check for the presence or absence of a sequence and to measure its size. In *Chapter 5* we will see examples of using PCR to check the actual nucleotide sequence.

Cases studied using a hybridization procedure

| CASE 11 | Kavanagh family | 81 | **97** | 156 | 389 |

- Healthy first baby boy
- Second child, Celia, pale with low hemoglobin levels
- Sickle cell disease

Sickle cell disease is caused by a single nucleotide substitution in exon 1 of the β-globin gene on chromosome 11. This changes a codon for glutamic acid into one for valine. Hemoglobin consists of two α-globin and two β-globin chains (plus four heme groups). The amino acid substitution in the β-globin affects the properties of the hemoglobin, causing it to aggregate and distort red blood cells. Heterozygotes have sickling trait, demonstrable in the laboratory, but they are normally healthy. Homozygotes have sickle cell disease, an autosomal recessive condition. Sickle cell disease and sickling trait are readily identifiable by standard hematological analysis; DNA tests are not needed to make the diagnosis. However, prenatal diagnosis requires testing of the DNA. Fetal blood sampling is difficult, not available in many centers and carries risks to the pregnancy; in any case, fetuses produce γ-globin instead of β-globin.

There are several alternative methods that could be used to check for the sickle cell mutation. The test used here is a dot-blot with two allele-specific oligonucleotides (ASOs) to distinguish the normal and sickle sequences. Some of the alternative methods that could have been used are discussed in *Chapter 5*.

The normal β-globin gene sequence reads (in part):

CTGACTCCTG**A**GGAGAAGTCTG

while the mutant version that is the cause of sickle cell disease reads:

CTGACTCCTG**T**GGAGAAGTCTG

Fetal DNA was obtained by chorion villus biopsy at 11 weeks of gestation (see *Chapter 14*). To increase the sensitivity of the test, a fragment containing the β-globin gene was amplified by PCR. The PCR product was denatured and spotted on to two slips of nitrocellulose film, together with control samples of known genotype (*Figure 4.11*). One slip was immersed in a solution containing each labeled probe. The result showed that the fetus was heterozygous for the mutation and therefore would not have sickle cell disease. Greatly relieved, Carol continued with the pregnancy and eventually delivered a healthy baby.

This case carries a lesson for health service planners. The genetic intervention achieved the best of all possible results: a worried couple were reassured, an abortion was avoided and a healthy child was born. It would be all too easy to

NORMAL SEQUENCE   SICKLE SEQUENCE   DOT BLOTS

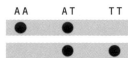

normal-specific oligo   A·C·T·G·A·G·G·A·C·**T**·C·C·T·C·T·T·C·A·G

C·T·G·A·C·T·C·C·T·G·A·G·G·A·G·A·A·G·T·C·T

sickle-specific oligo   A·C·T·G·A·G·G·A·C·**A**·C·C·T·C·T·T·C·A·G

A·C·T·G·A·G·G·A·C·**T**·C·C·T·C·T·T·C·A·G

C·T·G·A·C·T·C·C·T·G·**T**·G·G·A·G·A·A·G·T·C·T

A·C·T·G·A·G·G·A·C·**A**·C·C·T·C·T·T·C·A·G

Figure 4.11 – A dot blot test for sickle cell disease.
Denatured DNA from the fetus is immobilized on a sheet of plastic film and checked for hybridization to labeled oligonucleotides specific for the normal or sickle sequence.

record the outcome of the genetic intervention as 'no action'. Clinical geneticists are very concerned not to have their achievements measured by the number of abnormal fetuses detected and aborted.

| CASE 12 | Lipton family | 82 | **98** | 389 |

- Family history of learning difficulties
- Baby boy, Luke, with poor head control
- ? Fragile X syndrome
- Diagnosis confirmed by Southern blotting

Fragile X syndrome (OMIM 300624) was first described as a form of X-linked mental retardation, associated in affected males with a prominent high forehead, a long face, large jaw, large low-set ears and strikingly large testes (macroorchidism). When lymphocytes from patients were cultured in media deficient in folate (which disfavors DNA replication), the X chromosome in a proportion of the cells was seen to show a decondensed region (a 'fragile site') at Xq27.3, near the end of the long arm. The condition was not fully recessive because carrier women often had some degree of mental slowness, and occasional cells showed the 'fragile' X chromosome. Pedigrees showed several unusual features. The risk of being affected seemed to increase going down through the generations, while at the top of the pedigree there was often a mentally normal male who might have several carrier daughters, implying that he must have carried the pathogenic mutation but not been affected by it – a 'normal transmitting male'. The Lipton family pedigree (*Figure 4.2*) illustrates these features.

When the disease gene, *FMR1*, was cloned in 1991 it brought yet more surprises. The pathogenic change was an increased number of repeats in a run of tandemly repeated CGG trinucleotides in exon 1 of the gene. The repeats are in the 5′ untranslated region, so the repeats are present in the mRNA but do not affect the protein structure. Repeat numbers up to 55 were stable and non-pathogenic. Above 55 units, the repeats became unstable, both in mitosis and meiosis, and tended to increase in number down the generations. The classic Fragile X phenotype was seen when the repeat number exceeded 200. This behavior was unprecedented at the time, but subsequently a number of other diseases were found to depend on similar dynamic mutations; Huntington disease (**Case 1, Ashton family**) is one, and others are described in *Disease box 4*.

Alleles with 55–200 repeats are called premutation alleles: they do not cause the classic Fragile X syndrome, but they are unstable and risk expanding to cause the full syndrome in offspring. People with premutation alleles are at risk of other apparently unrelated conditions: 15–20% of female premutation carriers have premature ovarian failure (menopause before age 40), while male premutation carriers have a 1 in 3 risk of developing a neurodegenerative syndrome, FXTAS (fragile X tremor-ataxia syndrome, OMIM 300623) after age 50. Female premutation carriers also occasionally develop FXTAS. The problems in premutation carriers are thought to reflect a toxic effect of mRNA carrying the expanded CGG run. The classic Fragile X syndrome, on the other hand, is caused by lack of the FMR1 protein. *FMR1* genes carrying over 200 CGG repeats are not transcribed. The large repeat triggers methylation of promoter sequences upstream of the gene which affects the chromatin configuration so as to prevent transcription (see *Section 3.4*).

Fragile X syndrome is diagnosed by checking the size of the CGG repeat, but there are complications. Normal and premutation alleles can be amplified by PCR, much as in Huntington disease. However, as mentioned above, PCR does not work well for very long $(CGG)_n$ stretches, and the full mutation is normally confirmed by Southern blotting. The restriction digestion that is part of the Southern blotting procedure also allows the pattern of DNA methylation to be investigated. Either X-inactivation or a pathogenic repeat expansion cause methylation of the *FMR1* promoter, and this affects the ability of certain restriction enzymes to cut the DNA. For example, the enzyme *Ecl*X1 cuts a CGGCCG sequence in the promoter, but only if it is unmethylated. When genomic DNA is digested with a mixture of *Ecl*X1 and an enzyme that is insensitive to DNA methylation such as *Eco*RI, the size of fragment that hybridizes to a *FMR1* gene probe depends both on the size of the $(CGG)_n$ repeat and on whether or not the chromosome is methylated (*Figure 4.12*).

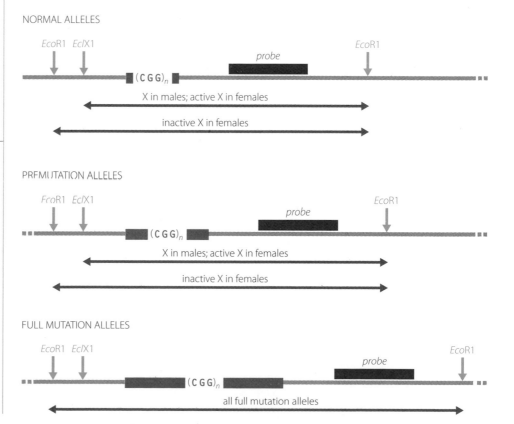

Figure 4.12 – Principle of using Southern blotting to diagnose Fragile X syndrome.
The restriction endonuclease *Ecl*X1 will only cut the DNA when its target sequence is unmethylated. When the $(CGG)_n$ run is over 200 repeats long (a full mutation) the DNA is methylated. It is also methylated on the inactive X chromosome in females regardless of the size of the CGG repeat. The black lines show the size of fragment that will hybridize to an *FMR1* gene probe. The drawing is not to scale.

Analysis in the Lipton family (*Figure 4.13*) confirmed the diagnosis:

- baby Luke had a full expansion of *c*. 800 CGG repeats
- Linda herself was heterozygous with a premutation allele with 145 repeats and a normal allele with 38 repeats
- Linda's mother Maria was heterozygous with a premutation allele with 80 repeats and a normal allele with 43 repeats
- Linda's cousin Lydia was heterozygous with a full expansion of *c*. 550 repeats and a normal allele with 32 repeats
- Lydia's mother Claudia was heterozygous with a premutation allele of 140 repeats and a normal allele of 30 repeats
- Luigi, the patriarch of the family, was a premutation carrier (a 'normal transmitting male') with 78 repeats
- Lucia (Claudia's mother) and Laurence (Linda's husband) show the patterns of normal females and males, respectively

In the female premutation carriers the band intensities on the Southern blot showed that in Claudia X-inactivation had been strongly skewed, with mainly the premutation allele being methylated and inactive. Linda and her mother each had a slight bias towards inactivating the normal X. These differences reflect the random variability of X-inactivation, and had no effect on the phenotype.

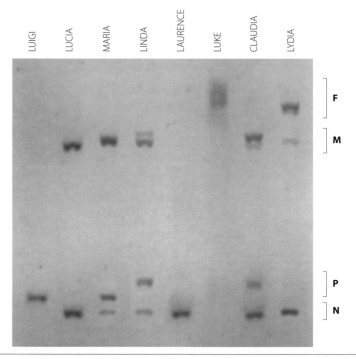

Figure 4.13 – **Southern blot analysis of the *FMR1* gene in members of the Lipton family.**
N: < 55 CGG repeats, unmethylated (the normal X in males and active normal X in females). **P:** 55–200 repeats, unmethylated (premutation allele in males and premutation-bearing active X in females). **M:** < 200 CGG repeats, methylated (normal or premutation allele on the inactive X of females; in fragments of this size the normal and premutation alleles are not clearly resolved from each other). **F:** > 200 repeats, methylated (full mutation alleles in either sex). See text for interpretation.

Linda and Laurence asked about the risks to other children they might have. There was a 1 in 2 chance any child would inherit Linda's premutation allele – the question was, how likely was it to expand, and by how many repeats? Empirical data suggest that the risk of expansion to a full mutation is quite high because Linda's premutation is at the higher end of the repeat range. The geneticist therefore told them that there was 'up to a 50% chance that a child would inherit a full mutation'. They then asked what the implications were if the child was a girl; they had already worked out that a boy might be similarly affected to Luke. This was a simple question but difficult to answer. The geneticist gave them the following information: 'only about one-third to one-half of affected females have learning problems, and they are usually less severe overall than affected males. However, even some affected girls with normal intelligence have areas of difficulty in learning due to poor attention span, and they can have poor social skills.' The geneticist suggested that if the family were going to have more children and wanted to consider prenatal diagnosis, because of the uncertainties in the clinical interpretation of laboratory results, they might wish to have a longer session with a genetic counselor to help them decide what course of action they would choose in the various scenarios that might occur.

| CASE 7 | Green family | 25 | 38 | 68 | **101** | 389 |

- Girl (Gillian) aged 3 years
- Slow to develop
- ? Chromosome abnormality
- Order tests to check for microdeletion at 22q11

Although conventional cytogenetic analysis showed a normal karyotype (*Figure 2.9*), this did not rule out a chromosomal deletion or duplication smaller than the 5 Mb resolution of standard preparations. Gillian's appearance was suggestive of a deletion of band 22q11. This is caused by recombination between misaligned low-copy repeat sequences on 22q11, as explained in *Disease box 3*. The usual deletion covers about 3 Mb and includes over 20 genes. One of these is the *TUPLE1* gene. A probe containing the *TUPLE1* sequence was used for FISH on a preparation of Gillian's chromosomes. The result showed a deletion on one copy of chromosome 22, confirming the diagnosis (*Figure 4.14*).

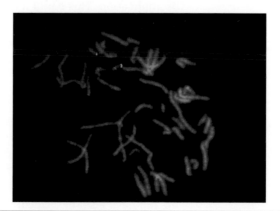

Figure 4.14 – 22q11 metaphase FISH.
The green spots are a control probe, used to identify the two copies of chromosome 22 and confirm that hybridization has taken place. The red spots are the *TUPLE1* probe. Only one of the two copies of chromosome 22 contains the sequence that hybridizes to this probe.

| CASE 8 | Howard family | 26 | 38 | 69 | **102** | 277 | 389 |

- Helen – new-born daughter of Henry and Anne (33 years old)
- Down syndrome
- Risk of recurrence if they have more children?

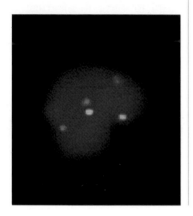

Helen's mother was offered a prenatal test in her next pregnancy. Although the risk of a recurrence of Down syndrome is low, someone who has already had one affected child is naturally extremely anxious in subsequent pregnancies. Waiting for the test result is also stressful. The fetal sample is cultured, but it takes two weeks for the cells to divide in sufficient numbers for conventional chromosome analysis. Two methods are available that give a rapid result on uncultured cells: QF–PCR is described in the final section of this chapter; in this case interphase FISH was used (*Figure 4.15*). As described above, DNA was denatured in non-dividing cells on a microscope slide and hybridized to a fluorescently labeled probe from chromosome 21. The average number of fluorescent dots, averaged over 50 cells, was 1.8. This suggests that the fetal cells had two copies of chromosome 21, although the hybridization failed in a few cases.

Figure 4.15 – **Interphase FISH test showing trisomy 21.**
The chromosome 21 probe is labeled with a red fluorochrome and a control probe (for chromosome 18) is labeled in green. The two green dots show that the hybridization has worked for this cell, and the three red dots show that there are three copies of chromosome 21. The clinical report is based on examining a large number of cells. For prenatal diagnosis a mix of differently colored probes from chromosomes 13, 18, 21, X and Y is often used.

| CASE 13 | Meinhardt family | 83 | **102** | 389 |

- Baby girl, Madelena, with small head, large ears and needing to be tube fed
- Normal 46,XX karyotype
- ? Underlying chromosome problem
- *De novo* 2.8 Mb deletion of a region of chromosome 16 found by SNP chip analysis

As with Gillian Green, the Meinhardts' daughter Madelena had features that suggested a chromosomal abnormality, but no abnormality was detectable on conventional karyotyping. Madelena's combination of mental retardation and dysmorphic features did not suggest any specific syndrome, so it was not possible to decide on one FISH probe that would give a useful test. Instead, her whole genome was scanned for copy number variations that would indicate a deletion or duplication. This could have been done by array-CGH, as shown in *Figure 4.8*, but in this case a high-resolution SNP chip was used. In about 10% of similar cases array-CGH or SNP chips identify submicroscopic chromosomal deletions or duplications. The precise abnormality seen varies widely between different cases.

DNA was extracted from a blood sample and sent for analysis. Madelena's DNA showed a decreased dosage for a series of contiguous clones from position 16p13.11–12.3 on the SNP chip. The data showed that the deletion involved 2.8 Mb of material, including a number of genes, as shown in *Figure 4.16*. The short arm of chromosome 16 is particularly rich in low-copy repeats that predispose to deletions and duplications by non-allelic homologous recombination, as explained in *Disease box 3*. As a result, several different recurrent microdeletions of sequences on 16p have been described. Madelena's deletion overlapped one of these but was larger, 2.8 Mb rather than the 1.5 Mb of the previously described deletions.

Before communicating this result to Madelena's parents, it was important to try to decide whether or not the deletion was the cause of her problems. This seemed highly likely since Madelena's deletion included a 1.5 Mb region, recurrent deletions of

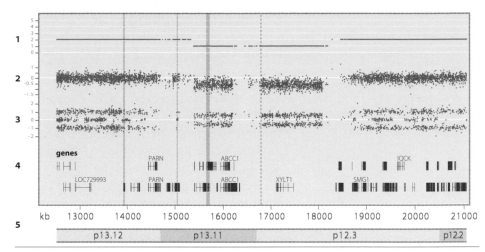

Figure 4.16 – SNP array data showing a microdeletion.
Across the bottom is an ideogram of chromosome 16, showing the bands and physical distance from 16pter. Track 2 shows the gene dosage for each SNP, as measured by the intensity of the hybridization signal summed across both alleles of each SNP. Track 1 shows the interpretation: there is only a single copy of the central part of the sequence, between positions 15 400 and 18 200. Track 3 shows the genotype at each SNP. In the non-deleted regions there are three possible genotypes, 1-1, 2-1 or 2-2, while in the deleted region there are only two, 1 or 2. In summary, there is a 2.8 Mb deletion encompassing the genes shown in track 4. Data generated using an Affymetrix SNP 6® microarray, courtesy of Lorraine Gaunt, St Mary's Hospital, Manchester.

which were known to be pathogenic. A necessary check was to see whether either parent carried the deletion, or whether it arose *de novo* in Madelena. If the deletion was *de novo* this would strengthen the case for it being pathogenic. The converse is less decisive: finding the variant in one of the clinically normal parents does not completely exclude a role in the pathogenesis, although clearly any role could be only contributory, not completely causative. Several variants (for example microdeletions at 1q21 or 15q13.3) have been described that are unquestionably more frequent in people with mental retardation, autism or schizophrenia, but that are also sometimes found in a clinically unaffected parent. It appears that these variants act as susceptibility factors, increasing the chances of a range of psychiatric conditions, but not inevitably causing any one. For a good discussion of the complexities see Girirajan *et al.* (2010).

It turned out that this was a *de novo* event. That did not prove that it is pathogenic, but made it more likely. Combined with the known pathogenicity of smaller deletions of the same region of 16p, the strong balance of probabilities was that this was the cause of Madelena's problems. This was an important conclusion because it suggested that the recurrence risk was very low. The deletion was a *de novo* event, and there was nothing to suggest any factor in either parent that might predispose to a recurrence. Counseling highlighted that the recurrence risk was not zero but was very low. Because of all the unknown factors, it was not possible to give a precise figure; however, it was small compared to the general risk of a problem that attaches to any pregnancy. It would be possible to test for this specific abnormality in future pregnancies if the parents so wished.

Cases studied using PCR

CASE 9	Ingram family	26	41	69	**104**	187	389	

- Isabel – *first daughter of Irene and Ian*
- *Small stature despite tall parents*
- *? Turner syndrome*

The diagnosis in Isabel has been clearly established from her karyotype (*Figure 2.13*). However, as explained in *Chapter 2*, it is important to check whether she has any 46,XY cells, as such cells in the gonads have the potential to become malignant. Such cells might be present if the cause of the syndrome in Isabel's case were loss of the Y chromosome during an early mitotic division of a 46,XY embryo. To check for the presence of XY cells a PCR reaction using Y-specific primers is performed to see if there is any product. This is a very much more sensitive method than looking for XY cells in a conventional cytogenetic preparation. Ideally the test would be done on tissue from her streak gonads, because that is the tissue we are concerned about developing a malignancy, but usually this is done on blood samples.

In Isabel's case, no Y chromosome sequence could be amplified, reassuring us that it is unlikely she has XY cells in her gonads.

CASE 4	Davies family	4	10	67	**104**	155	186	281	389

- *Boy (Martin) aged 24 months, parents Judith and Robert*
- *Clumsy and slow to walk*
- *Family history of muscular dystrophy*
- *Pedigree shows X-linked recessive inheritance*
- *Order diagnostic DNA test*

As we saw in *Chapter 1*, Martin had features (muscle weakness and calf pseudohypertrophy) suggestive of DMD. The pedigree reinforced the suspicion because there were two uncles who had a progressive neuromuscular disease. The geneticist had obtained their clinical notes. Their clinical course and muscle histology results were all consistent with DMD. The neurologist took a muscle biopsy from Martin and a blood sample to measure the level of creatine kinase (CK). CK is an enzyme present within muscle cells. If there is damage to the external cell membrane CK leaks out. The level is often raised in normal people after vigorous exercise, and tends to be permanently raised in female carriers of DMD (it can be used to give a probabilistic indication of a woman's carrier status). In affected boys it is strongly and unambiguously elevated.

These tests confirmed the bad news: Martin had Duchenne muscular dystrophy. At present there is no cure for this disease, only symptomatic treatment, and his prognosis was grave. Martin is unlikely to live much beyond age 20 unless in the meantime some new effective treatment is developed (the prospects for therapy are considered in *Chapter 14*). Initially Martin's parents Judith and Robert were entirely taken up with the emotional shock, and with planning how best to cope with a child with a severe progressive disability. But of course the diagnosis also had implications for any future pregnancies and for the wider family. When they were ready to consider such matters, the geneticist arranged a discussion. It seemed highly likely that Judith was a carrier, in which case any subsequent son would be at 1 in 2 risk. Other female relatives might very well also be carriers. To resolve all these questions it was necessary to identify the dystrophin gene mutation in Martin.

As we saw in *Chapter 3*, the dystrophin gene is huge, but about two-thirds of all mutations are deletions of one or more complete exons (see *Figure 3.9*). These deletions are relatively easy to detect in an affected male. If no deletion is found, this would not rule out the diagnosis because one-third of DMD cases have point mutations or duplications that would not be detected by this test. Further, more complex, tests would be necessary.

This is an X-linked condition, so a boy has only a single copy of the dystrophin gene. To check for partial deletions, individual exons of the gene are amplified by PCR. The 79 exons are all under 300 bp long (except for exon 79, the last exon, which is 2703 bp long – the last exon in a gene is often large, but consists mainly of the 3′ untranslated region). Thus individual exons are a suitable size for amplification by PCR. Primers are designed to match sequences in the introns flanking an exon, so that the product contains the complete exon and some intronic sequence. Experience shows that testing 18 carefully chosen exons picks up 98% of all deletions. By varying the amount of intron included, primers are designed so that each exon gives a differently sized product. A series of PCR reactions can then be performed in one operation (multiplexed), using all the primer pairs together in one reaction tube. The mix of products from all the PCR amplifications is run on an electrophoretic gel and shows a ladder of bands (*Figure 4.17*). An alternative technique, MLPA, is illustrated in *Figure 5.9*. MLPA is the most widely used general method for checking a given gene for deletions or duplications of one or a few exons.

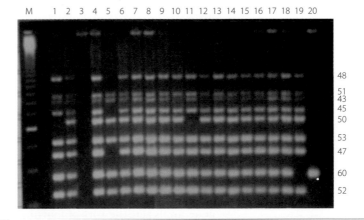

Figure 4.17 – PCR deletion screen in Duchenne muscular dystrophy.
Nine selected exons of the dystrophin gene have been amplified from the DNA of a panel of 20 affected boys. When the product is run on an electrophoretic gel each exon gives a band of a characteristic size. Because a boy has only a single X chromosome, any deletion shows up as missing bands. Different exon deletions can be seen in lanes 1, 5, 11, 12, 19 and 20. Lane 3 may be a large deletion or a technical failure. The boys with no deletion on this gel may have others of the 79 dystrophin exons deleted, or may have point mutations or duplications to cause loss of function of the gene.

The result (*Figure 4.17 Lane 5*) showed that Martin has a deletion of exons 45, 47 and 48. Exons 43 and 50 are present. Exons 44, 46 and 49 were checked in individual PCR tests, which showed that exons 44 and 46 were deleted but exon 49 was present. Thus Martin's deletion encompasses exons 44–48. The implications of this deletion for function of the dystrophin gene are considered in *Chapter 6*.

Now that we know exactly what mutation is segregating in this family, women can be offered an accurate carrier test, and if necessary accurate prenatal diagnosis. Judith and her mother are obligate carriers (see the pedigree in *Figure 1.10*) and the family includes at least eight women or girls who may be carriers. Judith's two daughters and her sister's daughter are all too young for any intervention at present. They will be re-contacted in their late teens. Through Judith, her three sisters and her two cousins (her mother's sister's daughters) were invited to contact the geneticist now. Carrier testing in women is more difficult than testing a boy because a carrier would be heterozygous and every exon of the dystrophin gene would amplify from her normal X chromosome. A quantitative test is required, as described in the final section of this chapter and in *Chapter 5*. Before this test was available, many carrier women opted for fetal sexing and aborted all male fetuses, even though there was only a 1 in 2 chance of them being affected. With prenatal diagnosis they can be confident, if the tests are normal, of delivering boys free of the disease.

| CASE 1 | Ashton family | 1 | 7 | 65 | **106** | 154 | 389 |

- John – 28-year-old son of Alfred Ashton
- ? Huntington disease
- Other family members with similar symptoms
- Autosomal dominant inheritance shown in pedigree
- Diagnostic test ordered

The next step in investigating this family is to perform a diagnostic test on John's father Alfred. Alfred is already showing signs of disease. Although it seems highly probable that the family disease (see the pedigree in *Figure 1.7*) is Huntington disease, this needs to be proved before John can be given accurate counseling or offered a predictive test. His doctor takes a 3 ml blood sample from Alfred and sends it to the laboratory, where DNA is extracted.

As mentioned in the previous chapter, the laboratory will want to check the size of a run of glutamine codons (CAG) in exon 1 of the *HTT* gene on chromosome 4. The normal range is 5–35 codons (15–105 bp) and anything over 35 codons is pathogenic (although some people with 36–39 repeats are apparently unaffected). Expansions are normally in the 40–60 codon range, but are virtually never over 100 codons or 300 bp. This sort of test is easy to perform by PCR. Primers are designed that flank the region of interest and the size of the product is measured. The products might be sized on a manual gel; more commonly, an automated gene analyzer (the sort of machine shown in *Box figure 4.1b*) would be used. The result shows two peaks because a genomic DNA sample includes DNA from both copies of the *HTT* gene. We see that Alfred's two copies of the gene have 18 and 41 CAG repeats, respectively (*Figure 4.18, Lower trace*). A repeat size over 35 is pathogenic. This result therefore confirms the diagnosis.

Now that Alfred's diagnosis was definite, it followed that John was at 50% risk of developing Huntington disease himself. If he wished, a PCR test on his DNA would tell him for sure whether or not he had inherited the *HTT* gene mutation. Over several sessions with the genetic counselor, John and his wife pondered long and hard over whether or not to take the test. Initially John thought it would be a bad idea because having a genetic test could affect his ability to get insurance and maybe his job.

On discussion, he became convinced that these anxieties were misplaced. If he applied for insurance in the UK he would have to reveal his family history of

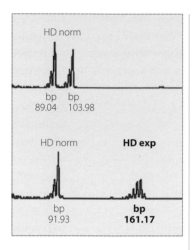

Figure 4.18 – Testing for the Huntington disease mutation.
This is a typical PCR application, amplifying a sequence a few hundred bp long using specific primers, and sizing the product by capillary electrophoresis. Smaller molecules move faster through the capillary so the position of a peak is a measure of the size of the PCR product. One of the PCR primers carried a fluorescent label to allow the machine to detect the product. The PCR primers used total 38 nt in length, so the number of CAG repeats is calculated by subtracting 38 from the fragment size and dividing by 3. So, for example, the 161 bp product in the lower trace contains (161-38)/3 = 41 CAG repeats. Each sample shows two peaks, corresponding to the different sized PCR products produced by the two copies of chromosome 4. Upper trace: a normal result (17 and 22 repeats); lower trace: an abnormal result (18 and 41 repeats). The upper limit of normal is 35 repeats. Courtesy of Dr Simon Ramsden, St Mary's Hospital, Manchester.

Huntington disease, and many companies would see this as a reason for heavily loading the premium. In fact a genetic test might help John: if it was negative, the family history would no longer count, while in the UK if it was positive he wouldn't have to declare the result for life policies up to a certain ceiling under a moratorium agreed by the insurance industry; in any case most of the bad news was already present in the family history. In the US, the Genetic Information Nondiscrimination Act (GINA) provides wide-ranging protection against genetic discrimination in health insurance including prohibiting the use of family history information. Unless John developed symptoms that prevented him doing his job properly, his genotype would be of no interest to any employer. John's wife was then worried about his existing insurance policy. He had a life insurance policy to pay off the mortgage on his house should he die. But when John took out that insurance he was unaware of the nature of the family problem. He had, however, answered all the questions on the form honestly, to the best of his then knowledge, and so that policy was valid and was not affected by later developments.

Having disposed of those concerns, the discussion returned to the basic question of whether or not John and his wife wanted to know. This is a very personal and difficult decision, but about 70% of people in John's position make the choice not to know. Of course a negative test would be a great relief, and a positive test would at least allow John and his wife to start planning for the future. But most of us like to see our lives as open-ended. Few of us would wish to know, at the age of 28, when and how we will die. After long reflection, John and his wife chose not to know. The counselor would have supported them whichever way they chose. Now she arranged to see them over the coming months to continue her support, and assured them that she would always be available at any time for further discussion. She also pointed out that if, over the coming years, a treatment was developed that could slow the very early development of the disease, it might be in John's interest to have the test, and she promised to contact them should any such development occur.

The final discussion concerned what to do about John's other at-risk relatives. His sister Helen, her two young sons, and his aunt Alice in Australia were all at risk as a result of the positive test on Alfred. It was agreed that John should contact Helen and Alice, explain the situation and give them contact details of their local genetics service. Whether or not they chose to take up the contact was then up to them. Had John chosen to take the test, the geneticist would not have revealed that fact or the result to any other family member. Since John was close to Helen, he might choose to discuss with her his own thoughts and decisions, but there was absolutely no obligation on him to do this.

4.4. **Going deeper ...**

Table 4.1 summarizes the techniques covered in this chapter and the type of problem for which each is appropriate. Considering the cases that involved small-scale changes to the DNA (sickle cell disease, Huntington disease and Fragile X syndrome), in each case the location and/or nature of the suspected genetic lesion was known in advance. Often this is not the case, and then other techniques are needed, in particular DNA sequencing. These are discussed in *Chapter 5*. Some additional techniques are considered below.

Table 4.1 – **Summary of the methods described so far, and their main applications**

Principle	Method	Application
Hybridization	Dot blotting with oligonucleotide probe	Checking for presence / absence of a sequence; checking for a specified single nucleotide change
	Southern blotting	Checking for large-scale changes (inversions, deletions, etc.) that alter the pattern of restriction fragments and for trinucleotide repeat expansions that are too large to amplify by PCR
	FISH on a chromosome spread	Checking for presence / absence and chromosomal location of a sequence at least several kb long
	FISH on interphase cells	Checking for copy number of specific chromosome(s)
	Comparative genomic hybridization	Scanning the entire genome for any copy number change involving sequences of a few kb or longer
	SNP arrays	Scanning the entire genome for copy number changes, with higher resolution than array-CGH; also, the genotypes of the patient can be compared with those of the parents to reveal some unusual types of variants
Amplification	Cloning in *E. coli*, etc.	Obtaining an inexhaustible supply of one specific DNA fragment, 2 kb–300 kb long depending on the vector used
	PCR	Checking the presence / absence and size of a specific 50 bp–5 kb sequence

Quantitative PCR

The cases in this chapter include two that might have been investigated using quantitative PCR.

- Females in Case 4 (Davies family, Duchenne muscular dystrophy) could be checked to see if they are heterozygous carriers of a deletion in the dystrophin gene (an alternative method, MLPA, is discussed in *Chapter 5*).
- In Case 8 (Howard family, Down syndrome) quantitative PCR of sequences on chromosome 21 could have been used in place of interphase FISH for a rapid prenatal check for Down syndrome.

When sequences are amplified using standard PCR protocols the results are not strictly quantitative – that is, the amount of product does not necessarily closely reflect the amount of template that was present in the original sample. This makes standard PCR unreliable for detecting duplications or heterozygous deletions. Various modified protocols overcome this limitation. Often these involve **real-time PCR**. Quantitative PCR is more reliable when it is based on measuring the rate of accumulation of product rather than the total amount at the end of a fixed number of cycles. Several commercial systems (e.g. TaqMan®) use ingenious tricks to label just the product, and not the primers or the pool of monomers, so that a special machine can follow the accumulation of the product in real time through each cycle of the reaction.

QF–PCR (quantitative fluorescence PCR; Verma *et al.*, 1998) is often used in place of interphase FISH for rapid diagnosis of chromosomal trisomies. This is not a real-time method; it depends on using a gene analyzer to compare the relative amounts of product from a multiplexed series of microsatellite markers (see *Chapter 9*) from chromosomes 13, 18, 21, X and Y. A current debate among geneticists concerns the relative merits of screening older women for chromosomal abnormalities by conventional karyotyping or by this technique. QF–PCR is much quicker and cheaper, but would miss any abnormality that was not a copy number variation of one of the five chromosomes tested. Arguably it may be positively beneficial to miss many of these other abnormalities (see *Chapter 11* for more information and discussion).

Detecting balanced abnormalities

Array-CGH or SNP chips are powerful tools for detecting deletions or duplications that are too small to be seen by standard karyotyping. However, they are unable to detect balanced abnormalities, where there is no extra or missing material. These can include 'cryptic' translocations of subtelomeric sequences and small inversions. *Figure 4.19* shows how interphase FISH can detect a relatively large inversion. Smaller inversions that disrupt a gene can be very hard to spot, because each exon of the gene has the correct sequence and will amplify normally by PCR. About 50% of mutations that cause severe hemophilia A are caused by a recurrent inversion that disrupts the *F8* (clotting factor VIII) gene (*Figure 4.20*). This eluded detection and baffled investigators for several years before Southern blotting revealed an abnormal pattern of hybridizing restriction fragments.

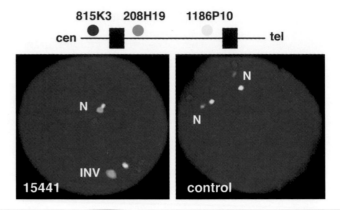

Figure 4.19 – Detecting an inversion by interphase FISH.
Case 15441 is heterozygous for a 1.5 Mb inversion between the sequences on 7q11.23 represented by black boxes at the top of the figure. The colored circles show the FISH probes used. The normal chromosome 7 shows hybridization spots with the sequence red–green–yellow, while the inverted chromosome shows red–yellow–green. A normal control is shown for comparison. Reproduced from *Nat. Genet.* 2001; **29**: 321–325 with permission from the Nature Publishing Group.

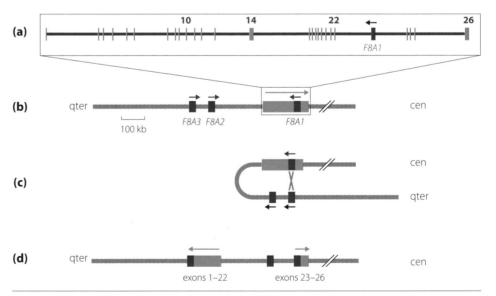

Figure 4.20 – An inversion that disrupts the *F8* gene.
(a) The *F8* gene has 26 exons spanning 187 kb of genomic DNA on the X chromosome at location Xq28. (b) The red boxes show a sequence present in intron 22 of the *F8* gene, of which two additional copies are located 360 kb and 435 kb away from the start of the *F8* gene. The red arrows show the orientation of the repeats. Note that these are inverted repeats (compare with the repeats in *Disease box 3*, which are direct repeats). (c) During male meiosis this part of the X chromosome has no matching partner. The DNA may loop round to allow two copies of the repeated sequence to pair in the same orientation. Occasionally there is recombination between the paired sequences. (d) The result is a chromosomal inversion of about 500 kb of DNA that disrupts the *F8* gene. Blue arrows show the 5′ → 3′ orientation of the *F8* gene.

Chromosome painting

This technique is a variant of FISH in which the fluorescently labeled probe is a whole cocktail of sequences from one particular chromosome. In a metaphase spread the whole length of that chromosome appears brightly colored. Its use is in identifying the origin of abnormal chromosomes seen on standard karyotyping. For example, if we used a chromosome 1 paint on cells from Elizabeth Elliot (Case 5, *Figure 2.15*), the paint would highlight both copies of her normal chromosome 1 plus that part of her translocated chromosome that was derived from chromosome 1. In this particular case we don't need chromosome painting to understand the karyotype, but patients sometimes show small extra 'marker' chromosomes, or extra material inserted into a chromosome, whose origin can be impossible to identify without chromosome painting. Extending the concept, M-FISH or SKY uses a mix of paints, one for each chromosome, each labeled with a different mix of fluorescent dyes, so that each chromosome is painted a different color. We will meet this technique when considering the very complex chromosomal changes typical of leukemia and cancer cells (*Chapter 12*).

Testing RNA: Northern blotting

Sometimes it is desirable to study RNA rather than DNA. For example, a basic question about any gene is when and where (in which tissue or organ) is it expressed? Also, hunting for mutations is sometimes easier if the mRNA rather than the genomic DNA can be studied. Partly this is because the mature mRNA is usually very much smaller than the gene (*Table 3.1*). Additionally, mutations that produce abnormal splicing of exons and introns are rather more obvious at the RNA than at the DNA level. However, RNA is much harder to obtain and handle than DNA. The appropriate tissue has to be sampled, for example, dystrophin mRNA would be obtained by a muscle biopsy, and RNA is unstable, requiring stringent precautions in the laboratory.

Among the techniques described above, an adaptation of Southern blotting can be used directly to identify mRNA molecules. This variant of the technique is called **Northern blotting**. (The name is a joke: Southern blotting was developed by Dr Ed Southern in Oxford, UK.) mRNA is extracted from the relevant tissue, run out on a gel and blotted on to nitrocellulose. The probe is a labeled DNA corresponding to exons of the gene in question. The result shows whether an mRNA is present, and if so, how big it is. Absence of the expected transcript might show that the gene is somehow being silenced, while an unexpected size could indicate a disturbance of normal splicing.

Making cDNA

RNA cannot be cloned, amplified by PCR or sequenced like DNA. Most RNA studies therefore first make a DNA copy of the RNA, and study the copy. This is a reversal of the normal DNA → RNA flow of information, as described in the Central Dogma (*Figure 3.3*). Some viruses encode an enzyme, reverse transcriptase, that makes DNA copies of a template RNA. The final product is a double-stranded **cDNA** (complementary DNA). In **RT-PCR** (reverse transcriptase–polymerase chain reaction), reverse transcription is performed on total extracted mRNA, and gene-specific primers are then used in a PCR reaction on the total cDNA to amplify the chosen gene. RT–PCR can be performed as a single operation and is a powerful tool, provided a tissue can be sampled where the gene of interest is expressed. **cDNA libraries** are made by reverse transcribing total mRNA and cloning the resulting population of cDNAs *en masse*. Tissue-specific cDNA libraries are a very important resource for identifying genes and their pattern of expression.

The complete mRNA repertoire of a cell type or tissue can be studied by hybridizing the bulk mRNA (or more usually, bulk cDNA) to a microarray. Suitable **expression arrays** carry anchored oligonucleotides corresponding to exons of a whole number of genes – maybe the entire genome. The mRNA or cDNA is labeled with a fluorescent dye and allowed to hybridize to the array. Usually a protocol of competitive hybridization is used, as described for CGH (*Figure 4.7*). The test sample is labeled with one color dye and mixed with a control sample labeled with a different color. The ratio of the two dyes bound to each cell of the array shows the ratio of expression of that gene in the test tissue compared to the control. An example is shown in *Chapter 12*.

Testing protein

If a disease is caused by absence of a particular protein, which in turn may be the result of any one of a large number of mutations in the relevant gene, might it not be simpler to test directly for the protein rather than hunting through the whole gene for any possible mutation? In principle the answer should be yes. However, while DNA from any sample can be used to test any gene, the relevant protein may be present only in an inaccessible tissue. Also DNA tests are generic while protein tests are specific. That is, a laboratory can apply the same well-tried techniques to test the DNA of any gene, whereas each protein needs a specific assay that must be developed, set up and optimized. Protein testing is best done using commercial kits, where the company will optimize the reagents and protocol. However, companies will only develop these for relatively common conditions. *Figure 1.4* shows an example, using an antibody to test for dystrophin protein rather than looking for the many possible mutations that can affect the huge dystrophin gene. We will see examples of protein testing used for population screening in *Chapter 11*, and used for diagnostic testing in *Chapter 12*.

Diseases caused by expanding nucleotide repeats

The mutation in Huntington disease is unusual but it is not unique. Starting with Fragile X syndrome in 1991, a growing list of human diseases have been identified that are caused by expansions of a nucleotide repeat. Mostly the repeats are trinucleotides, as in Huntington disease, but examples are known that involve 4, 5 and 12 nucleotide repeats. In every case the repeat is present in normal people, where it is stable and non-pathogenic. The number of repeat units varies among normal people as a result of occasional rare mutations, but is always below some threshold number. If one of these rare mutations creates a repeat that is above the threshold, it becomes unstable and has a high probability of expanding yet further on transmission from parent to child. The higher the repeat number, the more unstable it is. Separately from this, repeats above a certain size cause disease. Repeats that are big enough to be unstable but not big enough to cause disease are called **premutations**. People carrying premutations are healthy but are at high risk of having affected children. The main examples are shown in *Box table 4.3* below.

DISEASE BOX 4

Box table 4.3 – **Diseases associated with pathogenic expanded nucleotide repeats.**

Disease	OMIM no.	Mode of inheritance	Location of gene	Location of repeat	Repeat sequence	Normal range (repeats)	Pathological range (repeats)
Huntington disease	143100	AD	4p16	Exon 1	$(CAG)_n$	5–35	37–120
DRPLA	125370	AD	12p13	Exon 5	$(CAG)_n$	7–34	58–88
SCA1	164400	AD	6p23	Exon 8	$(CAG)_n$	19–38	40–81
SCA2	183090	AD	12q24	Exon 1	$(CAG)_n$	15–29	35–59
SCA3 (Machado–Joseph disease)	109150	AD	14q24-q31	Exon 10	$(CAG)_n$	14–40	68–82
SCA6	183086	AD	19p13	Exon 49	$(CAG)_n$	6–17	21–30
SCA7	164500	AD	3p21-p12	Exon 3	$(CAG)_n$	7–17	38–130
SCA17	607136	AD	6q27	Exon 3	$(CAG)_n$	25–44	50–55
SBMA	313200	Xl R	Xq11	Exon 1	$(CAG)_n$	11–33	38–62
Fragile X site A (FRAXA)	309550	XL	Xq27.3	5'UTR	$(CGG)_n$	6–54	200–>1000
Fragile X site E (FRAXE)	309548	XL	Xq28	Promoter	$(CCG)_n$	6–25	>200
Friedreich ataxia (FRDA)	229300	AR	9q13-q21.1	Intron 1	$(GAA)_n$	7–22	200–1700
Myotonic dystrophy 1 (DM1)	160900	AD	19q13	3'UTR	$(CTG)_n$	5–35	50–4000
Myotonic dystrophy 2 (DM2)	602668	AD	3q21	Intron 1	$(CCTG)_n$	12	75–11000
SCA8	603680	AD	13q21	Untranscribed RNA	$(CTG)_n$	16–37	110–>500
SCA10	603516	AD	22q13	Intron 9	$(ATTCT)_n$	10–22	Up to 22 kb
SCA12	604326	AD	5q31	Promoter	$(CAG)_n$	9–18	66–78
Progressive myoclonic epilepsy (PME)	254800	AR	21q22.3	Promoter	$(CCCCGCCCCGCG)_n$	2–3	40–80

SCA, spino-cerebellar ataxia; DRPLA, dentatorubral pallidoluysian atrophy; SBMA, spinobulbar muscular atrophy.

A feature of many of these diseases is **anticipation**. This describes the way a disease may get more severe going down the generations. It happens because the expanded repeats are very unstable and tend to expand still further on transmission. The size of expansion is often correlated with the severity of symptoms and/or with onset at younger ages. Thus an expanding repeat is suspected to lie at the root of any genetic disease that shows anticipation. However, reports of anticipation must be viewed with considerable skepticism. If a dominant disease is naturally very variable, as many are, then clinicians will often see severely affected children born to a mildly affected parent. Mildly affected children born to a severely affected parent will be seen less frequently. This is because severely affected people may not have children, and if they do, they may not feel there is anything wrong with a mildly affected child. Thus a common bias of ascertainment often mimics anticipation.

The first nine diseases in the table all involve expanding $(CAG)_n$ runs within the coding sequence of a gene. CAG is the codon for glutamine (see *Table 6.1*) so the effect is to encode a protein with an expanded polyglutamine tract. These proteins are in some way toxic to neurons. The cumulative death of neurons leads to a late onset neurodegenerative disease. SBMA is described in more detail in *Disease box 6*. For most of the other diseases in the table the expanded repeat prevents expression of a gene, and the disease is the result of lack of the gene product. The two forms of myotonic dystrophy, however, are the result of the toxicity of mRNA containing the expanded repeat. Toxic RNA may also be part of the molecular pathology of FRAXA, SCA8 and perhaps other diseases. Thus although all these diseases are caused by expanded repeats, the mechanisms by which they cause disease are quite diverse and for the most part, poorly understood.

Clinically, the polyglutamine diseases are all late onset neurodegenerative conditions. The precise symptoms probably depend on the pattern of expression of the mutant gene and of genes whose products interact with the mutant protein. Friedreich ataxia is also a result of progressive death of neurons, with die-back affecting cerebellar function. FRAXA was described in **Case 12 (Lipton family)**; FRAXE is very similar. The gene products are RNA-binding proteins that assist with the transport and translation of selected mRNAs. Finally, the two forms of myotonic dystrophy are multisystem diseases with muscle myotonia, cataracts, testicular atrophy and frontal balding. Myotonic dystrophy shows especially striking anticipation (*Box figure 4.4*).

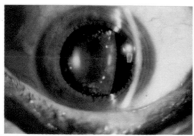
(a)

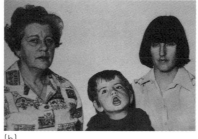
(b)

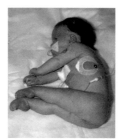
(c)

Box figure 4.4 – Anticipation in myotonic dystrophy.
(a) A 'blue-dot' cataract may be the only sign of the disease in the first affected generation. (b) A three generation family showing the grandmother who has bilateral cataracts but no muscle symptoms or facial weakness; her daughter has moderate facial weakness with ptosis and cataracts; the child has the congenital form. Reproduced from *Myotonic Dystrophy* by Peter Harper (Saunders, 3rd edition, 2001) with permission. (c) A baby with the congenital form showing hypotonia. The congenital form is seen only when the child inherits the disease from its mother. It is caused by very large expansions of the CTG repeat, which are never found in sperm.

4.5. **References**

General descriptions of the techniques covered here can be found in many textbooks, for example Strachan T and Read AP (2010) *Human Molecular Genetics, 4th edn.* Garland, New York.

Girirajan S, Rosenfeld JA, Cooper GM, *et al.* (2010) A recurrent 16p12.1 microdeletion supports a two-hit model for severe developmental delay. *Nat. Genet.* **42**: 203–209.

La Spada AR and Taylor JP (2010) Repeat expansion disease: progress and puzzles in disease pathogenesis. *Nat. Rev. Genet.* **11**: 247–258.

Mefford HC, Sharp AJ, Baker C, *et al.* (2008) Recurrent rearrangements of chromosome 1q21.1 and variable pediatric phenotypes. *New Engl. J. Med.* **359**: 1685–1699.

Verma L, Macdonald F, Leedham P, McConachie M, Dhanjal S and Hultén M. (1998) Rapid and simple prenatal DNA diagnosis of Down's syndrome. *Lancet,* **352**: 9–12. *Describes the QF–PCR method.*

Useful websites

The University of Utah Genetic Science Learning Center has an excellent animated explanation of gel electrophoresis at http://learn.genetics.utah.edu/content/labs/gel/

The Access Excellence Resource Center has elementary descriptions of Southern blotting (www.accessexcellence.org/RC/VL/GG/ecb/southern_blotting.php) and other techniques – lacking detail at this level, but good for graphics.

For a large amount of detailed information and pictures of FISH see Tavi's Multicolor FISH Page at http://info.med.yale.edu/genetics/ward/tavi/FISH.html

4.6. **Self-assessment questions**

(1) Design 10-nucleotide-long primers to amplify each of the 50 bp sequences underlined so as to produce a 50 bp product.

(a) - guidance provided.

```
CCACTCCCCTCGGCCAGGGCCGCGTCAACCAGCTCGGCGGTGTTTTTATCAACGGCAGGTACCAGG
AGACTGGCTCCATACGTCCTGGTGCCATCGGCGGCAGCAAGCCCAAGGTGAGCGGGCGGGCCTTGC
```

(b)

```
AAGAGAGAACCCGGGCGTGCCGTCAGGTACTAGGCCCATTAACCTCTCCCCGCTTCCTTCCTCCTC
CCGCCCCCAGTGAGTTCCATCAGCCGCATCCTGAGAAGTAAATTCGGGAAAGGTGAAGAGGAGGAG
```

[Note that real primers would be 16–25 nucleotides long and would be designed to give a product of a few hundred bp; this is an exercise in getting the position and orientation of your primers correct. Do it by hand even if you have access to a primer design program.]

(2) Extend *Box table 4.2* to show the progress of the PCR reaction up to cycle 10. (It would be neat to make a spreadsheet to do this). How many cycles would it take to produce 100 000 copies of Product B?

(3) There are four different nucleotides in DNA, 16 different dinucleotides, 64 different trinucleotides and 4^n different sequences n nucleotides long. If a restriction endonuclease cuts DNA whenever it encounters a particular five-nucleotide sequence, and assuming these occur at random throughout the human genome, into how many fragments might it cleave the DNA of a human cell?

(4) Assuming the human genome consisted entirely of unique sequence DNA, how long would an oligonucleotide probe need to be in order to hybridize to just one sequence in the genome? [Guidance provided.]

(5) For each of the following sequence changes or effects, choose possible testing methods from the list below that could be used to check for the presence of the change or effect (more than one method may be appropriate for some cases):

- a G>A change in exon 2 of the *PAX3* gene that results in replacement of valine 60 by methionine in the gene product
- a heterozygous 3 bp deletion in exon 6 of the *BRCA1* gene
- an A>T nucleotide substitution that changes the codon for arginine 214 (AGA) into a stop codon (TGA) in exon 7 of the *MITF* gene
- a GT>GA change in the donor splice site at the end of exon 4 of the *PAH* gene, which encodes the liver enzyme phenylalanine hydroxylase
- a C>A change in an intron near a splice site in the ubiquitously expressed actin gene: the question is whether or not it affects splicing of the primary transcript
- deletion of several contiguous genes on one copy of chromosome 17 in a child with suspected Smith–Magenis syndrome
- a duplication of one or more exons in the dystrophin gene in a boy with Duchenne muscular dystrophy
- deletion of one or more exons of the *HYP* gene in a boy with hypophosphatemia (an X-linked dominant condition)
- insertion of three nucleotides in the promoter of a gene – the question is whether this affects expression of the gene
- any material extra or missing on a copy of chromosome 7 in a patient – the cytogeneticist reported that the banding pattern on one copy of chromosome 7 was abnormal but could not work out exactly what events had produced the change

Options:

(a) PCR amplification, check for the presence / absence of product
(b) PCR amplification, check the size of the product
(c) PCR amplification followed by sequencing
(d) PCR amplification followed by dot-blot hybridization to an allele-specific oligonucleotide
(e) RT–PCR
(f) real-time quantitative PCR
(g) Southern blotting
(h) FISH
(i) chromosome painting
(j) array-CGH

05 | How can we check a patient's DNA for gene mutations?

After working through this chapter you should be able to:

- Describe the principle of DNA sequencing and read a straightforward DNA sequencer trace
- Describe the circumstances in which a DNA test involves scanning a gene for mutations or checking for a specific change
- Describe briefly the principles of two methods (apart from sequencing) by which a gene can be scanned for mutations
- Describe briefly the principles of two methods by which a person's DNA can be checked for a specified mutation
- Describe briefly the principles of two methods by which a person's DNA can be checked for deletion or duplication of exons of a gene

5.1. Case studies

CASE 14	Nicolaides family	**117**	135	157	389

- ? β-thalassemia carriers

Spiros Nicolaides is an IT graduate who was born in the UK but whose family originally came from Cyprus. He is healthy, and on a recent trip to see his grandparents in Cyprus met and fell in love with Elena, who recently returned there from the USA where she was studying. Both of the families are delighted and a big engagement party is planned. However, Elena's older sister tells her that before she married she was advised to have some blood tests to see if she was a carrier for β-thalassemia. Luckily, although Elena's sister was shown to be a carrier, her future husband was not and they now have a healthy son. Naturally Elena and Spiros are concerned and request an appointment in the genetic clinic to discuss their risks.

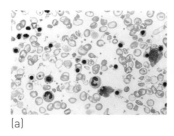
(a)

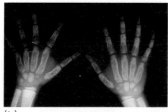
(b)

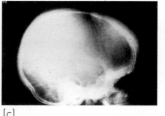
(c)

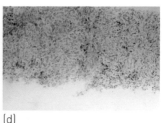
(d)

Figure 5.1 – Effects of thalassemia.
(a) Blood film with very marked hypochromia and many nucleated red cells.
(b) Osteoporotic appearance of hands due to bone marrow extension. (c) 'Hair on end' skull. (d) Liver biopsy with Perl's stain, showing iron overload. Courtesy of Dr Andrew Will, Royal Manchester Children's Hospital.

5.2. **Science toolkit**

In the previous chapter we saw how PCR or various hybridization methods can be used to examine any chosen small piece of the DNA in a sample. Sometimes no further investigation is needed. That was the case for several of the families:

- for Case 4 (Davies family), PCR identified and characterized a partial deletion of the dystrophin gene, confirming the diagnosis of Duchenne muscular dystrophy.
- in Case 1 (Ashton family), the size of the PCR product identified the pathogenic Huntington disease allele.
- for Case 12 (Lipton family), Southern blotting confirmed the Fragile X mutation and identified premutation carriers.

But many disease mutations are substitutions of one nucleotide for another somewhere within the DNA of a gene, which would not generate any visible difference in a PCR product or Southern blot. Insertion or deletion of a nucleotide or two would also not make a noticeable difference to the size of a PCR product. We need therefore to consider how to check a gene for such point mutations.

The available methods fall into three classes:

- DNA sequencing
- methods that check for a specific sequence change
- methods that rapidly scan a gene for any change, without identifying the nature of the change

DNA sequencing – the ultimate test

For almost all of the past 30 years all DNA sequencing has been based on a single basic technique: dideoxy or Sanger sequencing. Just recently several revolutionary new sequencing technologies have arrived on the scene. Collectively called 'Next Generation' or 'Massively Parallel' sequencing, these new techniques are changing the way genetics research is carried out. They generate previously unthinkable amounts of sequence for quite modest costs. This makes all sorts of sequencing-intensive applications possible that would previously have been prohibitively expensive; indeed, sequencing whole genomes is rapidly becoming routine. In clinical service their immediate impact is less dramatic, because most of the clinical questions that are currently answered by sequencing are about whether a patient has a mutation in a given gene; such investigations involve relatively modest amounts of sequencing and are well addressed by dideoxy sequencing. However, in the medium term the new technologies are likely to have major impacts on genetic services as they allow questions to be answered that were formerly intractable. The cost of sequencing is still falling rapidly, driven by intense competition between the companies promoting the various technologies. It is entirely likely that within a few years the standard approach to most clinical service questions will be to sequence the patient's entire genome and look for significant variants.

In this section we will describe the current clinical technology, dideoxy sequencing, in some detail, and then discuss the capabilities and potential of the new technologies without going in to technical details. Readers who would like to know more should consult a review: we recommend the paper by Tucker and colleagues (2009) but, because of the breakneck speed of development, the most recent possible review should be used.

Rather like PCR, dideoxy sequencing uses a DNA polymerase to make many copies of the fragment of interest. The starting material is a collection of identical DNA molecules – usually a PCR product, or sometimes a cloned copy of the fragment of interest. Unlike in PCR, for sequencing we want to make copies of just one of the DNA strands. Therefore a single primer is used (as in *Figure 4.9*). Rather than denaturing the template DNA to make it single-stranded, a special cloning procedure is often used. This involves using a specialized vector, M13, that reels off copies of just one of the two DNA strands.

Having got our single-stranded template, we add the primer, the four nucleotide monomers A, G, C and T, and a DNA polymerase enzyme to synthesize the complementary strand. However, the pool of monomers is spiked with chain-terminating molecules. This is the key to the sequencing technique. The idea was developed by Fred Sanger, and earned him a share of the 1980 Nobel prize for chemistry (his second! – he had already won the 1958 Nobel prize for determining amino acid sequences of proteins).

The chain terminating molecules are modified versions of the standard A, G, C and T nucleotides (*Figure 5.2*). They are incorporated into a growing polynucleotide chain just like their regular counterparts, but they then prevent the chain growing any further. The chemical trick that does this is the removal of the hydroxyl group on position 3 of the deoxyribose sugar: chain terminators are *dideoxy* nucleotides. Since this hydroxyl group provides the link to the next nucleotide in the chain, its absence means that no new nucleotide can be added to that particular chain.

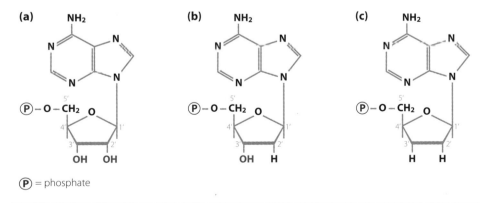

Figure 5.2 – Formulae of (a) a ribonucleotide, (b) a deoxyribonucleotide, (c) a dideoxynucleotide. The dideoxynucleotide can be added to a growing DNA chain through its 5′ phosphate, but because it lacks a 3′ hydroxyl group, no further growth of the chain is then possible. In sequencing reactions the dideoxynucleotides are normally labeled, either radioactively or by tagging with a fluorescent dye.

To make the whole thing work, we need to add just the right amount of chain terminators. When it is incorporating an A into the growing chain the polymerase will randomly pick a normal or a dideoxy version of the A nucleotide. If there is 1% as much dideoxy-A as normal A, then at each A position around 1% of the growing chains will incorporate the chain terminator and grow no further. As a result, a series of nested fragments accumulate, each terminated by a dideoxy-A. Putting this into a concrete example: suppose we use a 20-nucleotide primer and the DNA we are copying has Ts 27, 30, 35, 41, etc. nucleotides from the 5′ end of the primer. Opposite each T in the template strand, the polymerase will incorporate an A in the growing strand. A proportion of growing strands will terminate at each of these positions. Thus there will be fragments of length 27, 30, 35, 41, etc. nucleotides. When the product is size-separated by electrophoresis, if we can read off the lengths of the fragments, we can read off the positions of the As in the newly synthesized strand. If dideoxy-A was the only dideoxy nucleotide used, there would not be fragments 28, 29, 31, 32, etc. nucleotides long, because at those positions the polymerase would not be incorporating an A into the growing chain, and so there would be no risk of a dideoxy-A preventing the chain from growing further.

The original version of the Sanger sequencing technique worked exactly as we have just described, using four parallel reactions, each with one radiolabeled chain terminator. Nowadays most sequencing is done using fluorescent labeling of the dideoxynucleotides, as shown in *Figure 5.3*. This brings several benefits, apart from avoiding the inconvenience of radioactive work. The four dideoxynucleotides are tagged with four different colored fluorescent dyes; the standard nucleotides are unlabeled. Now small amounts of all four terminators can be included in a single reaction mix. Each fragment that ends with an A will be (say) green, each fragment ending in C will be blue, and so on. An automated DNA analyzer (see *Box figure 4.1b*) separates the fragments by length using electrophoresis through a gel or fine capillary and reads the color. The result is displayed as a series of colored peaks (*Figure 5.4*). Sophisticated software interprets the sequence and can provide other information, such as quantitating each peak and defining the length of each fragment. These features make automated sequencers useful for other tasks as well as sequencing. Increasingly, PCR-based tests are formatted to use fluorescently labeled primers, so that the PCR product can be sized and quantitated on a sequencing machine, rather than run on a manual electrophoretic gel. A number of the tests illustrated below by photographs of gels are nowadays commonly run on a sequencer (we used the gel photos here to give a more direct feel for the process).

Figure 5.3 – Principle of DNA sequencing.
(a) Each time a nucleotide is incorporated into the growing chain, there is a small chance that it will be a dideoxynucleotide, which will terminate growth of the chain. The result is a series of nested fragments.
(b) The result of running the reaction products on an automated gene analyzer such as that shown in *Box figure 4.1b*. Electrophoresis separates the fragments by length. Each dideoxynucleotide carries a different colored fluorescent dye.

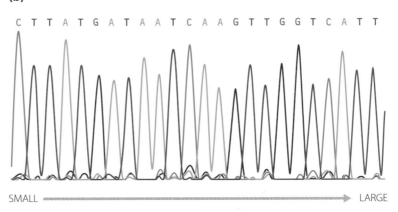

(a)

sequence to be copied

5′ AGCTTGAAGACTTAATGACCAACTTGATTATCATAAGTACGGCTAGC 3′
                    ← direction of growth   3′ ATGCCGATCG 5′ primer

CATGCCGATCG
TCATGCCGATCG
TTCATGCCGATCG
ATTCATGCCGATCG
TATTCATGCCGATCG
GTATTCATGCCGATCG
AGTATTCATGCCGATCG
TAGTATTCATGCCGATCG
ATAGTATTCATGCCGATCG
AATAGTATTCATGCCGATCG
TAATAGTATTCATGCCGATCG
CTAATAGTATTCATGCCGATCG
ACTAATAGTATTCATGCCGATCG
AACTAATAGTATTCATGCCGATCG
GAACTAATAGTATTCATGCCGATCG

Products of the reaction: a nested set of fragments, each terminated by a color-labeled dideoxynucleotide

(b)

C T T A T G A T A A T C A A G T T G G T C A T T

SMALL ⟶ LARGE

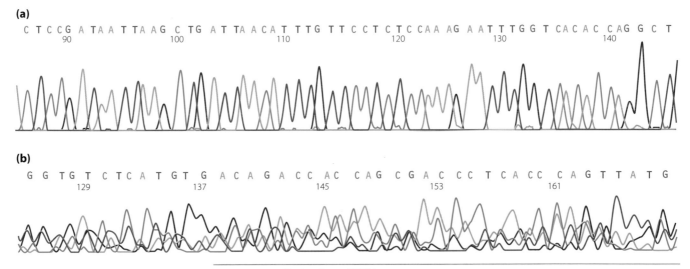

(a)

C T C C G A T A A T T A A G C T G A T T A A C A T T T G T T C C T C T C C A A A G A A T T T G G T C A C A C C A G G C T
    90   100   110   120   130   140

(b)

G G T G T C T C A T G T G A C A G A C C A C C A G C G A C C C T C A C C C A G T T A T G
      129   137   145   153   161

Figure 5.4 – Examples of DNA sequencer traces.
(a) Sequence of part of exon 15 of the *OCRL* gene. (b) Sequencing requires high quality DNA. If the DNA used is not carefully purified, the result may be a trace that cannot be reliably interpreted. (Track (a) courtesy of Dr Andrew Wallace, University of Manchester; track (b) anonymous.)

Massively parallel sequencing

Four different 'next generation' sequencing technologies were brought to market during 2006–10 (*Table 5.1*), and even more advanced 'third generation' technologies are already being piloted. The key novelty of all these is that, as the name suggests, they are massively parallel and simultaneously perform millions of independent sequencing reactions. Compared to Sanger sequencing, they generate a staggering amount of data per run at a far lower cost per base sequenced. However, they lack a key feature of the Sanger method – they are not targeted. In Sanger sequencing the choice of primer determines the sequence to be read. The massively parallel techniques all simply sequence everything in the test sample. This is ideal for sequencing whole genomes or for any job that requires mass sequencing, and for such purposes they have completely supplanted Sanger sequencing. But clinicians usually want to check the sequence of just one or a few exons in a patient's DNA; for those purposes Sanger sequencing is still the method of choice.

A second feature of the massively parallel technologies (with the exception of the 454 method) is that they sequence only short stretches of DNA at a time – typically 50–100 bp. This is a limitation for sequencing whole genomes, because the final sequence must be assembled by computer from millions of short runs – but for clinical purposes it could well be an advantage, because most exons are much shorter than the 500–800 bp sequenced in a single Sanger run. Additionally, individual sequences determined by the new methods are less accurate than the best Sanger sequencing. High overall accuracy is achieved by using a high sequencing depth – that is, many independent copies of each fragment are sequenced – but this does mean that the amount of finished sequence generated per run is correspondingly less than the raw figure in *Table 5.1*.

Table 5.1 – **A comparison of sequencing technologies**

Technology	Read length (bp)	Run time	Throughput per run	Read base error rate** (%)	Cost per Mb
Dideoxy sequencing	500–800	4 h	80 kb*	<0.01	$500
Roche / 454	400	10 h	400–600 Mb	0.5–1.5	$84
Illumina / Solexa	75+	7 days	17 Gb	0.2–2	$6
ABI SOLiD	50	3–7 days	10–15 Gb	<0.1	$5.80
Helicos Biosciences	32	7 days	17 Gb	4–5	$0.70

Data from Tucker *et al.* (2009) and Li and Wang (2009). All these figures are likely to change given the rapid pace of technical development.

1 Gb = 1000 Mb. *On a machine with 96 capillaries. **Final reported sequence has a much higher accuracy after quality filtering and comparison of multiple reads.

As yet more advanced 'third generation' sequencing technologies mature, sequencing may become so cheap (*Figure 5.5* illustrates the tumbling cost of genome sequencing) and routine that everybody will arrive at the genetics clinic with their full diploid genome sequence on a memory stick. Until that day, the potential of the new methods to change clinical services depends on the ability to select a subset of a patient's DNA for sequencing. The key to doing this is to use capture methods. Genomic DNA from the patient is fragmented, denatured and exposed to a cocktail of probes that, between them, represent all the sequences it is desired to check. Hybridizing fragments are isolated and used for massively parallel sequencing. The capture may use a custom-designed microarray or it can be done in solution. The immediate impact on clinical services is likely to be with conditions that can be caused by mutations in any one of a large number of genes. Deafness (see the Choudhary family, Case 3), blindness and mental retardation are prime examples. In each case it might be desirable to sequence each exon of, say, 50 or 100 candidate genes. In cancer, the ability to check a biopsied tumor for changes in a few hundred key genes could allow much better targeted treatment. Preliminary estimates suggest such investigations might involve consumables costs in the order of only $1000 per case, although the need for extensive bioinformatic analysis might be a limiting factor. These are exciting times for clinical geneticists – but meanwhile life goes on, and the rest of this chapter will illustrate the ongoing and very substantial importance of the current methods for checking a patient's DNA for mutations.

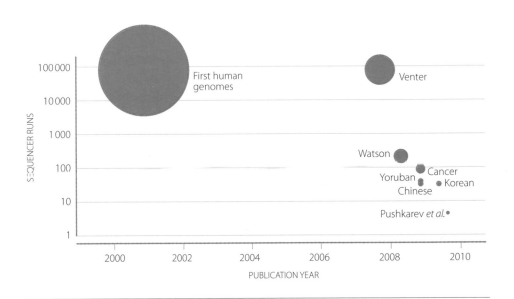

Figure 5.5 – The rapidly falling costs of genome sequencing.
The diagram shows the estimated costs of some published human whole genome sequences. The size of each circle represents the estimated cost of consumables, and the vertical axis shows the number of machine runs required, as an indicator of the labor costs. Reproduced from *Nature Biotechnology*, 2009; **27**: 820 with permission from the Nature Publishing Group (see that article for references to the individual sequences).

Methods for detecting specific sequence changes

It often happens that the laboratory is looking for the presence or absence of one specific sequence variant in a sample. This happens under various circumstances.

- The disease in question may always be caused by exactly the same sequence change. The prenatal test for sickle cell disease in the Kavanagh family (Case 11) relied on the fact that sickle cell disease is always caused by precisely the same sequence change. The reasons why some diseases are always caused by one specific mutation are discussed in *Chapter 10*.

- A disease may be caused by various different mutations, but one or a few mutations may be so frequent in a particular population that it is worth first checking for these before going on to a more general search. An example is cystic fibrosis. Over 1000 different mutations have been reported, but 80% of all mutations in Northern Europeans are one particular deletion of three nucleotides (see *Table 11.1*); 80% of all β-thalassemia mutations in Greek Cypriots are c.93–21G>A (see *Table 5.3*).

- The test may be to check a patient for a family mutation that has already been identified and characterized in other family members.

- The test may be to check samples from healthy controls to make sure a variant found in a patient is not a non-pathogenic variant present in the normal population.

The same techniques are also used for genotyping people for non-pathogenic single nucleotide polymorphisms (SNPs), for example, in linkage and association analysis (*Chapter 9*) and in anthropological investigations.

Many methods are available to detect a specific sequence change. These include:

- Sequencing the DNA, usually in the form of a PCR product. A standard Sanger sequencing run as described above delivers several hundred nucleotides of sequence, which is not what is required here. A special variant method, Pyrosequencing®, sequences just a few nucleotides from a given starting point. Pyrosequencing requires a special machine and reagents but, once set up, it is good for checking one specific nucleotide in samples from a large collection of individuals. *Figure 5.17* shows an example.

- Hybridizing the PCR-amplified sample to an allele-specific oligonucleotide (ASO) probe, as was done for sickle cell disease (*Figure 4.11*).

- Digestion with a restriction enzyme. If the mutation happens to either create or destroy a sequence that is the recognition site for a restriction enzyme, this allows an easy test. The relevant region is PCR amplified, the product is digested with the appropriate restriction enzyme and then run out on a gel. The size of the fragments shows whether the restriction site was present. Heterozygotes show both the cut and uncut fragments. Examples are illustrated below for LHON (Case 6 – Fletcher family, *Figure 5.16*) and β-thalassemia (Case 14 – Nicolaides family, *Figure 5.15*).

- Performing an allele-specific PCR reaction. PCR primers may work even if there are slight mismatches to their target, provided the primer is long enough to hybridize, but the 3′ end nucleotide of the primer is critical. Unless it correctly base-pairs to the template the reaction will not work. We can therefore check whether a given nucleotide is A or G by setting up a PCR reaction where this nucleotide must pair with the 3′ end nucleotide of one of the primers. A primer ending in T will amplify only the A allele, while one ending in C will amplify only the G allele. As with ASOs, two parallel reactions are run with the two different primers, or alternatively the primers are differently labeled (e.g. with different dyes) so as to give identifiable products in a single mixed reaction. *Figure 5.6* shows the principle; *Figures 5.11* and *5.14* show applications.

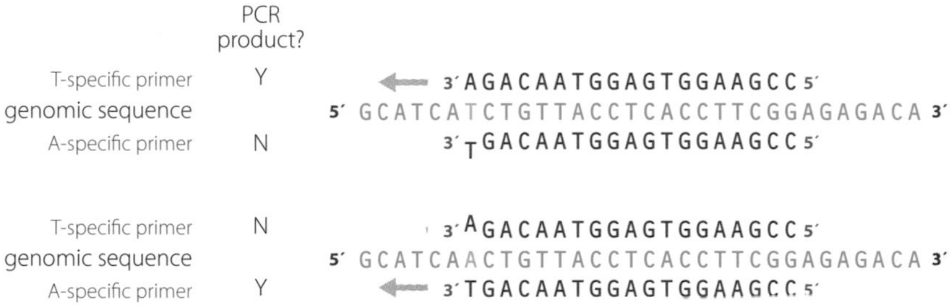

Figure 5.6 – Principle of allele-specific PCR reaction.
A PCR reaction will not yield product if the 3′-most nucleotide of a primer is not correctly base-paired. Mismatches elsewhere in the primer sequence may be tolerated, but the 3′ end must match. One primer (not shown, off to the left) is standard; the second primer is specific for one allele of a T/A single nucleotide polymorphism (green). Two reactions are set up, one using the common plus T-specific primers, the other using the common plus A-specific primers. See *Figures 5.11* and *5.14* for examples.

- Oligonucleotide ligation analysis (OLA). The enzyme DNA ligase was mentioned in *Box 4.5*. This enzyme will covalently seal a single-strand gap in a DNA double helix. To test for a C/T change by OLA, three oligonucleotides are hybridized to the test DNA. Two allele-specific oligos have their 3′ end at the variable position, one ending with G, the other with A. The two have different sized 5′ extensions, or are labeled with different colored dyes. The third oligo is a common oligo which has its 5′ end at the next nucleotide and carries a 5′ phosphate group. DNA ligase will join two oligonucleotides if they perfectly match the test strand, but not if either of the two end nucleotides to be linked is not correctly base-paired with the test DNA. The size or color of the ligation product is checked to see which of the allele-specific oligos has taken part in the ligation reaction. OLA has been developed commercially as a convenient kit for checking for a panel of specific sequence changes in a single operation. *Figure 5.7* shows the principle.

The choice of method depends to a large extent on how many samples require the test. Allele-specific oligonucleotides and oligonucleotides for OLA have to be custom-synthesized. This makes those methods unattractive for a one-off test.

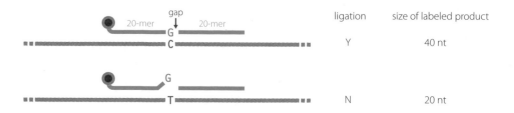

Figure 5.7 – Using the oligonucleotide ligation assay to genotype a C/T variant. DNA ligase can only seal the gap between the two abutting oligonucleotides if the two ends are correctly base-paired with a template strand. The allele-specific oligonucleotides are different sizes, while the common oligonucleotide is labeled with a fluorescent dye. After the ligation reaction the size of the labeled product is measured on a DNA sequencer. OLA tests can be multiplexed by designing oligonucleotides to give different sized ligation products, and/or by labeling them with different fluorescent dyes.

Primers for allele-specific PCR also have to be custom-synthesized, but this is less of an extra expense because whatever technique is used, primers for PCR amplification will be needed. Restriction enzyme digestion is simple in principle, but if the particular sequence change requires the use of an unusual enzyme this can be expensive. Also, not all changes create or remove a restriction site. Pyrosequencing is a good general method for testing many samples, but it requires expensive special equipment.

Methods for scanning a gene for any sequence change

The most common task for a diagnostic DNA laboratory is to check the entire sequence of a gene for any possible mutation. Increasingly, the laboratory will simply sequence every exon and splice junction of the gene. Sequencing provides the gold standard for such mutation scanning – but it is not the method of choice in every case. Although costs keep falling, it is still a relatively expensive technique. Skill and good quality DNA are needed to get results clear enough to detect heterozygotes reliably. The structure of genes also makes scanning by dideoxy sequencing relatively inefficient. Individual human exons average only 145 bp, well below the 500–800 bp that can be read in one sequencing run. But most introns are too large to allow more than one exon to be amplified from genomic DNA as a single PCR product. Thus testing a gene usually involves a separate PCR reaction and sequencing run for each exon. For a gene like fibrillin (see **Case 10, Johnson family**) with 66 exons, this is a lot of work. Studying mRNA by RT–PCR would solve that problem (see *Chapter 4*), but RNA is hard to handle, and obtaining it may be excessively invasive (what if the relevant gene is expressed only in the brain?).

For these reasons, a variety of other methods are used as adjuncts to sequencing. These perform a quick scan of a DNA fragment such as a PCR-amplified exon, and report whether its sequence differs in any way from the normal version. Using these can save time and money. The commonest methods are based on either of two principles:

- *Properties of heteroduplexes.* If a person is heterozygous for a sequence variant in an exon, PCR amplification of the exon will give a mix of the mutant and normal sequences. If the mix is heated to denature the DNA and then slowly cooled, some of the resulting double helices will be **heteroduplexes**, containing one strand from each of the two alleles (*Figure 5.8a*). Heteroduplexes denature more easily than fully matched duplexes. This can be noted in various ways, for example, by their altered mobility on a <u>d</u>enaturing <u>h</u>igh <u>p</u>erformance <u>l</u>iquid <u>c</u>hromatography (dHPLC) column. An alternative technique, melting curve analysis, follows the denaturation by monitoring the fluorescence of a dye such as SYBR Green, which fluoresces strongly in the presence of double-stranded, but not single-stranded DNA. Heteroduplexes also have bulges or kinks compared to perfectly matched DNA. This makes them run slower through an electrophoretic gel than the corresponding homoduplexes. Their presence can be revealed as extra bands on the gel.
- *Properties of single-stranded DNA.* Single-stranded DNA ties itself into knots as bases in different parts of the strand pair with each other. The precise shape of the knot depends on the sequence, and affects the rate at which the knot migrates through an electrophoretic gel. <u>S</u>ingle <u>s</u>trand <u>c</u>onformation <u>p</u>olymorphism (SSCP) analysis looks for any differences between the migration of the test sequence and a normal sequence (*Figures 5.8b* and *5.12*). Compared to dHPLC or melting curve analysis, SSCP requires no expensive equipment and is simple to set up, but probably misses more mutations (claimed sensitivity is 80–90%). It is particularly useful for testing small numbers of samples.

Laboratories often use these or similar methods for a preliminary scan of each exon of a gene. Any exon showing a departure from the normal version is then sequenced. Compared to simply sequencing every exon, this two-stage approach saves the cost and labor of sequencing the normal exons. However, none of these methods picks up 100% of the changes in a sequence, and as the cost of sequencing keeps falling, the use of these alternatives is diminishing.

Methods for detecting deletion or duplication of whole exons

As described in *Chapter 3* (*Figure 3.9*), large deletions or duplications in genomic DNA usually cause deletion or duplication of whole exons. Exons form only a very small part of the whole human genome sequence, so a random breakpoint is unlikely to fall within an exon. Even if the breakpoint is within a gene, it is much more likely to be within an intron than an exon. In a heterozygous person, a deletion or duplication of one or more whole exons would not be detected using any of the methods described above. For example, Judith Davies (Case 4) is heterozygous for a deletion of several exons of the dystrophin gene. But if we individually PCR-amplified each exon of her dystrophin gene, the appropriate sequence would amplify from her normal X chromosome, and the PCR product would appear entirely normal by any of the tests described above. Special techniques are needed to detect whole exon deletions or duplications.

(a)

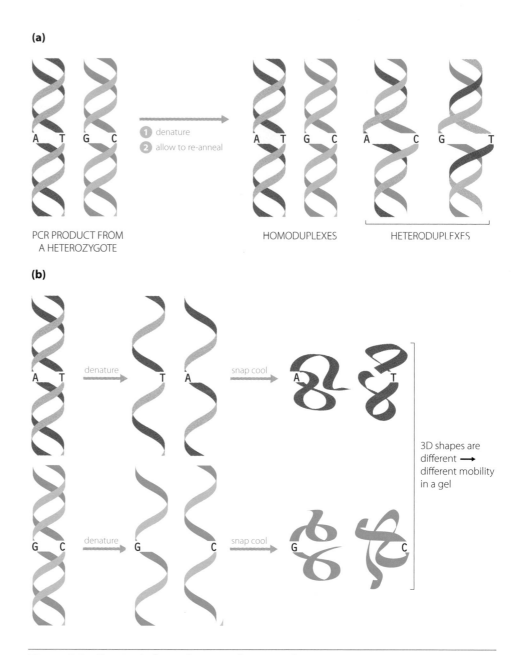

(b)

Figure 5.8 – Two techniques for mutation scanning.
(a) Heteroduplexes are formed when the PCR product from a heterozygous person is heated then allowed to re-anneal. Heteroduplexes can be detected by their lower denaturation temperature or by their slower rate of migration on an electrophoretic gel. (b) Single-stranded DNA adopts a conformation that depends on its sequence. Samples from people with different sequence variants may fold in different, though unpredictable, ways and have different mobilities in a gel. A real example is shown in *Figure 5.12.*

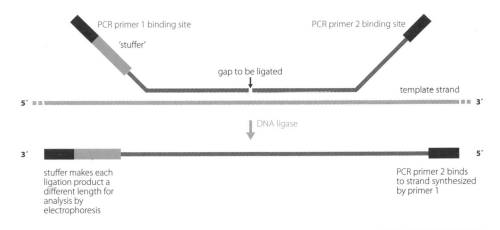

Figure 5.9 – Principle of the multiplex ligation-dependent probe amplification (MLPA) method for detecting deletions or duplications.
Each probe consists of a pair of oligonucleotides that can be ligated only if their matching sequence is present in the test sample, as in the oligonucleotide ligation assay (*Figure 5.7*). In MLPA, unlike in OLA, the chosen target sequence may be variable in copy number but hopefully not in sequence. Thus only two oligonucleotides are used per sequence tested. Ligation creates a PCR-amplifiable molecule. The mixed ligation products are amplified using a single pair of primers that hybridize to sequences present on the ends of every probe pair. One of the primers is fluorescently labeled, and the reaction mix is analyzed on a fluorescence DNA sequencing machine. Each ligation product is a different length, giving a unique peak on the sequencer trace.

- *Quantitative PCR* was described in *Chapter 4*. When major life decisions hang on the result of a single test, as with the at-risk females in the **Davies family (Case 4)**, a very accurate and reliable test is essential. Various commercial systems using real-time quantitative PCR are used most often.

- *Multiplex ligation-dependent probe amplification (MLPA)* uses the specificity of the OLA (*Figure 5.7*) to increase the accuracy of simple quantitative PCR. *Figure 5.9* shows the principle and *Figure 5.10* an example. MLPA has rapidly gained acceptance in genetic diagnostic laboratories due to its simplicity compared to other methods, relatively low cost, capacity for reasonably high throughput and perceived robustness – although many laboratories prefer to use array-CGH or SNP chips for these purposes. MLPA is a multiplex procedure, testing up to 45 short (typically 60 bp) sequences simultaneously for copy number variation. This makes it well suited to checking a large multi-exon gene for any whole exon deletion, but equally it could be used to test selected exons from several different genes. Establishing a new MLPA assay is time-consuming because each individual probe needs to be carefully designed, so it is mostly used for frequently investigated genes, where probe sets are commercially available. MLPA probes are expensive because they are much longer than normal PCR primers, but overall the technique is cheaper than most alternatives.

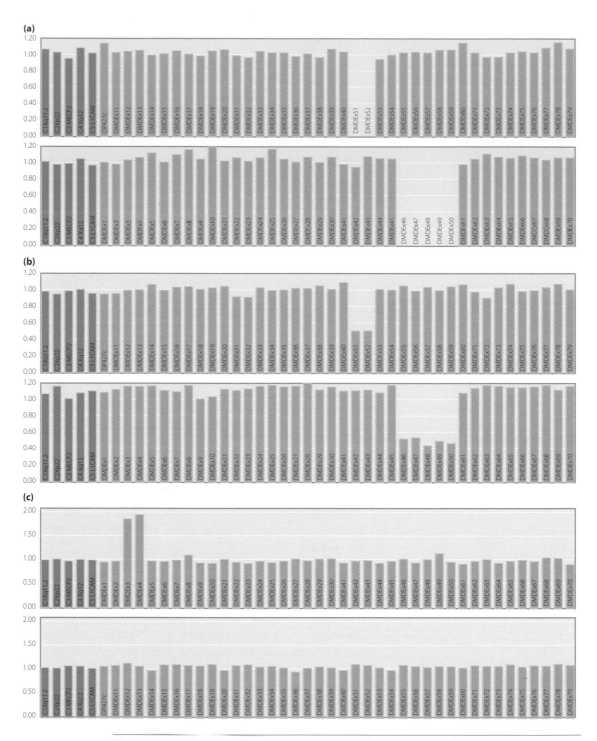

Figure 5.10 – Using MLPA to detect exon deletions or duplications in the dystrophin gene.
A multiplex MLPA assay tests every exon of the dystrophin gene. The bar charts show peak intensities for each product, as measured on a capillary sequencer. Numbers in each bar show the exon involved. Bars in blue are from unrelated control sequences. (a) This boy has a deletion of exons 46–52; (b) his sister is heterozygous for the deletion. (c) This patient has a duplication of exons 3 and 4. Courtesy of Dr Simon Ramsden, St Mary's Hospital, Manchester.

5.3. **Investigations of patients**

The stories so far...

Table 5.2 summarizes the achievements and requirements for testing in the cases described so far. This section describes the further tests performed on **Cases 2, 6 and 14**, which illustrate the various techniques described above.

Table 5.2 – **Summary of testing performed to date in the cases featured, and further tests required**

Case	Problem	Tests so far	Tests needed
1	Huntington disease	Size of expansion checked by PCR	None needed
2	**Cystic fibrosis**		**Check *CFTR* gene for mutations**
3	Deafness		Identify gene and mutation (see *Chapter 9*)
4	Duchenne muscular dystrophy	Deletion of exons 44–48 defined by PCR	None needed
5	Chromosomal translocation	Identified by karyotyping	None needed
6	**Leber's hereditary optic neuropathy**		**Check for mitochondrial mutation**
7	? Deletion of 22q11	Deletion confirmed by FISH	None needed
8	Down syndrome	Confirmed by karyotyping. Prenatal test by FISH	None needed
9	Turner syndrome	Confirmed by karyotyping. Check for Y sequences by PCR	None needed
10	Marfan syndrome		Molecular testing not undertaken – clinical diagnosis suffices
11	Sickle cell disease	Prenatal test using allele-specific oligonucleotides	None needed
12	Fragile-X	Check size of trinucleotide repeat by PCR and Southern blotting	None needed
13	? Chromosomal abnormality	Check for chromosomal imbalances on SNP chip; check if it is *de novo*	No further routine investigation
14	**β-thalassemia**		**Identify mutation**

CASE 2   Brown family   2   8   66   **132**   154   281   389

- Girl aged 6 months, parents David and Pauline
- ? cystic fibrosis
- Order molecular test?
- Define mutations in *CFTR* gene

David and Pauline indicated that they might consider having more children in the future but would definitely wish for prenatal tests because they felt that coping with the extra needs of one child with cystic fibrosis was as much as they could do. Before that could be done, it would be necessary to define both mutations in Joanne. Additionally, after discussion at family reunions, other members of the large extended family became concerned about their own carrier risk and several relatives expressed a desire for carrier testing. Again, this has to be done by checking for the mutations present in Joanne. Although over 1000 different mutations in the *CFTR* gene have been described in cystic fibrosis patients, most of these have been seen only in one or a very few cases. A small number of mutations are relatively common. Mutation testing in cystic fibrosis therefore starts by checking for these common mutations. Several commercial kits are available for this purpose. Joanne's DNA was screened using a multiplex allele-specific PCR assay (see *Figure 5.6* for the principle). The result (*Figure 5.11*) shows that she has the p.F508del mutation (see *Box 5.1* for a brief explanation of this nomenclature – though this one is often called by the non-standard name delta-F508). This mutation is the commonest cystic fibrosis mutation in Northern Europeans, comprising 70–80% of all cystic fibrosis mutations in many populations.

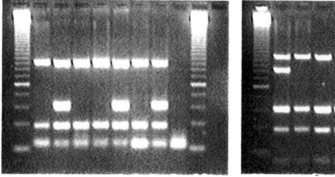 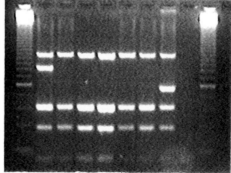

Figure 5.11 – A multiplex allele-specific PCR test for 29 common *CFTR* mutations. The same seven samples are amplified with different cocktails of primers in the two gels. No mutation is detected in lanes 3, 4 or 6. Extra bands in the other lanes define particular mutations by their presence and size. Courtesy of Victoria Stinton and Roger Mountford, Liverpool Women's Hospital.

Joanne is heterozygous for the p.F508del mutation because the test shows that she also has the corresponding normal allele. No second mutation was detected. Given her diagnosis she should have a second mutation, but it might be anywhere in the gene. Rather than immediately sequencing all 27 exons of the *CFTR* gene, the laboratory PCR-amplified each exon and used the SSCP method (see *Figure 5.8b*) to identify exons containing sequence variants. The result (*Figure 5.12*) showed that something was different in exons 3 and 14b in Joanne's DNA compared to a normal control. Either or both of these may well be non-pathogenic sequence variants. (For historical reasons, in the main mutation database the 27 exons of

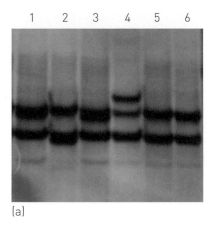

(a)

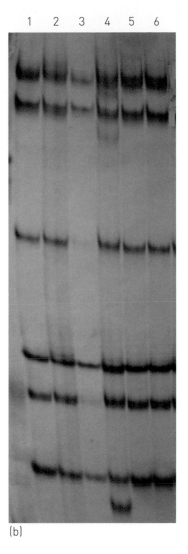

(b)

Figure 5.12 – SSCP analysis of exons of the *CFTR* gene.
Each exon was amplified in separate PCR reactions from each of a series of samples from cystic fibrosis patients. Results from exons 3 (a) and 14b (b) are shown. In Joanne's sample the products (lane 4 on each gel) show a different band pattern from the other samples, indicating that they have some difference in their sequence. The samples in lanes 2 and 3 (from other cystic fibrosis patients) also show abnormalities. It is then necessary to sequence (*Figure 5.13*) in order to identify the change and decide whether it is pathogenic. Using this procedure reduced the sequencing requirement for Joanne from 27 to 2 exons.

the gene are numbered 1–5, 6a, 6b, 7–13, 14a, 14b, 15, 16, 17a, 17b, 18–24; the genome browsers number them 1–27.)

Figure 5.13 shows one of the sequencer traces. The following changes were identified:

- exon 3   c.368G>A
- exon 14b   c.2752–15C>G

In *Chapter 6* we will see how the laboratory attempted to decide whether either of these changes was likely to be pathogenic.

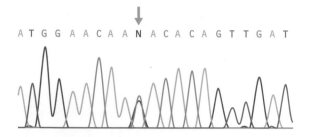

ATGGAACAANACACAGTTGAT

Figure 5.13 – DNA sequencer trace of part of the exon 14b PCR product from Joanne Brown's *CFTR* gene.
At the arrowed position G and C nucleotides are both present, showing that Joanne is heterozygous for a nucleotide substitution (remember that the products of PCR and sequencing are normally a mix of the products from the two alleles). Control samples show only the G. It is usual to sequence both strands of the DNA separately to confirm any change. In this case the sequence shown is of the reverse strand, so in the sense strand the change in Joanne is C>G.

A brief guide to nomenclature of mutations

BOX 5.1

A mutation can be described in terms of the change in the genomic DNA, the cDNA or the encoded protein. The description is prefixed with g., c., or p. according to which of these it describes.

For DNA, > means 'changes to'. Thus G>A means the normal G is replaced by an A nucleotide. Deletions and insertions are symbolized by del and ins respectively. The affected nucleotide is numbered from an agreed starting point and database file. For cDNA, nucleotides are counted from the A of the AUG start codon. A nucleotide in an intron is given the number of the last nucleotide of the preceding exon, a plus sign and the position in the intron, such as c.77+1, c.77+32, etc. If it is near the end of a large intron it may be given the number of the first nucleotide of the following exon, a minus sign and the position (*Tables 5.3* and *11.1* show examples). For genomic DNA, the start nucleotide position must be specified.

For protein level changes the one-letter or three-letter amino acid abbreviations are used (see *Box 3.6*). X means a stop codon. Amino acids are counted from the initiator methionine of the protein (even though this is usually removed in post-translational processing).

Examples:

c.76A>C means that at nucleotide 76 an A is changed to a C
c.76–78del means a deletion of 3 nucleotides, from nucleotides 76 to 78 inclusive
p.Ala26Val or p.A26V means that amino acid alanine-26 is changed to a valine
p.Cys318X or p.C318X means the codon for cysteine 318 is changed to a stop codon

This level of detail is sufficient for understanding everything in this book. Nomenclature has been defined for describing every possible sequence variation. You can find full details at the Human Genome Variation Society website:
www.hgvs.org/mutnomen

- ? β-thalassemia carriers
- Check mutations

Hemoglobinopathies are the most intensively studied of all genetic diseases, and rightly so, because they affect millions of people in many countries. Children homozygous for β-thalassemia have a difficult life. They require endless blood transfusions, but then have major problems with iron overload. Among Greek Cypriots, it has been estimated that one person in seven is a carrier of β-thalassemia. Thus we would expect one in 49 marriages to be between carriers. This has triggered a national population screening program. The reasons why hemoglobinopathies are so remarkably common in some populations are discussed in *Chapter 10*. Carrier testing is carried out using routine hematological methods. This indicated that both Spiros and Elena were carriers, though entirely healthy in themselves. They were offered molecular tests to identify their precise mutations, and because they thought they might wish for prenatal diagnosis in any pregnancy, they took up the offer. It was better to do it now, when there was no urgency, than to wait until Elena was pregnant and would require urgent testing.

Spiros and Elena each provided a mouthwash sample from which DNA was extracted. Five specific mutations in the β-globin gene make up 98.4% of all β-thalassemia mutations among Greek Cypriots (*Table 5.3*). Their DNA was therefore first tested for each of these mutations. Had the results been negative, their β-globin genes would have been sequenced to look for the mutations. The β-globin gene is small (3 exons and 2 introns; only about 1500 bp in total), so it is not difficult to sequence the exons, introns and promoter to check for mutations.

Table 5.3 – **Common β-thalassemia mutations among Greek Cypriots**

Mutation	Location	Percentage of all β-thalassemia mutations in Greek Cypriots	Sequence change: (normal, mutant)
c.93–21G>A	Intron 1	79.8	ctatt**gg**tctattttccc ctatt**ag**tctattttccc
c.92+6T>C	Intron 1	5.5	AGgttggt**a**t AGgttgg**c**at
c.92+1G>A	Intron 1	5.1	AG**g**ttggtat AG**a**ttggtat
c.316–106C>G	Intron 2	5.1	cag**c**taccat cag**g**taccat
p.Gln39X	Exon 2	2.9	TGGACC**CAG**AGGTTC TGGACC**TAG**AGGTTC

Exon sequences are in upper case, intron sequences in lower case. See *Box 5.1* for the nomenclature of mutations and *Chapter 6* for discussion of how these mutants cause disease. Data from HbVar database: http://globin.cse.psu.edu/globin/hbvar

Neither of them carried the most common Cypriot mutation, c.93–21G>A, so the DNA was then checked for the other four common mutations. Spiros turned out to be carrying the p.Gln39X mutation while Elena carried the c.316–106C>G mutation. All these mutations could be checked by sequencing, allele-specific PCR or by hybridization to allele-specific oligonucleotides; the c.316–106C>G mutation also creates a restriction site for the enzymes *Rsa*I (GTAC) and *Kpn*I (GGTACC). A convenient general method would be a **reverse dot blot**, in which a panel of allele-specific oligonucleotides is spotted onto a nitrocellulose filter, which is then hybridized to dye-labeled product of PCR – amplifying the patient's β-globin genes. *Figures 5.14* and *5.15* illustrate the use of different methods for detecting these mutations.

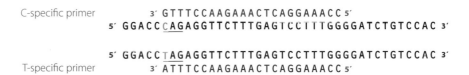

C-specific primer   3′ GTTTCCAAGAAACTCAGGAAACC 5′
    5′ GGACC CAGAGGTTCTTTGAGTCCTTTGGGGATCTGTCCAC 3′

    5′ GGACC TAGAGGTTCTTTGAGTCCTTTGGGGATCTGTCCAC 3′
T-specific primer   3′ ATTTCCAAGAAACTCAGGAAACC 5′

Figure 5.14 – Identification of the p.Gln39X mutation by allele-specific PCR.
The C>T change converts a codon for glutamine (CAG) into a stop codon (TAG). The C-specific and T-specific primers are used with a common primer that hybridizes to a sequence to the left of the region shown. A deliberate mismatch at position 3 of each primer increases the specificity of the reaction.

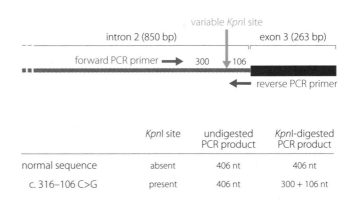

	*Kpn*I site	undigested PCR product	*Kpn*I-digested PCR product
normal sequence	absent	406 nt	406 nt
c. 316–106 C>G	present	406 nt	300 + 106 nt

Figure 5.15 – Identification of the c.316–106C>G mutation.
The mutation creates a *Kpn*I restriction site (GGTACC) in intron 2 of the β-globin gene. A suitable size fragment including the mutation site is PCR amplified and the product incubated with the restriction enzyme.

- Frank, aged 22, with increasingly blurred eyesight
- Family history of visual difficulties
- Pedigree suggests X-linked recessive inheritance but not conclusive
- ? LHON
- Order blood test to check for mutation in mtDNA
- Check mutations by Pyrosequencing

LHON (OMIM 535000) is the result of inadequate function of the mitochondria, caused by mutations in the mitochondrial DNA (mtDNA). Confirming the diagnosis in Frank depends on demonstrating the presence of a mutation. The molecular genetics of LHON is quite complicated. Eighteen different point mutations in the mtDNA have been associated with this one disease. Presumably there are many ways in which mitochondrial function can be impaired, leading to the disease. Five of the 18 have a sufficiently serious effect to cause LHON by themselves; the others are found in combination with each other and presumably cause disease by an accumulation of smaller effects.

Three point mutations cause the great majority of cases, at least in people of European origin (we use the usual mtDNA nomenclature here):

- G11778A – substitution of A for G at nucleotide 11778 of the 16.5 kb mitochondrial genome. This results in replacement of arginine 340 by histidine in the ND4 protein that is part of the oxidative phosphorylation machinery.
- G3460A – the G→A nucleotide change replaces alanine 52 in the ND1 protein with tyrosine.
- T14484C – this nucleotide substitution causes methionine 64 in the ND6 protein to be replaced by valine.

The usual diagnostic procedure is first to test for these three specific mutations. If none is present, then a wider search is needed, which may include sequencing parts of the mtDNA.

Any of the methods described previously could be used for checking for the common mutations. *Figure 5.16* shows a restriction enzyme-based method for the G11778A mutation. An alternative method uses Pyrosequencing (*Figure 5.17*); this has the advantage that the result is quantitative. As explained in *Chapter 1*, people can be homoplasmic or heteroplasmic for mitochondrial mutations, so a full mutation test includes checking the relative amounts of normal and mutant mitochondria. The result showed that Frank was homoplasmic for the G3460A mutation, thus confirming the diagnosis of LHON.

	SEQUENCE			FRAGMENT SIZES	
				*Sfa*NI	*Mae*III
	11770	11780	11790		
normal	CGAACGCACT	CACAGTCGCA	TCATAATCCT	417 + 91	233 + 218 + 57
	11770	11780	11790		
G11778A	CGAACGCACT	CACAGTCACA	TCATAATCCT	508	233 + 131 + 87 + 57

Figure 5.16 – Detecting the G11778A mutation by its effect on restriction enzyme recognition sites.
The mutation abolishes a site for the enzyme *Sfa*NI (GCATC) but creates one for the enzyme *Mae*III (GTNAC, where N is any nucleotide). The assay shown here involves PCR amplifying a 508 bp portion of the mtDNA that includes nucleotide 11778. Separate samples of the PCR product are digested with the two enzymes and the fragments sized on an electrophoretic gel. Restriction sites are underlined, the changed nucleotide is highlighted in color and the sizes of fragments are shown.

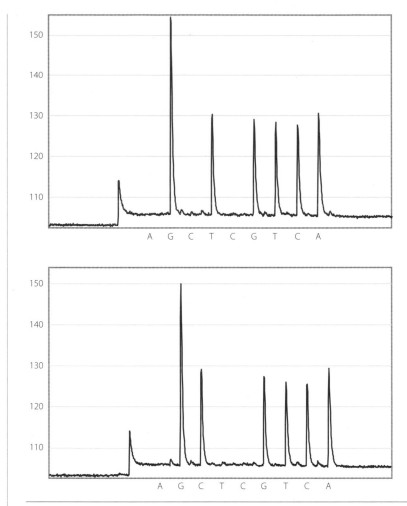

Figure 5.17 – Detection of the G3460A mtDNA mutation by Pyrosequencing.
The Pyrosequencing machine tries adding each nucleotide in turn to the end of a primer. Successful addition triggers a bioluminescent reaction, recorded by the machine as a peak. Upper trace: mutant sequence GTGTCA; lower trace: normal control GCGTCA (the sequences are of the reverse strand).

5.4. **Going deeper ...**

The three questions

The feasibility and methodology of mutation testing depends crucially on the precision of the question being asked. Consider these three possible questions:

(1) Does Joanne Brown (Case 2) have any mutation in any gene that would account for her condition?
(2) Does Joanne Brown have any mutation in the *CFTR* gene?
(3) Does Joanne Brown have the p.F508del mutation in the *CFTR* gene?

Question (3) is quick and cheap to answer, using any of the methods described in the section on detecting specific sequence changes. That section also describes the circumstances under which it is possible to ask such a specific question.

Question (1) is not answerable in a service context. *Disease box 9* shows how the new massively parallel sequencing technologies may make an answer technically feasible, given several patients with the same phenotype, but this represents the cutting edge of research, not a current diagnostic service. Even if the technology becomes cheap and routine, answering such a question would almost certainly depend on having a reasonably short hit list of candidate genes, based on knowledge of the patient's condition. There are just too many differences between genomes to pick out the one pathogenic variant in a single patient, from among the millions of variants present in every genome, without some pointers to the correct answer. However, for copy number variants this question can be answered, using array-CGH or SNP chips (see *Chapter 4*).

Question (2) is always answerable in principle but the cost depends on the total number of exons to be screened. For Nasreen Choudhary (Case 3) there were over 50 known candidate deafness genes, totaling many hundreds of exons. Next generation sequencing technology will allow a screen of every exon for mutations, though such a development is still a little way in the future, and the bioinformatic analysis might be laborious and expensive. With Sanger sequencing, mutation screening is not feasible unless the field can be narrowed down to one or a few genes. How this was done in that particular case is described in *Chapter 9*. For Joanne Brown (Case 2) there is only a single candidate gene: cystic fibrosis is always caused by mutations in the *CFTR* gene. Testing that whole gene would still involve testing 27 exons. How far a laboratory will go in trying to answer question (2) depends on how much expense could be justified by the clinical importance of the answer. Increasing automation, and the use of some of the technologies described in this chapter are rapidly increasing the size of mutation screen that a diagnostic laboratory can undertake for a given cost.

Mutation detection using microarrays

Microarrays offer a way of performing a large number of hybridization tests in parallel. As described in *Chapter 4*, SNP chips contain hundreds of thousands of different allele-specific oligonucleotide probes. SNP chips are designed to genotype specific single nucleotides that commonly vary between normal healthy people. However, the same principle can be used to test for any set of sequence variants. Two possible designs of microarray could be used:

• The probes can be oligonucleotides that systematically cover the sequence of a gene. Oligo #1 might match nucleotides 1–25 of the cDNA, oligo #2 would match nucleotides 2–26, and so on right through one or more genes. Any deviation from this sequence in the test DNA would be revealed by a pattern of reduced or absent hybridization to certain oligos. These 'resequencing chips' also carry oligos matching all possible single-nucleotide substitutions in the target gene. In a single experiment, the complete coding sequence of a large gene can be checked for single base substitutions.
• The probes might be oligonucleotides chosen to detect a whole series of specific mutations in all the candidate genes for a certain disease. This might provide a solution to the problem of looking at 50 candidate

genes for deafness, for example, or looking for mutations in all the genes identified as possible causes of Long QT syndrome (see *Disease box 5*). However, they would only test for a limited predefined set of mutations in those genes. If a patient had a novel mutation it would probably be missed. These chips would therefore be used as a first screen to pick up the mutations in the majority of samples. Those samples negative on this screen would need to be investigated by other methods.

Each chip is used just once, to analyze one sample. This is expensive, but when labor costs are taken into consideration, using chips may be cost-effective compared to amplifying and sequencing every exon of a large gene. Start-up costs are high: the company must develop, manufacture and validate an appropriate array and the laboratory must buy the equipment needed to use and read arrays. For this reason, the main application of chips to diagnostics would be for analyses that need to be done many times – mutation testing for breast cancer or other relatively common diseases, for example. However, the rapid progress in sequencing technology has put the future of microarray-based mutation screening in question. It may turn out to be cheaper just to sequence everything.

High-throughput technologies, particularly next generation sequencing, are changing the face and pace of genetic research and this includes clinical research. But beyond extending the scope of mutation screening, how far will these technologies also change the face of clinical genetics services? Services focus on individual patients, so the question is, how far will it be useful to generate huge amounts of genotype or sequence information on individual patients? Sequencing tumor genomes to identify the most effective anticancer treatment seems one likely service application, as described in *Chapter 12*. Will it go further? Undoubtedly the time is soon coming when many healthy people who do not have tumors will carry around with them an electronic record of their own genome sequence. How far this will simply serve personal curiosity or vanity, and how far it will serve any useful clinical purpose, is a wide open question – and one to which clinical geneticists would dearly love an answer.

5.5. **References**

Choi G *et al.* (2004) Spectrum and frequency of cardiac channel defects in swimming-triggered arrhythmia syndromes. *Circulation,* **110**: 2119–2124.

Church GM (2006) Genomes for All. *Sci. Amer.* **294**: 47–54.

Li Y and Wang J (2009) Faster human genome sequencing. *Nat. Biotech.* **27**: 820–821.

Tucker T, Marra M and Friedman JM (2009) Massively parallel sequencing: the next big thing in genetic medicine. *Am. J. Hum. Genet.* **85**: 142–154.

The January 2006 edition of *Clinica Chimica Acta* (**363** nos.1–2) consists of a series of reviews on 'Present and Future of Rapid and/or High-throughput Methods for Nucleic Acid Testing'. These are quite technical, but they cover all the advanced methods mentioned here, and many more.

Long QT syndrome

It has long been recognized that sudden death can occur in apparently healthy young people without there being any clue on post-mortem examination as to why the tragedy happened. Occasionally more than one person in a family is affected. In recent years two main groups of conditions have been recognized that cause sudden adult death without obvious signs on post-mortem: Long QT syndromes and cardiomyopathies. In the latter group there may be preceding symptoms and, in some individuals, obvious hypertrophy at post-mortem. However, some individuals may have no symptoms and histological signs detectable only by experts in the field.

Long QT syndromes are characterized by ECG abnormalities (*Box figure 5.1*). These consist of QT prolongation (indicating prolonged or disordered ventricular repolarization) and T-wave abnormalities associated with a tendency to tachycardia (rapid beating of the heart) which may cause syncope (fainting). Twitching occurring during the syncope may lead to the misdiagnosis of epilepsy. Often these episodes self-terminate, but they can progress to ventricular fibrillation where the heart ceases to pump blood effectively and sudden death occurs. In 10–20% of all cases of drowning, Long QT or other genetic pro-arrhythmic conditions may be the cause (see Choi *et al.*, 2004). Long QT syndrome may also explain some cases of Sudden Infant Death Syndrome.

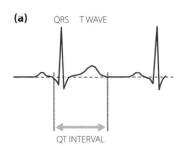

(a)

QRS T WAVE

QT INTERVAL

Box figure 5.1 – (a) the QT interval and (b) part of an exercise electrocardiogram showing a long QT interval (535 ms). Courtesy of Dr Kay Metcalfe, St Mary's Hospital, Manchester.

(b)

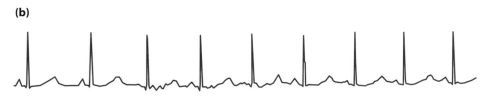

Families have been described where the condition is compatible with dominant inheritance but others are reported where affected individuals have sensorineural deafness and autosomal recessive inheritance. The dominant types (*Box figure 5.2*) are collectively called Romano–Ward syndrome (OMIM 192500) and the recessive types Jervell and Lange–Nielsen syndrome (JLN; OMIM 220400). JLN-affected individuals have profound sensorineural hearing loss and a long QT interval. Half of those untreated die before the age of 15 years.

The underlying problem is a malfunction of one or another of the ion channels that are important for regulating cardiac rhythm. Linkage studies revealed that both Romano–Ward and JLN syndromes are heterogeneous, with different loci implicated in different families. Mutations have been found that implicate the following ion channel genes.

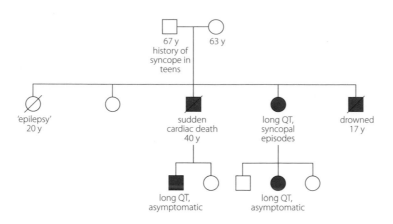

Box figure 5.2 – A typical pedigree of a family in which dominant Long QT syndrome is segregating.

- *KCNQ1* and *KCNE1* – these encode components of the IKs potassium channel. Romano–Ward patients can be heterozygous and JLN patients homozygous for mutations in either gene. Syncope and sudden death are particularly triggered by physical exertion, especially swimming.
- *KCNH2* and *KCNE2* – these encode components of the IKr potassium channel. Heterozygous mutations in either gene have been described in some Romano–Ward patients. Emotional excitement or loud noise (especially noises that wake somebody up) are the commonest triggers of sudden death.
- *SCN5A* – encodes a cardiac sodium channel. Heterozygous mutations have been described in some Romano–Ward patients. Death most commonly occurs during quiet rest or sleep.

In *Chapter 6* we discuss the reason why mutations in *KCNQ1* and *KCNE1* can cause either of these syndromes, with different modes of inheritance. Up to 30% of families do not have a detectable mutation in any of these genes. The genotype–phenotype relationship is further complicated by the fact that an apparently separate condition, Brugada syndrome (OMIM 601144) can be caused by mutations in *SCN5A*. In this condition, ventricular fibrillation and sudden death occur but the ECG abnormalities are different (resembling right bundle branch block with variable ST segment elevation), or they may be absent without provocation.

After a catastrophic event such as sudden death, particularly in a young person, close relatives are usually anxious. Screening and genetic counseling can provide reassurance and help these individuals cope with the risk of sudden death. A detailed family history should be taken, particularly noting a history of syncope or unexplained 'seizures'. First degree relatives should be assessed for evidence of Long QT syndrome. It is highly desirable to identify a causative mutation, so that at-risk relatives can be clearly identified and those not at risk reassured. Treatment for all the Long QT syndrome disorders is directed at avoiding known precipitating factors, reducing the tendency to tachycardia by the use of beta-blocker medication, and, for some, the use of implantable cardioverter defibrillators. Knowledge of the specific mutation may enable anticipatory guidance about avoiding specific precipitating factors. However, because any one of several genes may be involved, molecular diagnosis encounters similar problems to those for families with deafness (see **Case 3, Choudhary family**).

5.6. **Self-assessment questions**

(1) For each of the following sequence changes or effects, choose possible testing methods from the list below that could be used to check for the presence of the change or effect (more than one method may be appropriate in many cases).
   - A point mutation in any of the 26 exons of the *F8* gene
   - Duplication of exons 50–54 of the dystrophin gene in a boy with Duchenne muscular dystrophy
   - Expansion of the $(CAG)_n$ repeat in the *SCA3* gene in a woman suspected of having Machado–Joseph disease
   - Identifying a small additional 'marker' chromosome seen in a dysmorphic baby
   - Insertion of 4 nucleotides in exon 7 of the dystrophin gene in the sister of a boy known to have this mutation
   - Deletion of any of 20 exons of the dystrophin gene in a boy with Duchenne muscular dystrophy
   - An A>G mutation in exon 4 of the *OCRL* gene
   - Deletion of any of 20 exons of the dystrophin gene in the mother of a boy who died of Duchenne muscular dystrophy
   - A 1.5 Mb deletion at 7q11.23 in a child suspected of having Williams–Beuren syndrome
   - Lack of expression in lymphocytes of an apparently intact gene that is normally expressed in these cells
   - Deletion of exons 5–6 of a gene on chromosome 15 in a mentally retarded boy
   - A point mutation anywhere (exons or introns) in the β-globin gene

Possible methods:
   - Karyotyping
   - FISH
   - Array-CGH
   - Southern blotting
   - Northern blotting
   - Multiplex ligation-dependent probe amplification
   - PCR – check for presence / absence of product
   - PCR – size product
   - PCR – sequence product
   - PCR – check for restriction digestion of product
   - Allele-specific PCR
   - Reverse transcriptase–PCR
   - SSCP (single-strand conformation polymorphism)
   - Hybridization to allele-specific oligonucleotide
   - Sanger sequencing
   - Pyrosequencing

(2) For each of the following tests, note whether it uses a property of single-stranded or double-stranded DNA:
- Checking for heteroduplexes by gel mobility
- Dot-blotting with an allele-specific oligonucleotide
- Conformation-sensitive gel electrophoresis
- Checking for creation / abolition of a restriction site
- Allele-specific PCR
- Denaturing high-performance liquid chromatography
- Sequencing using a microarray
- FISH

(3) The restriction enzyme *Eco*RI cuts the sequence GAATTC. Part of the coding sequence of a certain gene reads as follows:

```
CAA   AAC   CTC   AAG   TCA   ACG   AGT   TCG   GTA   ACG   TAC
Gln   Asn   Leu   Lys   Ser   Thr   Ser   Ser   Val   Thr   Tyr
```

This part of the gene is PCR amplified from DNA of a patient with a disease that is often caused by mutations in this gene. It is noted that the PCR product, which in normal people is not cut by *Eco*RI, is now cut into two fragments. Assuming the mutation changes a single nucleotide in the segment shown, identify it.

06 | What do mutations do?

After working through this chapter you should be able to:

- Describe and identify silent, mis-sense, nonsense and frameshift changes in coding sequences and splice site mutations
- Use a table of the genetic code to define the effect on the gene product of a change within a coding sequence
- Explain and give examples of loss of function, gain of function, haplo-insufficiency, dominant negative effects, nonsense-mediated decay and dosage sensitivity
- Discuss how far genotype–phenotype correlations can be established
- List ways in which a change in non-coding DNA may affect expression of a gene

6.1. Case studies

| CASE 15 | O'Reilly family | **145** | 158 | 389 |

- Family history of myopia and hip problems
- Orla has severe myopia, is short, and has hip problems
- ? Stickler syndrome

Orla O'Reilly, who is married to Raymond, has worn glasses for severe myopia since she was a young child. She is also only 4′ 11″ (150 cm) tall. Her brother Oliver is also short and myopic and he was born with a cleft palate. He also wears hearing aids. They take after their father who is short and stocky and has recently needed bilateral hip replacements; when he was 35 years old he underwent surgery for a retinal detachment in one eye, and laser treatment to prevent a detachment in the other eye. Orla went for a medical check for an insurance policy and mentioned that she had been getting some hip pain. The doctor doing the medical had just been on a genetics course and, after taking a family history, thought there might be a connection between Orla's and Oliver's medical problems and those of their father, so he referred her to the genetics clinic. There Orla had a detailed examination including an eye test which, in addition to the myopia, showed she had paravascular lattice retinopathy. The doctor also noted she had a short nose with a flat nasal bridge and rather knobbly joints. He told Orla he suspected she might have a condition called Stickler syndrome. This condition is due to mutations in genes encoding components of either type II or type XI collagen. See Snead and Yates (1999) for a review.

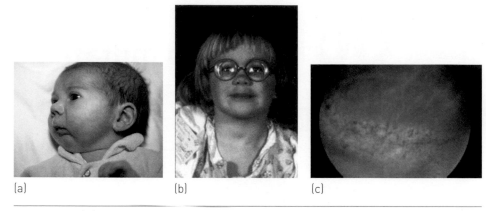

(a)   (b)   (c)

Figure 6.1 – (a) A baby with Stickler syndrome; note the small jaw (often associated with cleft palate) and rather flat face with prominent eyes. (b) Facial features of a 4-year-old child with Stickler syndrome. (c) Typical pigmented paravascular retinal lattice degeneration. (b) and (c) reproduced from Snead and Yates (1999) with permission from the BMJ Publishing Group.

6.2. **Science toolkit**

The word '**mutation**' can be used to describe either the event that produces a DNA sequence variant, or the resulting variant, whether produced then and there, or inherited maybe through many generations. In other words, it can describe the process or its product. Here we are using it to mean the product. Note, incidentally, that in genetic counseling the term 'mutation' is rarely used in discussion with patients, partly to avoid technical jargon but also because it has pejorative connotations (*mutants...*). A mutation may be described as a 'gene change', 'alteration', or 'fault'.

In the last two chapters we have seen some of the methods used to detect DNA sequence variants, and in some cases considered their effects. In this chapter we will look more systematically at the effects of sequence changes. There are two aspects to this:

- on the one hand we need to understand how a sequence change can affect the basic processes of transcription and translation
- on the other hand we want to think in terms of overall gene function – is there a loss of function or a gain of function, and how far does the genotype predict the phenotype?

In this section we will consider transcription and translation. If a protein-coding sequence is to function as proposed in the Central Dogma (*Figure 3.3*), a series of steps is necessary. Any of these steps might be affected by a mutation. *Box 6.1* summarizes the types of change discussed. *Section 6.3* provides a series of examples that lead on to a discussion of molecular pathology in the last section of the chapter, including loss and gain of function and the prospects for genotype–phenotype correlations. *Disease box 6* illustrates a particularly striking example of how loss, modification or gain of function in the same gene can produce a set of very different phenotypes.

Summary of types of mutation considered in this section

In terms of the DNA, mutations can be classified as:

- deletions of a whole gene
- duplications of a whole gene
- disruption of a gene by a chromosomal rearrangement
- deletions or duplications of one or more exons of a gene
- mutations in the promoter or other *cis*-acting regulatory sequence
- mutations that affect splicing by altering an existing splice site
- mutations that affect splicing by activating a cryptic splice site
- mutations that alter the triplet reading frame (frameshifts)
- mutations that introduce a premature stop codon (nonsense mutations)
- mutations that replace one amino acid in the protein with another (mis-sense mutations)
- mutations that alter one codon for an amino acid into another codon for the same amino acid (synonymous substitutions)

Alternatively, mutations can be classified as null or amorphic (no product is made, or there is no function), hypomorphic (too little product, or too little function) and hypermorphic (too much product or excessive function).

Deletion or duplication of a whole gene

These would be expected to decrease or increase the amount of gene product proportionally to the change in gene number, though this may be modified by feedback controls regulating the level of expression according to the need for the gene product. Not all deletions or duplications are pathogenic. It has recently become apparent that there is considerable variation among normal people in the copy number of some genes. Comparative genomic hybridization (*Figure 4.7*) has revealed unexpected large-scale copy number variants that are common and not evidently pathogenic (see *Section 2.4*). Other examples of common non-pathogenic duplications or deletions include the following:

- people vary in the number of tandemly repeated green color vision pigment genes on the X chromosome
- people vary in the number of beta-defensin genes at 8p23
- some major histocompatibility complex haplotypes at 6p21 (see *Chapter 8*) contain different numbers of HLA genes

For most genes, however, copy number changes are abnormal and often pathogenic. A gene is called **dosage-sensitive** if a 50% decrease or increase in copy number (having 1 or 3 copies of a gene that is normally present in 2 copies) causes a phenotypic change. Duplications are much less common than deletions and are less likely to be pathogenic (although chromosomal trisomies must produce their pathogenic effect through increased dosage of genes on the relevant chromosome – see *Section 6.4*).

Disruption of a gene

If a gene is disrupted by a chromosomal rearrangement, the 5′ fragment of the gene retains the promoter and may still be transcribed, but there can be no production of the normal full-length transcript. The Factor VIII inversion that causes half of all cases of severe hemophilia A (see *Figure 4.20*) is an example. Stability of an mRNA is largely mediated by the 3′ untranslated region, and a partial mRNA is unlikely to be stable or to encode any product. Occasionally a chromosomal rearrangement may create a novel chimeric gene by bringing together exons of two different genes. Changes of this sort are important in cancer (see *Chapter 12*) and form a partial exception to the rule that disruptions prevent expression of a gene.

Mutations that affect the transcription of an intact coding sequence

Here we are concerned with *cis*-acting effects – changes in DNA sequences that regulate expression of an immediately adjacent gene. In *Section 3.4* we noted that transcription of a gene can depend both on the promoter immediately upstream of the coding sequence and on more distant *cis*-acting regulatory elements (enhancers). These sequences bind proteins so as to assemble the transcription initiation complex on the promoter. Enhancers influence the process because the DNA loops round to bring them physically close to the promoter. Changes in any of these sequences can directly affect expression of the gene they control. That change in expression may in turn have all sorts of downstream effects on other genes, which may be far away or on other chromosomes (*trans*-acting effects). For example, mutations in genes encoding transcription factors can affect expression of many of their target genes. Similarly, mutating genes whose products control chromatin conformation can cause wide-ranging changes in gene expression (see *Disease box 2*).

Unfortunately it is very difficult to predict the likely effect of a sequence change in non-coding DNA. For this reason, diagnostic laboratories seldom search for such changes. Even if they found a change, they would not usually know how to interpret its significance. Programs are available that identify likely transcription factor binding sites, but these tend to report large numbers of possible binding sites and they do not take account of the protein–protein interactions between the various factors, so they have limited predictive power. A large collaborative project, the ENCODE project (Encyclopedia of DNA Elements, http://genome.ucsc.edu/Encode/), is using a variety of methods to try to identify every regulatory DNA sequence in the human genome. Ultimately this may provide the knowledge necessary to evaluate the effect of any change in the 99% of our DNA that does not code for protein – but that goal is a long way off. Promoter changes can be investigated in the laboratory using a so-called transient transfection assay. A gene whose activity is easily monitored (β-galactosidase is often used) is placed in a vector where its expression is governed by the promoter under investigation. The recombinant vector is introduced into a cell and the level of expression is measured. This can be compared to the level seen when the wild-type promoter is used. Transient transfection assays are valuable research tools, but their results must be viewed with great caution because the experimental system is quite artificial. Such tests are not part of routine diagnostic investigations.

Despite these problems, some regulatory mutations are known, and no doubt many more remain to be discovered because they are undoubtedly under-diagnosed – but for most mendelian diseases, careful studies of coding sequences and splice sites can usually identify the causative mutation in the great majority of cases. Thus regulatory changes may have their main relevance in complex multifactorial disease (*Chapter 13*), where susceptibility may depend on combinations of subtle changes in gene expression, rather than mendelian diseases, which usually have single mutations of large effect.

Mutations that affect splicing of the primary transcript

Abolition or modification of existing splice sites. Any change to the (almost) invariant GT...AG dinucleotides that mark the beginning and end of introns will prevent the affected site from being used. What the cell will do in response to this is hard to predict. The exon involved may be skipped, or sequence from the intron may be retained within the mature mRNA. Often some other nearby site is used as a replacement splice site, with consequent changes to the sequence of the mature mRNA. Other changes close to an exon–intron junction also often affect splicing, but less predictably. As mentioned in *Section 3.2*, GT...AG sequences only function as splice sites when they are embedded in a loosely defined consensus sequence. Additionally, correct functioning of a splice site depends on splicing enhancer or suppressor sequences nearby that bind components of the splicing machinery. Again these are not rigidly defined. They may be located in the intron near a splice site, but they may also lie in the exon. If a change within a coding sequence alters an exonic splicing enhancer, it may be pathogenic for reasons unconnected with any predicted amino acid sequence change. Two examples will illustrate these effects.

- Near the 3′ end of intron 8 of the *CFTR* gene is a run of T nucleotides. In different people there may be 5, 7 or 9 Ts. The 5T variant causes inefficient use of the nearby splice site; exon 9 is often skipped, leading to loss of function. The loss of function is only partial because a proportion of transcripts are correctly spliced. Thus the 5T variant is associated with mild and atypical forms of cystic fibrosis.
- Spinal muscular atrophy (SMA or Werdnig–Hoffmann disease, OMIM 253300) is caused by loss of function of the *SMN1* gene on 5q13. A duplicate copy of the gene (*SMN2*) lies only 500 kb away on the same chromosome, and at first sight should be able to replace the function of the mutated gene. The two genes have only apparently insignificant sequence differences. One of these is a C>T change in exon 7, six nucleotides downstream of the 5′ splice site. The substitution apparently only replaces one phenylalanine codon with another (TTC>TTT). But in fact this change disrupts splicing, probably by inactivating an exonic splicing enhancer, so that exon 7 is skipped in about 90% of transcripts. Thus the *SMN2* gene is largely non-functional. Interestingly, some SMA patients have several copies of this gene. Although each one produces very little protein, together they make enough to render the disease in these patients milder and of later onset.

Creation of novel splice sites. Some sequence changes affect splicing by activation of a **cryptic splice site**. That is, there is a sequence that by chance has many of the features of a splice site, but is sufficiently different for the cell not to mistake it for a real splice site. A change may increase the resemblance to the point where the cell does start using it. The cryptic site can be either in an exon or an intron, as the following examples show.

- In hemoglobin E the β-globin gene has a G>A substitution 14 nucleotides upstream of the 3′ end of exon 1. This would be predicted to cause an amino acid substitution Glu26Lys. However, the pathogenic effect is on splicing. Changing this one nucleotide causes the changed sequence to be used as an alternative splice site. Transcripts that use this site are non-functional, and the effect is β-thalassemia.
- One cause of cystic fibrosis is a single base change c.3849+10kb C>T, 10 kb inside intron 19 of the *CFTR* gene. This activates a cryptic splice site, causing aberrant splicing and loss of function of the gene.

Changing the balance of splice isoforms. Rather than prevent production of any functional transcript, splicing mutations may simply alter the balance between isoforms. Many transcripts are subject to alternative splicing, as illustrated in *Figure 3.11*. The average number of different transcripts per locus found by the ENCODE project is 5.4 (although some of these are due to the use of alternative promoters and first exons, rather than to alternative splicing of a single transcript). If a change in a consensus splice sequence or a splicing enhancer changes the efficiency of a splice site, it may affect the balance of splice isoforms, and this may produce a phenotype. Again, such changes are more likely to act as susceptibility factors for common disease rather than mendelian disease mutations.

In summary, effects on splicing are widespread but, apart from changes to the invariant GT…AG dinucleotides, hard to predict. Undoubtedly they are under-reported because they may only be recognized if mRNA is studied, rather than genomic DNA. Computer programs are available that try to predict the effect of a sequence change on splicing. The best ones, used in combination, are probably right 90% of the time, but they are far from infallible.

Mutations that cause errors in translation

Effects on translation of a sequence change in a protein-coding sequence need to be considered in relation to the genetic code (*Table 6.1*).

Frameshift mutations. Insertion or deletion of any number of nucleotides that is not a multiple of three produces a **frameshift mutation**. The effect is to change completely the reading of all the message downstream of the mutation (see *Box 3.3*). In principle, a completely novel polypeptide might be produced by translation of the frameshifted mRNA. Even if such a protein were produced, it would probably be unstable. Only a very small subset of all the myriad possible polypeptide chains can fold so as to produce a stable protein. Cells detect and degrade those that fail to fold correctly. More commonly, however, no novel polypeptide is produced. It is usually not long before the frameshifted message includes a stop codon. As explained below, mRNAs containing premature termination codons are normally

Table 6.1 – **The genetic code**

1st base in codon	2nd base in codon				3rd base in codon
	U	**C**	**A**	**G**	
U	Phe	Ser	Tyr	Cys	**U**
	Phe	Ser	Tyr	Cys	**C**
	Leu	Ser	STOP	STOP	**A**
	Leu	Ser	STOP	Trp	**G**
C	Leu	Pro	His	Arg	**U**
	Leu	Pro	His	Arg	**C**
	Leu	Pro	Gln	Arg	**A**
	Leu	Pro	Gln	Arg	**G**
A	Ile	Thr	Asn	Ser	**U**
	Ile	Thr	Asn	Ser	**C**
	Ile	Thr	Lys	Arg	**A**
	Met	Thr	Lys	Arg	**G**
G	Val	Ala	Asp	Gly	**U**
	Val	Ala	Asp	Gly	**C**
	Val	Ala	Glu	Gly	**A**
	Val	Ala	Glu	Gly	**G**

Some amino acids such as serine and arginine have multiple codons, whereas tryptophan and methionine have only one each. AUG doubles as the initiator codon and as the codon for internal methionines. Note the three stop codons.

degraded and do not produce protein. Thus one way or another, no protein is produced. *Figure 6.2* shows an example of a common frameshift mutation that produces a premature stop codon.

Whole exon deletions or duplications. When one or more complete exons of a gene are deleted or duplicated, the effect will partly depend on whether or not this produces a frameshift. Whole-exon deletions in the dystrophin gene

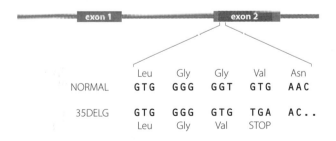

Figure 6.2 – The c.35delG mutation in the connexin 26 (*GJB2*) gene.
This mutation is a frequent cause of autosomal recessive congenital deafness. One G nucleotide out of a run of 6 Gs is deleted. Reading the frameshifted message the ribosome quickly hits a stop codon. The *GJB2* gene has only two exons. Coding sequence is shown in black; the colored parts of exons 1 and 2 encode the 5' and 3' untranslated regions of the mRNA. Diagram is not to scale.

provide a classic example. *Table 6.2* lists the sizes of the exons shown in *Figure 3.9*. Exons 41, 42, 47, 48 and 49 have exact multiples of three nucleotides. Deleting any one of those exons will not cause a frameshift. The other exons have either one nucleotide more than a multiple of three (+1) or one fewer (–1). Deleting any one of these will cause a frameshift. The dystrophin protein is still partly functional if an internal segment is missing or duplicated, but a frameshift will of course completely wreck it. As a result, non-frameshifting deletions or duplications cause a milder disease, Becker muscular dystrophy (BMD, OMIM 300376), while frameshifting deletions or duplications (and other major mutations) cause the severe Duchenne muscular dystrophy (DMD, OMIM 310200) as in Case 4 (Davies family). Because of the frameshift effect, deletions of several exons can have a counter-intuitive effect: combining a lethal mutation with a second lethal mutation can produce a non-lethal mutation. For example, deleting either exon 43 or 44 causes the severe DMD, yet somebody who has both these exons deleted has a frame-neutral deletion and will have the milder BMD.

Table 6.2 – **Sizes of exons of the dystrophin gene**

Exon	Size (bp)	Frame	Disease
41	183	0	BMD
42	195	0	BMD
43	173	–1	DMD
44	148	+1	DMD
45	176	–1	DMD
46	148	+1	DMD
47	150	0	BMD
48	186	0	BMD
49	102	0	BMD
50	109	+1	DMD

Deletions of exons produce the severe Duchenne muscular dystrophy (DMD) or the milder Becker muscular dystrophy (BMD) depending whether or not the deletion produces a frameshift. See text for further explanation.

Nonsense mutations. The three codons UAG, UAA and UGA in mRNA are stop codons (*Table 6.1*). A single nucleotide change that converts any other codon into a stop codon (TAG, TAA or TGA in the DNA) causes the ribosome to detach and protein synthesis to terminate at that point. Such mutations are called **nonsense mutations**. Contrary to common belief, mRNAs containing nonsense mutations do not normally produce truncated proteins. Cells have a very interesting mechanism (**nonsense-mediated decay**) for detecting and degrading mRNAs that contain premature termination codons (*Figure 6.3*). In some cases a certain amount of a

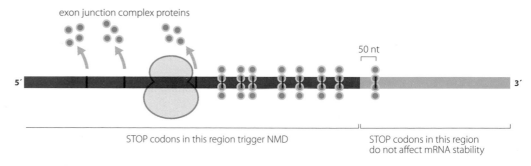

exon junction complex proteins

50 nt

5′   3′

STOP codons in this region trigger NMD

STOP codons in this region
do not affect mRNA stability

Figure 6.3 – Nonsense-mediated decay.
When a spliced mRNA is exported from the nucleus to the cytoplasm certain components of the splicing machinery (the exon junction complex, EJC) remain attached to each splice site. As the first ribosome moves along the mRNA it displaces each EJC until it reaches the stop codon and detaches. If this happens in the red segment of the mRNA, one or more EJCs will remain in place. This triggers degradation of the mRNA. Thus mRNA molecules are only stable if the first stop codon lies within the green segment. Equally, nonsense mutations in the red segment are detected and no truncated protein is produced, but any mutation in the green zone is able to direct production of a truncated protein that may be pathogenic.

truncated protein may be produced, but the usual effect of a nonsense mutation is the same as a complete deletion of the gene.

Nonsense-mediated decay probably evolved to protect cells against possibly toxic dominant negative effects of truncated proteins (see below). It presumably also explains why the last exon of many genes is very large – you can't split the 3′ untranslated region between several exons. Some rather mystifying differences between the effects of nonsense mutations in different parts of the same gene are the result of nonsense-mediated decay operating in the red zone (*Figure 6.3*) but not in the green zone (see OMIM 602229 for an example). For further details see the review by Holbrook *et al.* (2004).

Mutations that cause amino acid substitutions

A single nucleotide change within a coding sequence will change one codon into another. Assuming the changed codon is not a stop codon, there are two possible results.

- *Synonymous substitutions* are single nucleotide changes that replace a codon with a different one that encodes the same amino acid – for example, a T>G change in the DNA that converts a UUU codon in the mRNA to UUC. Both code for phenylalanine.
- *Mis-sense mutations* replace one amino acid with another by changing a codon. Use *Table 6.1* to identify the effect of a codon change on the amino acid sequence.

It is important to remember, as mentioned above, that seemingly innocuous synonymous or mis-sense changes may have a major pathogenic effect by disrupting splicing.

Table 6.3 in *Section 6.4* gives a general guide to the likely effect of the various types of mutation.

6.3. Investigations of patients

Here we consider the molecular pathology of the mutations that have already been identified, as well as the investigation of Case 15 (O'Reilly family).

| CASE 1 | Ashton family | 1 | 7 | 65 | 106 | **154** | 389 |

- John – 28-year-old son of Alfred Ashton
- ? Huntington disease
- Other family members with similar symptoms
- Autosomal dominant inheritance shown in pedigree
- Diagnostic test ordered

The trinucleotide repeat expansion was described in *Chapter 4*. Formally this is an insertion in the coding sequence of the *HTT* gene. The mutant gene is transcribed and translated. The expansion adds CAG triplets, thus it does not disrupt the reading frame. The protein product is the normal 3142 amino acid huntingtin protein with an expanded run of glutamines near the N-terminal end (CAG is a codon for glutamine). Affected people are normally heterozygotes, but rare homozygotes have been described and they are usually clinically indistinguishable from heterozygotes. This suggests that it is the presence of the mutant protein, rather than the absence of the normal protein, that is causing the problems. No Huntington disease patients have been described who have deletions, nonsense mutations or other changes in the gene. Additionally at least one person has been described who does not have Huntington disease despite having a chromosomal rearrangement that disrupts one copy of the Huntington disease gene. Together, these observations make it clear that Huntington disease must be caused by a gain of function. The mutant protein is somehow toxic to neurons, especially in the striatum and caudate nucleus of the brain. Gradual cell death leads to the late-onset disease. Exactly why the mutant protein is toxic is controversial. It forms aggregates inside neurons but it is not clear that the aggregates are themselves harmful. More probably an intermediate in the aggregation process is toxic. The normal protein interacts with many other proteins – it probably functions as some sort of scaffold for assembling multiprotein complexes – making it very difficult to identify one key altered function.

| CASE 2 | Brown family | 2 | 8 | 66 | 132 | **154** | 281 | 389 |

- Girl (Joanne) aged 6 months, parents David and Pauline
- ? Cystic fibrosis
- Order molecular test?
- Define mutations in *CFTR* gene

Cystic fibrosis is a recessive disease caused by complete loss of function of the chloride channel encoded by the *CFTR* gene. Being affected, Joanne must have no functional copy of the gene (what matters is having no functional copy, rather than having two mutant copies, although of course normally these amount to the same thing). DNA testing (*Chapter 5*) revealed three sequence changes: c.368G>A in exon 3, p.F508del in exon 10 and c.2752–15C>G in the exon 14b PCR product. Of these, p.F508del is very well understood, being by far the commonest mutation in Europeans with cystic fibrosis (see *Table 11.1*). The mutation is an in-frame deletion of three consecutive nucleotides in the coding sequence. A virtually full-length protein is produced with 1479/1480 correct amino acids – but the one missing amino acid affects the structure. The mutant protein is not correctly processed after synthesis, and fails to locate to the apical cell membrane where it is needed. The result is a complete loss of function (see *Table 6.4*). Joanne's other two mutations were not common and required further analysis. The exon 14b change was thought to be non-pathogenic for two reasons.

(1) The C>G change was in intron 14a, 15 nucleotides before the start of exon 14b. Intronic changes can sometimes be pathogenic by affecting splicing. This mutation did not have any features suggesting it might do so, but without RNA studies an effect on splicing could not be ruled out. However, in this case there was a second line of evidence.

(2) When DNA from Joanne's parents David and Pauline was checked, both the p.F508del and c.2752-15C>G mutations came from David. They must both be in the same gene copy. Even if the c.2752-15C>G mutation was pathogenic, it would not explain Joanne's disease, because the gene she inherited from Pauline must also be mutated.

Joanne's other mutation, c.368G>A did come from her mother. The nucleotide change is within exon 3 and converts the codon for tryptophan 79 (TGG) into a stop codon (TAG). This is an unambiguously pathogenic change. Because of nonsense-mediated mRNA decay (see above) it is unlikely that the mutant gene would produce any protein, and any that it did produce would certainly be non-functional since the stop codon occurs very early in the sequence. Additionally, a search of the *CFTR* mutation database at www.genet.sickkids.on.ca/cftr/ showed that it had previously been identified in other CF patients.

| CASE 4 | Davies family | 4 | 10 | 67 | 104 | **155** | 186 | 281 | 389 |

- Boy (Martin) aged 24 months
- Family history of muscular dystrophy
- Pedigree shows X-linked recessive inheritance
- Order diagnostic DNA test
- Frameshift mutation in the dystrophin gene

Martin has a deletion of exons 44–48 of the dystrophin gene (*Chapter 4*). The long dystrophin molecule functions within the muscle cell a bit like a rope with hooks at each end (*Figure 6.4*). The body of the rope consists of repeated units, the precise number of which is not critical to dystrophin function. If Martin simply made slightly smaller than normal dystrophin molecules, he would have a relatively good prognosis. But adding up the exon lengths in *Table 6.2*, we can see that his deletion produces a frameshift. Any protein produced would have a completely wrong amino acid sequence downstream of the frameshift – but in fact a ribosome reading the message in this novel reading frame would soon encounter a stop codon. As before, nonsense-mediated decay means that Martin's gene would produce no protein product, rather than a truncated protein. Studying a muscle biopsy with labeled dystrophin antibody would confirm the absence of dystrophin protein (see *Figure 1.4*). In Martin's case this adds no useful new information, but in boys where the PCR or MLPA deletion screen identifies no mutation it is a valuable diagnostic test. Searching all through the huge dystrophin gene (79 exons, 11 kb of coding sequence, 2.4 Mb of genomic DNA) for a point mutation can be impossibly laborious, and a muscle biopsy provides a much easier confirmation of the diagnosis.

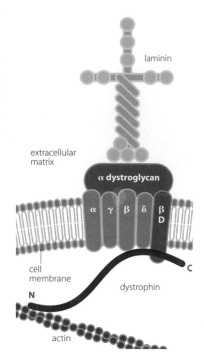

laminin

extracellular
matrix

α dystroglycan

cell
membrane

N

C

dystrophin

actin

Figure 6.4 – The dystrophin molecule anchors the cytoskeleton of muscle cells to the extracellular matrix, via the dystrophin glycoprotein complex.
This includes the α, β, γ and δ sarcoglycans (mutations in which cause limb-girdle muscular dystrophies) and the α and β (labeled βD) dystroglycans. Muscle cells that lack dystrophin are mechanically fragile, and fail after a few years, hence the progressive muscle weakness.

| CASE 6 | Fletcher family | 5 | 12 | 67 | 137 | **156** | 389 |

- Frank, aged 22, with increasingly blurred eyesight
- Family history of visual difficulties
- Pedigree suggests X-linked recessive inheritance but not conclusive
- ? LHON
- Order blood test to check for mutation in mtDNA
- Check mutations by Pyrosequencing
- G3460A mutation in mtDNA

The causative mutation was identified as G3460A in his mitochondrial DNA (*Chapter 5*). Most mitochondrial proteins are encoded by nuclear genes, synthesized on cytoplasmic ribosomes and then imported into the mitochondria, but the 13 protein-coding genes in mitochondrial DNA are transcribed and translated within the mitochondrion in a way closely similar to the way nuclear genes are expressed. They encode components of the electron transport chain of oxidative phosphorylation (*Figure 3.10b*).

Mitochondrial mutations can be classified in the same way as nuclear mutations (*Box 6.1*). Large deletions and duplications are relatively more common, and splicing mutations are absent because mitochondrial genes do not have introns. Heteroplasmy introduces an extra layer of variability between genotype and phenotype. The three common LHON mutations are all mis-sense mutations affecting three different proteins in the electron transport system: p.Ala52Tyr in the ND1 protein, p.Arg340His in ND4 and p.Met64Val in ND6. Frank's mutation is the first of these.

| CASE 11 | Kavanagh family | 81 | 97 | **156** | 389 |

- Healthy first baby boy
- Second child, Celia, pale with low hemoglobin levels
- Sickle cell disease
- Single nucleotide mutation, Glu→Val

The single nucleotide change in the coding sequence of the β-globin gene changes the codon for amino acid 6 from a codon for glutamic acid into one for valine (*Figure 6.5*). The effect of this change has been studied in great detail. Glutamic acid is, chemically, a polar amino acid. The carboxy (–COOH) group in its side chain is acidic. It readily loses a proton forming a –COO⁻ anion. When a soluble protein

	Val	His	Leu	Thr	Pro	Glu	Glu	Lys	Ser
NORMAL	GTG	CAT	CTG	ACT	CCT	GAG	GAG	AAG	TCT
SICKLE	GTG	CAT	CTG	ACT	CCT	GTG	GAG	AAG	TCT
	Val	His	Leu	Thr	Pro	Val	Glu	Lys	Ser

Figure 6.5 – Sickle cell disease nucleotide change.
In sickle cell disease an A>T nucleotide substitution causes glutamic acid to be replaced by valine at position 6 of the β-globin protein.

chain folds, such charged groups tend to be located on the outside of the molecule, in contact with the aqueous environment. Valine is non-polar and naturally associates with other non-polar amino acids in the interior of the folded protein, away from water. Having a valine on the outer surface makes the mutant β-globin molecules tend to stick together. The resulting protein aggregates distort the red cells into a sickle shape, cause clumping and subsequent vascular ischemia. Thus the sickle cell change might be considered a gain of function mutation, because the mutant protein does something positively harmful. However, gain of function mutations would normally be expected to be pathogenic in heterozygotes, and people with sickling trait are healthy.

CASE 14	Nicolaides family	117	135	**157**	389

- ? β-thalassemia carriers
- p.Gln39X nonsense mutation for Spiros
- c.316–106C>G mutation for Elena

Spiros has the p.Gln39X mutation. This is a classic nonsense mutation. A single nucleotide substitution converts a codon for glutamine (CAG) into a stop codon (TAG) (*Figure 6.6*). The mutated gene produces no product, causing a β⁰ thalassemia in homozygotes.

INTRON 1	Leu	Leu	Val	Val	Tyr	Pro	Trp	Thr	Gln	Arg	Phe	Phe	Glu
ccacccttagGCTG		CTG	GTG	GTC	TAC	CCT	TGG	ACC	CAG	AGG	TTC	TTT	GAG
ccacccttagGCTG		CTG	GTG	GTC	TAC	CCT	TGG	ACC	TAG	AGG	TTC	TTT	GAG
INTRON 1	Leu	Leu	Val	Val	Pro	Pro	Trp	Thr	STOP				

Figure 6.6 – The p.Gln39X mutation in the β-globin gene.
This mutation near the start of exon 2 converts a glutamine codon into a stop codon. Lower case letters represent intron, upper case exon.

Elena's mutation (*Figure 6.7*) is more subtle. The change, c.316–106C>G, is a single nucleotide change deep within intron 2 of the β-globin gene, 106 nucleotides upstream of the start of exon 3. It is an example of the sort of mutation that could only be characterized by studying mRNA. This apparently innocuous change activates a cryptic splice site that is then preferentially used compared to the normal donor splice site. The result is a β⁺ thalassemia – that is, the mutant gene produces some correct β-chains, using the normal splice site, but not a sufficient quantity.

Table 5.3 listed three other β-globin mutations that are common causes of thalassemia in Greek Cypriots. Interestingly, all three affect splicing.

- The commonest mutation, c.93–21G>A, again activates a cryptic splice site in an intron, intron 1 this time. Studies of the mRNA showed that

NORMAL INTRON 2	ctaatagcagctacaatccagctaccattctgct
MUTANT- part handled as exon, with new donor splice site	CTAATAGCAGCTACAATCCAGgtaccattctgct

Figure 6.7 – The c.316–106C>G mutation in β-globin.
This mutation activates a cryptic splice site deep within intron 2 of the β-globin gene. Lower case letters represent intron, upper case are the abnormal exon.

80% of the time the new splice site is used, so this allele produces only 20% of the normal quantity of β-globin. For many genes a 20% level of function would be sufficient, but β-globin is required in large amounts, so the result is a β$^+$ thalassemia.

- The second mutation, c.92+6T>C, is an example of a mutation that reduces the efficiency of a normal splice site. The changed nucleotide is in intron 1, six nucleotides from the start of the intron (GGCAGgttgg**t**atcaa.., where exon sequence is in upper case letters and the nucleotide that is mutated is underlined). The T nucleotide is not part of the invariant GT found at the 5′ end of every intron, but forms part of the context that is necessary for the splice site to be recognized efficiently. Again the result is a β$^+$ thalassemia.

- The third common Greek Cypriot mutation is c.92+1G>A. This directly changes the obligatory GT at the exon 1–intron 1 splice site to AT. No transcripts can be correctly spliced, so this mutation produces β^0 thalassemia.

CASE 15	O'Reilly family	145	**158**	389

- Family history of myopia and hip problems
- Orla has severe myopia, is short, and has hip problems
- ? Stickler syndrome
- Frameshift mutation in *COL2A1*

Orla's combination of high myopia and joint problems, inherited in autosomal dominant manner, is characteristic of people who have a mutation in Type II collagen (or occasionally Type XI collagen). As described in *Box 3.4*, there are at least 27 different human collagens, encoded by at least 30 genes. To recapitulate, each collagen gene encodes a polypeptide, preprocollagen, which is subject to extensive post-translational modification. The final processed collagen molecule contains tightly wound triple helices of polypeptide chains. Some are homotrimers, some are heterotrimers.

Collagen II is a homotrimer of polypeptides encoded by the *COL2A1* gene on chromosome 12q13. It forms fibrils that are major structural proteins of cartilage, and are also important in the vitreous humor of the eye and in the inner ear. *COL2A1* mutations cause autosomal dominant phenotypes of variable severity depending on how they interfere with collagen biogenesis. They are one cause of chondrodysplasias – a group of some 150 clinically defined phenotypes with defects of cartilage that often lead to defects of modeling of long bones. The *COL2A1* chondrodysplasias form a spectrum from achondrogenesis type II, an intrauterine or perinatal lethal condition, through hypochondrogenesis, spondyloepiphyseal dysplasia (SED) and Kniest dysplasia, to Stickler syndrome, a relatively mild condition that is often diagnosed late. Interestingly, the mutations with the most drastic effect on protein synthesis are not the ones that produce the most severe phenotypes.

- The most severe phenotypes are caused by mis-sense mutations that replace glycines in the Gly–X–Y units of the triple helical region (see *Box 3.4*). Only glycine, the smallest amino acid, can fit into the interior of the tight-packed triple helix, so replacements prevent proper assembly of the fibril. The triple helix assembles from the C-terminal end and, in general, substitutions near that end have a more severe effect than those in more N-terminal positions.
- Whole exon deletions and exon skipping due to splicing mutations are also associated with relatively severe phenotypes. Collagen genes are unusual in that all the exons encoding the triple helical region of the processed protein are frame-neutral. The *COL2A1* gene encodes a 1418-amino acid preprocollagen. It has 53 exons, of which exons 8–49 encode the triple helical region. These exons are mostly 54 or 108 bp, with a few of 45 or 99 bp. Thus deleting or skipping exons in this region does not cause a frameshift or nonsense-mediated decay; the mutant protein is just a little shorter. However, when heterozygous people try to combine chains of different lengths into the triple helix, this disrupts the structure. Mutations located in exons 12–24, towards the N-terminus, tend to cause Kniest dysplasia which, whilst not lethal, is associated with severe short stature, retinal detachment, deafness and disabling joint abnormalities.
- Nonsense mutations and frameshifts cause the mildest phenotype, Stickler syndrome. Because of nonsense-mediated decay there are no abnormal chains to interfere with assembly of the normal chains in a heterozygous person, but there is a quantitative deficiency of collagen II. The phenotype can be variable, with short, normal or tall stature.

This series shows that it is better (in a heterozygote) to make no protein than one that can interfere with the function of its normal counterpart. Mutations are called **dominant negative** if the mutant product prevents the normal product from functioning (*Figure 6.8*). If molecules are selected at random from a 50:50 mix of normal and abnormal polypeptide chains for incorporation into triple helices, only one triple helix in eight would consist of three normal chains, compared to a 50% level of normal triple helices in a heterozygote for a null mutation.

Orla's mutation might be anywhere within exons 8–49 that encode the triple helical domain of Type II collagen. Changes outside this region are not associated with her phenotype. Because of the large number of exons in this and other collagen genes, mutation screening is laborious and is available only in specialized laboratories. In Orla's case, sequencing of PCR-amplified exon 40 revealed a single nucleotide deletion. This would cause a frameshift, leading to a premature termination codon and nonsense-mediated decay of the mRNA. She will therefore produce no abnormal COL2A1 product, but a half quantity of the normal product, consistent with her phenotype.

Figure 6.8 – A dominant negative effect.
The mutant allele produces an abnormal protein that disrupts the construction of a multiprotein complex. In heterozygotes dominant negative alleles produce more severe phenotypes than null alleles.

6.4. **Going deeper ...**

A central ambition of clinical molecular genetics is to be able to predict the phenotypic effect of any DNA sequence change. This goal, of establishing genotype–phenotype correlations, can be divided into two tasks:

- deciding how a mutation affects the function of a gene – does it cause loss of function (partial or total), gain of function, or does it have no effect?
- deciding how loss or gain of function of a gene will affect the phenotype.

Loss of function and gain of function changes

A first question to ask concerning the effect of a mutation is, does it cause a loss of function or a gain of function? To put it differently, does the mutated gene product simply fail to do its normal job (partially or totally), or does it do something positively harmful? *Table 6.3* summarizes the likely effects of different types of mutation.

Many of the changes in *Table 6.3* are likely to abolish the gene function. Some mis-sense mutations and in-frame deletions or duplications will reduce but not abolish the function of the gene product, like the exon deletions in the dystrophin gene that produce Becker muscular dystrophy (*Table 6.2*). It is difficult to predict what effect a mis-sense mutation would have on a protein. Many amino acid substitutions affect the stability of the three-dimensional structure of the protein, rather than altering an active site or other directly functional part of the protein. Proteins are often cleaved, glycosylated, phosphorylated or otherwise modified after synthesis of the basic polypeptide chain. Any mis-sense mutation that replaces amino acids required for any of these modification steps will probably cause a loss of function. But as *Table 6.4* shows, mis-sense mutations can have a range of other effects.

Gains of function are less common. Generally we are not talking about a gain of a completely novel function, but of the product functioning when it should not. It may become insensitive to signals that should shut it off, or be expressed at too high a level. A cell surface receptor may become constitutionally active, transmitting a signal to the cell interior even when no ligand is present. Huntington disease is an example of a mutant protein having a toxic gain of function (see above). Gain of function mechanisms require the mutant allele to produce an abnormal protein (or sometimes a toxic mRNA). Gain of function is therefore seen with mis-sense or regulatory mutations, not nonsense or frameshift mutations.

Changes that create chimeric genes are a special class of gain of function mutation. As mentioned earlier, chromosomal rearrangements sometimes create a novel gene by juxtaposing exons of genes that are normally far apart in the genome. Such chimeric genes may gain novel functions. This type of exon shuffling has probably been important in evolution – many proteins can be seen to be made of varying combinations of a limited repertoire of functional domains, each encoded by separate exons (see *Figure 3.12*). Because chromosomal translocations cause major problems in meiosis (*Chapter 2*), such rearrangements are rarely the cause of inherited disease. However, cancers develop entirely by mitosis from mutant

Table 6.3 – **Common types of mutation and their likely effects**

Type of mutation	Likely effect on a gene
Large deletion or inversion	Most likely to completely abolish function
Duplication of whole gene	Will increase the amount of product by 50% (from 2 to 3 gene copies); this will generally have no phenotypic effect, unless the precise level of the gene product is critical (dosage-sensitive gene); see for example Aitman *et al.* (2006)
Change in promoter or regulatory sequence	May reduce or increase the level of transcription, or alter the response to control signals; any protein produced has the normal structure and function
Change in intron	Most likely to have no effect – but can sometimes affect splicing
Change in 5' or 3' untranslated region of mRNA	Most likely to have no effect – but can sometimes affect the stability or translation efficiency of the mRNA
Splicing mutation	Mutation of the canonical GT…AG splice sites is likely to abolish function of that allele. Other mutations may have more subtle effects, causing a proportion of transcripts to be incorrectly spliced or changing the pattern of alternative splicing. This can produce a partial loss of function. A change deep within an intron may activate a cryptic splice site
Frameshift mutation	Likely to abolish function of that allele. The polypeptide downstream of the frameshift bears no resemblance to the correct sequence. Usually a stop codon will be encountered quite soon as the ribosomes read the frameshifted codons. The effect will then be the same as a nonsense mutation
Nonsense mutation	Likely to abolish function of that allele. Most mRNAs containing premature termination codons are not translated to produce a truncated protein. Instead, they are degraded and not used at all (nonsense-mediated mRNA decay)
Mis-sense mutation	Effect very variable, depending on the nature and function of the amino acids concerned. Could be loss or gain of function, or no effect. Replacing an amino acid by a chemically very similar one is likely to have less effect than a more radical change. Some amino acids in a protein are essential to its structure or function, others are not. Apparent mis-sense mutations may actually be pathogenic because of an effect on splicing
Synonymous substitution	Most likely to have no effect – but can sometimes affect splicing

somatic cells, and so there is no obstacle to the propagation of chromosomal rearrangements. See *Chapter 12* for a much fuller discussion.

Dominant or recessive?

Dominance and recessiveness are properties of characters or phenotypes, not of genes. We should not really talk of 'dominant genes' and so on, though it is sometimes hard to avoid doing so. A character is dominant if it is seen in a heterozygote, and recessive if not.

Table 6.4 – **Mutations in the *CFTR* chloride channel gene reduce or abolish function of the gene product in different ways. A loss of function in both copies of the gene leads to cystic fibrosis.**

Class of mutation	Effect	Type of mutation	Example
I	No synthesis Reduced synthesis	Nonsense, frameshift or splicing Mutations that affect the efficiency of correct splicing	p.Gly542X c.3849+10kb C>T
II	Block in protein processing	Mis-sense or in-frame deletions	p.F508del
III	Chloride channel not correctly regulated	Mis-sense	p.Gly551Asp
IV	Altered conductance of chloride channel	Mis-sense	p.Arg117His

- Gain of function mutations are expected to produce dominant characters. The gain of function is present in a heterozygote, regardless of the presence of the normal allele.

- Loss of function mutations can produce either dominant or recessive characters, depending how sensitive the organism is to a partial loss of that particular function (*Figure 6.9*). For most genes the threshold for pathology is below 50% and loss of function mutations cause recessive phenotypes. Sometimes there is **haplo-insufficiency**, meaning that 50% of the normal function is not sufficient. In that case, a mutation causing complete loss of function will produce a dominant phenotype, because the normal allele in a heterozygote cannot provide sufficient function on its own.

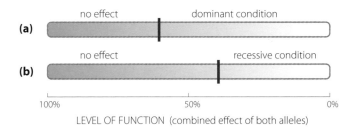

Figure 6.9 – **Whether a loss of function mutation causes a dominant or a recessive condition depends on how sensitive the organism is to loss of that function.** If the threshold for normal function is as shown in (a) a heterozygote with 50% function will be affected, and the condition will be dominant. This situation is called haplo-insufficiency. If the threshold is as in (b) the condition will be recessive.

- Dominant negative mutations are a special class of loss of function mutations, where the abnormal product interferes with the function of the normal product (see *Figure 6.8*). The Long QT syndromes (*Disease box 5*) are an example. Simple loss of function mutations in the ion channel genes produce the recessive Romano–Ward syndrome: a 50% level of the protein is adequate for normal function. The dominant JLN syndrome is the result of dominant negative mutations in the same genes. A single mutant allele produces more than 50% loss of function. Because dominant negative effects are so damaging, full-length but abnormal proteins are particularly dangerous to the organism. This probably provides the force that drove evolution of the nonsense-mediated decay mechanism.

Understanding the phenotype

There is often a wide gulf between the biochemical action of a gene product within a cell and the clinical result of mutations in the gene. Many of the cases discussed through this book illustrate this. Even when we know both the biochemistry and the phenotype it is often difficult to explain how the one leads to the other. Why, as one example among many, should lack of the FMR1 RNA-binding protein cause mental retardation, macro-orchidism and a long face in men with Fragile-X syndrome?

It is important to avoid thinking naively about 'the gene for...'. You would hopefully not describe your domestic freezer as a machine for ruining your stocks of frozen food. That is what happens when things go wrong. Similarly we don't have genes 'for' cystic fibrosis or muscular dystrophy. Many human genes were discovered through studies of the diseases that result when they go wrong, so there is a natural tendency to attach the disease name to the gene. It can be hard to avoid talking about 'the Huntington disease gene', etc. – but it is important not to be drawn into thinking that the disease defines the function of the gene.

Genotype–phenotype correlations

Accurately establishing predictive correlations between mutations and phenotypes is the Holy Grail of molecular pathology – highly desirable but seldom achieved. For the most part the chain of events between a DNA sequence change and a patient's problems is just too long to allow neat correlations. Genes do not act in a vacuum. All the other direct interactors with the gene and its product, the general biochemical milieu, the patient's history and lifestyle, and simple chance events – all conspire to prevent simple predictions of phenotypes. The mendelian diseases that have been the main topic of this book so far are simply the small subset of all diseases where the effect of a single genetic change happens not to be completely submerged by other genetic or environmental effects. Even mendelian diseases are seldom simple when investigated carefully. An excellent article by Scriver and Waters (1999) dissects the reasons why close correlations do not exist in one typical mendelian disease, phenylketonuria – see *Chapter 8* for further discussion.

In the light of this, diseases where a good genotype–phenotype correlation does exist appear as the interesting exceptions to the general rule.

- One such class is exemplified by the hemoglobinopathies. Sickle cell disease and thalassemia are defined in terms of the globin gene product, rather than by distant downstream effects of the mutations. Thus sickle cell disease is quite specifically the result of a p.Glu6Val mutation in β-globin, and other mutations lead predictably to β^0- or β^+-thalassemia.

- Gain of function mutations may produce highly specific effects that are not easily over-ridden by other genetic or environmental factors. The $(CAG)_n$ expansion in the Huntington disease gene always produces Huntington disease, and there is even a statistical (though not individually very predictive) correlation between repeat size and age of onset. Perhaps the most striking example of tight genotype–phenotype correlations in clinical genetics is seen with gain of function mutations in the fibroblast growth factor receptor genes (*Box 6.2*).

The concept of **syndrome families** has proved a productive way of exploring the relationship between genotypes and phenotypes. Before it was known which genes were involved in specific diseases, clinicians classified diseases by clinical signs and by the investigations that were then available. The clinicians themselves could be classified as 'splitters' or 'lumpers'. Splitters concentrated on the differences between conditions and divided them into sub-types, arguing that the underlying mechanisms might be different for the different sub-types. Lumpers concentrated on the similarities and classified conditions with similar clinical signs all together, arguing that there would be a single underlying mechanism. The latter approach was adopted in the 1980s by the German pediatrician J. Spranger for groups of skeletal dysplasias. He lumped many separately named syndromes together into a set of syndrome families based on the patterns of radiological and clinical findings and not on their severity. For example, he classified hypochrondroplasia (where affected individuals are short but otherwise healthy) and achondroplasia (where affected individuals are dwarfed and can have serious joint problems but normal intelligence) together with thanatophoric dysplasia which is lethal at birth because of severe shortening of bones and ribs. Other syndrome families he identified were the Stickler–Kniest family (characterized by varying degrees of shortening of limb bones, cleft palate and severe myopia) and the Oto-palato-digital and Larsen family (with joint deformities and dislocations and cleft palate). Now we know the molecular bases for these conditions, Spranger's approach is seen to have been insightful. The Stickler–Kniest family are all the result of *COL2A1* mutations (see Case 15, O'Reilly family), while achondroplasia and related disorders are all due to mutations in *FGFR3* (see *Box 6.2*).

Studies of normal development and exploration of genotype–phenotype correlations in developmental syndromes have been mutually beneficial. The cross-fertilization happens in two main ways.

- It often happens that mutations in one gene are found in most but not all patients with a particular developmental syndrome. Where there is already some knowledge of the pathway involved, it is logical to seek the missing mutations in other genes involved in the pathway. Often it turns out that the phenotypic spectrum of patients with these new mutations is somewhat different from the original cases, and this leads to clearer genotype-phenotype correlations. The overlapping clinical syndromes caused by mutations in various genes in the RAS–MAPK pathway (see *Disease box 8*) are a prime example. Other examples are shown in *Disease boxes 2* (Rubinstein–Taybi syndrome) and *7* (Rett syndrome).

Genotype–phenotype correlation in mutations of the *FGFR* genes

The nine fibroblast growth factors (FGFs) control the growth and differentiation of various mesenchymal and neuro-ectodermal cells. They act through four cell surface receptors. Each receptor consists of an extracellular portion with three immunoglobulin-like domains, a transmembrane segment, and an internal portion with two tyrosine kinase domains and a C-terminal transactivation region (see *Box figure 6.1*). On activation by the ligand, receptors dimerize. This triggers conformational changes that activate the intracellular tyrosine kinase. This in turn leads to activation of Stat1 signaling molecules and ultimately to cell cycle arrest.

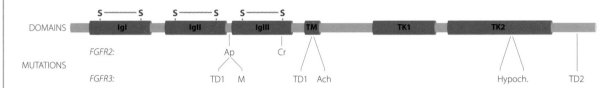

Box figure 6.1 – **Structure of a fibroblast growth factor receptor and position of major mutations.**
TM, transmembrane domain, TK, tyrosine kinase domain; Ap, Apert syndrome; Cr, Crouzon syndrome; TD, thanatophoric dysplasia; M, Muenke craniosynostosis; Ach, achondroplasia; Hypoch, hypochrondroplasia.

The four *FGFR* genes each encode at least 12 alternative splice isoforms. Receptors can heterodimerize as well as homodimerize, and they have different affinities for the nine FGFs. As a result they can mediate a large variety of subtly tuned responses to different combinations of FGFs in different cell types. Mutations cause a gain of function. The mutant receptor becomes constitutively active and transmits its signal, to a greater or lesser extent, even in the absence of ligand. The FGFR mutations show quite remarkably specific genotype–phenotype correlations (see *Box table 6.1*). Nearly all the mutations are in the *FGFR2* and *FGFR3* genes. They produce specific syndromes with craniosynostosis or skeletal dysplasias. Mutations occur particularly in the short linker between the second and third immunoglobulin domains, where they may affect the flexibility of the molecule and hence its dimerization potential, or in the transmembrane domain. Each immunoglobulin domain is held together by an S–S bridge. Other common mis-sense mutations either remove one of the cysteines or create another, and it is likely that these too make the molecules more likely to dimerize even in the absence of ligand.

Box table 6.1 – **Phenotypes and major mutations in the *FGFR2* and *FGFR3* genes**

Gene	Disease (OMIM number)	Mutations
FGFR2	Apert syndrome (101200)	p.Ser252Trp (65%), p.Pro253Arg (34%)
	Crouzon syndrome (123500)	p.Cys342Tyr or Arg (50%)
	Beare–Stevenson cutis gyrata (123790)	p.Ser372Cys (25%), p.Tyr375Cys (75%)
FGFR3	Achondroplasia (100800)	p.Gly380Arg (97%)
	Hypochondroplasia (146000)	p.Asn540Lys (50%), p.Asn540Thr, p.Ile538Val
	Thanatophoric dysplasia I (187600)	p.Arg248Cys (60%), p.Tyr373Cys (25%)
	Thanatophoric dysplasia II (187600)	p.Lys650Glu (100%)
	Muenke syndrome (see 134934.0014)	p.Pro250Arg (100%)

- Sometimes when the gene underlying a syndrome is identified through purely genetic means (mapping then cloning it without any prior knowledge of the gene product), the identification points to a hitherto unknown pathway. An example among many would be identification of the defect underlying Fragile-X syndrome (see Case 12, Lipton family). Studies of the DNA identified a novel mutational mechanism, and studies of the protein function highlighted new aspects of mRNA transport.

For further discussion and examples see Donnai and Read (2003) and Brunner and van Driel (2004).

By way of summary, *Table 6.5* lists the extent of genotype–phenotype correlations for the clinical cases considered so far in this book.

Predicting the phenotype: the problem of novel mis-sense changes

Diagnostic laboratories routinely check many kilobases of a candidate gene in patients with a disease, in the hope of finding a causative mutation. Nonsense or frameshifting changes are convincingly pathogenic – but if a mis-sense change is found, there is a problem of interpretation. Is this the cause of the patient's disease, or is it a harmless variant? To resolve the problem, various lines of evidence are considered.

- Has the change previously been reported as a cause of the disease? And if so, is there a reason to believe the report?
- Is the change found in unaffected people? If it is not present in a few hundred randomly selected unaffected people from the same ethnic background as the case, then at least it is not a common polymorphic variant, but it still might be a previously undescribed rare neutral variant.
- If the patient is from a large family with several affected members, is the change found in all the affected people? If not, then it is unlikely to be pathogenic. However, even if it is found in all the affected people in the family, it may be that the real mutation has not been found, and this is just an irrelevant rare variant that is in the same gene. The c.2752–15C>G change in Joanne Brown (Case 2) would be an example if the true mutation in the same gene had not already been discovered.
- Does the amino acid that is replaced have a vital role in the function or structure of the protein? There is rarely enough detailed knowledge of the protein to allow a certain answer. Computer programs such as POLYPHEN or SIFT try to answer this question. If all related proteins in humans and other animals have the same amino acid at this position (evolutionarily conserved residue), this would be evidence (but not proof) of a vital role.

After all these lines of inquiry have been exhausted, all too often the laboratory has to label the change as a 'variant of unknown significance'. This is of course deeply unsatisfactory for everybody concerned.

Table 6.5 – Genotype–phenotype correlations in the clinical cases discussed so far

Case	Condition	Extent of genotype-phenotype correlation
1	Huntington disease	All cases have >36 CAG repeats in the Huntington disease gene. The repeat size correlates statistically with the age of onset. Large repeats reproducibly cause juvenile-onset Huntington disease which has a rather different phenotype
2	Cystic fibrosis	Little correlation with severity in patients with classical cystic fibrosis, but certain 'mild' mutations are seen in related conditions such as congenital absence of the vas deferens, nasal polyps, etc.
3	Deafness	Considering the commonest cause, in patients with connexin 26 mutations, mis-sense mutations are associated statistically with less severe hearing loss than truncating mutations – but the association is not predictive for individuals
4	Muscular dystrophy	Frameshifting deletions almost always produce Duchenne muscular dystrophy, while in-frame deletions nearly always produce the milder Becker form
5	Chromosomal imbalance	Phenotype depends on the size and gene content of the region involved
6	Leber's hereditary optic neuropathy	Very little correlation, even when heteroplasmy is taken into account
7	22q11 deletion	Little correlation between size of deletion and severity of phenotype
8	Trisomy 21	Phenotype is readily recognizable but quite variable. Mosaic cases are likely to be less severe
9	Turner syndrome	It has been claimed that behavioral problems depend on whether the single X chromosome is of maternal or paternal origin (see *Chapter 7*)
10	Marfan syndrome	A variable condition; little genotype–phenotype correlation
11	Sickle cell disease	Always the same mutation; downstream effects vary
12	Fragile X	Large expansions (>200 repeats) cause the classic syndrome in males; effects in females are variable. Premutation alleles (50–200 repeats) may cause tremor ataxia syndrome, especially in males, and premature ovarian failure in females.
13	Chromosomal microdeletion	Probably correlations will eventually be established; insufficient cases at present
14	Thalassemia	Good correlations between mutation type and β^0 or β^+ phenotype; clinical result modified by variable persistence of fetal hemoglobin
15	Stickler syndrome	Nature of *COL2A1* mutation correlates fairly well with position along the spectrum of chondrodysplasias

Dosage sensitivity and the pathology of chromosomal abnormalities

Although some large-scale copy number variants are harmless, and may even be common population polymorphisms (see *Section 2.4*), most chromosomal imbalances are pathogenic. Presumably the cause is having wrong numbers of certain dosage-sensitive genes. Since there are on average around 1000 genes per chromosome, even a small imbalance can involve many genes. Most genes are not dosage-sensitive. Relatively few loss of function mutations produce dominant phenotypes through haplo-insufficiency, and it is still less common for a 50% increase in the number of copies or level of product to cause problems. Nevertheless, all autosomal monosomies and trisomies are embryonic lethals or cause major congenital abnormalities. We can consider two possible explanations.

- In some cases imbalance of just two or three dosage-sensitive genes may explain much of the pathology. For example, the major problems of Down syndrome may be caused by just two genes on chromosome 21, *DSCR1* and *DYRK1A*. The products of these genes regulate certain transcription factors, and so indirectly affect expression of many genes. Chromosomal phenotypes must, however, always involve more than one gene. Clinicians can usually recognize 'chromosomal' patients even when they can't predict which chromosome is involved. Their phenotypes involve multiple independent developmental abnormalities and, except for a few specific cases, are not seen in patients with single-gene abnormalities.
- In other cases the problem may be an accumulation of many lesser effects. Genes encoding functionally related proteins are seldom located close together on the same chromosome. The individual components of multi-chain proteins like hemoglobin are usually encoded by genes on separate chromosomes. Similarly, the genes for a transcription factor and its target are more often than not on different chromosomes. Whether this is the result of some principle that we don't understand, or just an example of the apparently chaotic nature of our genome is not known, but it means that chromosomal imbalances almost always cause imbalances in multiple interacting systems. Having 50% extra of one partner of an interaction might result in only a subtle imbalance, but the cumulative effect of dozens of such imbalances could well derail development. The fact that patients with all sorts of different chromosomal imbalances tend to have rather the same spectrum of abnormalities (mental retardation, growth retardation, fits and dysmorphic face) supports this view of the pathology.

It is noteworthy that the three autosomal trisomies that are compatible with survival to term (trisomies 13, 18 and 21) involve chromosomes that are small and relatively poor in genes. These three chromosomes have 3.50, 4.23 and 5.77 genes per Mb of DNA respectively, compared to a genome-wide average of 7.32, according to data from the ENSEMBL genome browser (release 35, November 2005). Similarly, the low number of genes on the Y chromosome helps explain why most 47,XYY men are within the normal spectrum and remain undiagnosed.

Nevertheless, the X chromosome carries large numbers of genes, and so the fact that normal people can have either one or two X chromosomes is unexpected and requires a special explanation. This is covered in the following chapter.

Somatic mutations

The case studies reviewed in this chapter have all involved inherited mutations. But mutations can affect any cell and so, by simple arithmetic, the majority happen in somatic cells and do not get passed on. As discussed in *Section 1.4*, somatic mutations are only a problem in two circumstances.

- If a somatic mutation arises very early in embryogenesis, the one mutant cell may give rise to a substantial clone. The person is mosaic for the mutation. Whether this matters depends on what cells are affected and what the mutation does.
- If a mutation causes a somatic cell to start multiplying out of control, the result could be cancer. These mutations are considered in *Chapter 12*.

How do mutations arise?

Mutations arise through DNA damage or replication errors. DNA is a fairly stable molecule, but it is not immune to chemical change. Cytosine bases are liable to deaminate spontaneously – the consequences of this are described in the following chapter. Reactive oxygen species generated within cells as part of normal oxidative metabolism cause chemical modifications of the bases. Strand breaks are happening all the time as a result of errors in replication, chemical changes or natural radiation. The great bulk of all this damage is unrelated to industrial pollution, nuclear power plants or any other human activity. Cells have enzymes that are able to repair many types of DNA damage, so that much damage passes unnoticed, but they are not infallible. If damage is limited to one strand of the double helix, the complementary strand can be used as a template to make a correct repair. Double strand breaks, however, pose more problems, and often the repair process leaves errors in the sequence.

DNA replication is also a fallible process. The likelihood of the polymerase incorporating a mispaired base into a growing chain is simply a function of the relative binding energies of correctly paired and mispaired bases. That thermodynamic calculation suggests an error rate orders of magnitude higher than the observed rate. The higher accuracy is the result of proof-reading and mismatch detection mechanisms. The polymerase checks the newly synthesized DNA for mispaired bases. If one is detected, the polymerase backs up, degrades a short stretch of the DNA and tries again. Interestingly, when mice were engineered to abolish the proof-reading capacity, but not the polymerase activity, of one minor DNA polymerase (specialized for replicating the mitochondrial DNA), they showed many features of accelerated aging (see Trifunovic *et al.*, 2004). One theory of aging ascribes it to accumulation of mutations. After the polymerase has moved on, special enzymes excise and repair mismatched bases in newly replicated DNA. In *Chapter 12* we will see what can happen when this mechanism fails. Even with all this, occasional errors persist. Runs of identical bases are

Molecular pathology of variants in the androgen receptor gene

Mammals, including humans, develop by default as females. A specific cascade of events is necessary to produce males. In normal development the cascade starts with the *SRY* gene on the Y chromosome. This causes the early indifferent gonad to develop as a testis. The testis secretes the androgen (male sex hormone) testosterone. An enzyme, steroid 5-α reductase, converts testosterone to dihydrotestosterone (DHT). DHT activates the androgen receptor, a nuclear Class I steroid receptor which then stimulates transcription of a variety of genes whose effect is to produce the male sexual anatomy. The androgen receptor is encoded by the *AR* gene on the proximal long arm of the X chromosome at Xq11–q12. The gene has eight exons covering 178 kb of genomic DNA and encodes a protein of 920 amino acids. Different mutations in this gene have a surprisingly wide range of effects (see *Box figure 6.2*).

Loss of function mutations result in the X-linked androgen insensitivity syndrome (OMIM 300068), previously called testicular feminization syndrome. XY embryos develop testes as normal, and these secrete testosterone as normal. But if there is complete loss of function of the receptor, the tissues of the embryo are unable to react to androgens, and so anatomical development proceeds along the default female line. Affected patients are phenotypically female, with female external genitalia and breast development, but a blind vagina and absent uterus. The testes are inguinal or abdominal, and patients often come to medical attention because of a presumed inguinal hernia. It is advisable to remove the testes surgically because they have a propensity to develop malignancy. Apart from this, and their inevitable infertility, most affected people lead normal female lives.

Partial loss of function of the androgen receptor can result in a variety of sexually ambiguous states, often including hypospadias and micropenis with gynecomastia (Reifenstein syndrome, OMIM 312300). Such pseudohermaphroditism can have many other causes. Perhaps the most intriguing of these is the recessive condition (PPSH, OMIM 264600) caused by loss of function of the *SRD5A2* gene that encodes steroid 5-α reductase. Being unable to convert testosterone to dihydrotestosterone, affected infants have ambiguous genitalia but are normally raised as girls. However, at puberty an alternative 5-α reductase gene, *SRD5A1*, kicks in, triggering a conversion to male phenotype. The patient's voice breaks, he grows a beard and usually takes on a male identity. It is reported that they live comfortably with their new male identity, which if true suggests that early masculinization of the brain by testosterone may be at least as important as social factors for determining a person's sexual identity.

Expansion of a (CAG)$_n$ repeat in exon 1 of the **AR gene** has very different effects. Spinal and bulbar muscular atrophy (SBMA, OMIM 313200) is one of the family of conditions caused by unstable repeat expansions (see *Disease box 4*). Like Huntington disease, the CAG repeat is in the coding sequence and encodes an expanded run of glutamines in the receptor protein. As in the other diseases caused by expanded polyglutamine runs, there is a gain of function: the mutant protein is toxic to neurons. The result is an X-linked adult-onset slowly progressive muscular atrophy. However, there is a second effect. The expanded polyglutamine run is located in the N-terminal part of the protein, which is the transactivation domain through which the activated (androgen-bound) receptor stimulates transcription of its target genes. Expansion of the polyglutamine tract decreases the efficiency of transactivation. Males with SBMA therefore show mild signs of androgen deficiency, in particular gynecomastia.

Normal variation in the (CAG)$_n$ repeat mediates normal variation in response to androgens. Short repeats promote a strong response and longer repeats (within the normal range) a weaker response. This shows up in the incidence of prostate cancer, an androgen-dependent condition. Though the distributions overlap strongly, the average repeat size is lowest in African–Americans, intermediate in non-Hispanic white Americans and highest in the Japanese and

Chinese. The incidence of prostate cancer varies between these groups in inverse proportion to the average repeat length. Repeats at the upper end of normal (>27 repeats), on the other hand, are associated with a fourfold increase in the risk of male infertility.

Androgen receptor variation as a susceptibility factor for male baldness. For almost a century geneticists have studied the inheritance of balding in middle-aged men (androgenic alopecia, OMIM 300710). One clear conclusion is that though balding can run in families it is not a simple mendelian character. However, it has recently been shown that a major susceptibility factor lies somewhere within the androgen receptor locus. Variation at this locus may explain about half the overall genetic susceptibility. Precisely what variant confers susceptibility is not certain, but a strong candidate is variation in a run of glycines in exon 1. Unlike the polyglutamine run described above, this is variable but stable. A likely reason for the stability is that at the DNA level it is not a pure repeat, but includes various different glycine codons $(GGN)_n$, where N can be any nucleotide. This variation reduces the risk of slippage during DNA replication.

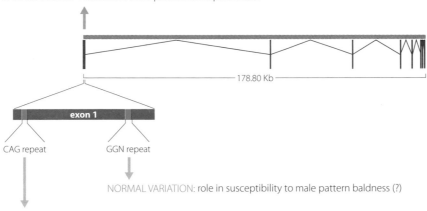

COMPLETE LOSS OF FUNCTION: androgen insensitivity syndrome, M>F sex reversal (OMIM 300068)

PARTIAL LOSS OF FUNCTION: male pseudohermaphroditism

178.80 Kb

exon 1

CAG repeat

GGN repeat

NORMAL VARIATION: role in susceptibility to male pattern baldness (?)

NORMAL VARIATION: low copy number increases susceptibility to prostate cancer
(11–33 repeats)   high copy number associated with some cases of male infertility

ABNORMAL EXPANSION: spinal and bulbar muscular atrophy (OMIM 313200)
(38–62 repeats)

Box figure 6.2 – Different variations in the *AR* gene lead to a wide variety of different effects.
Loss of function or gain of function mutations cause distinct mendelian conditions, while normal variation affects susceptibility to several different common non-mendelian conditions.

particularly liable to lose or gain a base by slipped-strand mispairing. The 35delG mutation in the *GJB2* gene (*Figure 6.2*) is an example.

Mutations can affect any piece of DNA at any time. We have focused on mutations affecting coding sequence because these are the ones studied in relation to genetic diseases, and where we can often predict the effect on the gene product. Because only around 1% of our DNA is coding, these are actually a very minor subset of all mutations. Most mutations in non-coding sequence are unlikely to have any phenotypic effect. Very little of this sequence is conserved between humans and other species, implying that it could mutate over evolutionary time without the mutants suffering any selective disadvantage. No doubt certain changes are pathogenic but at present, with a few fortuitously discovered exceptions, we are unable to identify them.

6.5. References

Aitman TJ, Dong R, Vyse TJ, *et al.* (2006) Copy number polymorphism in *Fcgr3* predisposes to glomerulonephritis in rats and humans. *Nature* **439**: 851–855.

Brunner HG and van Driel MA (2004) From syndrome families to functional genomics. *Nat. Rev. Genet.* **5**: 545–51.

Donnai D and Read AP (2003) How clinicians add to knowledge of development. *Lancet,* **362**: 477–484.

Holbrook JA, Neu-Yilik G, Hentze MW and Kulozik AE (2004) Nonsense-mediated decay approaches the clinic. *Nature Genetics,* **36**: 801–808.

Scriver C and Waters PJ (1999) Monogenic traits are not simple: lessons from phenylketonuria. *Trends Genet.* **15**: 267–272.

Snead MP and Yates JRW (1999) Clinical and molecular genetics of Stickler syndrome. *J. Med. Genet.* **36**: 353–359.

Trifunovic A *et al.* (2004) Premature ageing in mice expressing defective mitochondrial DNA polymerase. *Nature,* **429**: 357–359.

Useful websites

For more discussion of molecular pathology see Chapter 13 of Strachan and Read (2010), *Human Molecular Genetics* (4th edn, Garland).

For the nomenclature of mutations see www.hgvs.org/mutnomen/

POLYPHEN (http://genetics.bwh.harvard.edu/pph) and SIFT (http://sift.jcvi.org) are web-based programs that attempt to marshall all available data to decide whether a coding sequence change is likely to be damaging.

6.6. Self-assessment questions

(1) Cystic fibrosis is caused by the absence from apical cell membranes of functional chloride ion channels that are encoded by the *CFTR* gene. Which of the following mutations might be a cause of cystic fibrosis?

(a) Deletion of the *CFTR* gene.
(b) A mutation in the gene encoding arginine-specific tRNA that causes the protein synthesis machinery to incorporate arginine in growing polypeptide chains in response to serine codons. Substitution of arginine for serine in the CFTR protein makes it non-functional.
(c) A mutation in the promoter of the *CFTR* gene that abolishes its ability to recruit the RNA polymerase machinery.

(d) A mutation in the coding sequence of the *CFTR* gene that replaces an essential serine with a non-functional arginine.

(e) A mutation in one of the small non-coding RNA molecules in the spliceosome that causes the splicing machinery to treat GA...AG as the signal for the start and end of introns, instead of GT...AG.

(f) A mutation in the RNA polymerase II gene that renders the polymerase non-functional.

(g) A mutation in the coding sequence of the *CFTR* gene that causes the ion channel to transport excessive quantities of chloride ions.

(2) *Box 6.3* shows the sequence of two exons (upper case), with flanking intron sequence (lower case), as amplified by PCR for mutation detection in the *PAX3* gene. For exon 1, only part of the 5′UT is included in the PCR product. Nucleotides are numbered as in the cDNA (with the first nucleotide of the initiator codon numbered +1), and the protein sequence is shown using single-letter codes (see *Box 3.6*).

BOX 6.3

Partial sequence of *PAX3* gene for Self-assessment questions

Exon 1 (451 nt)

```
                 ..CCGTTTCGC CCTTCACCTG GATATAATTT CCGAGCGAAG TGCCCCCAGG
  1  ATG ACC ACG CTG GCC GGC GCT GTG CCC AGG ATG ATG CGG CCG GGC CCG GGG
  1   M   T   T   L   A   G   A   V   P   R   M   M   R   P   G   P   G
 52  CAG AAC TAC CCG CGT AGC GGG TTC CCG CTG GAA Ggtaagggagg gcctcagcgc..
 18   Q   N   Y   P   R   S   G   F   P   L   E
```

Exon 2

```
                      ..tgactttttcc cttgcttctc tttttcacct tcccacag
 86   TG TCC ACT CCC CTC GGC CAG GGC CGC GTC AAC CAG CTC GGC GGC GTT TTT
 29    V   S   T   P   L   G   Q   G   R   V   N   Q   L   G   G   V   F
136  ATC AAC GGC AGG CCG CTC CCC AAC CAC ATC CGC CAC AAG ATC GTG GAG ATG
 46   I   N   G   R   P   L   P   N   H   I   R   H   K   I   V   E   M
187  GCC CAC CAC GGC ATC CGG CCC TGC GTC ATC TCG CGC CAG CTG CGC GTG TCC
 63   A   H   H   G   I   R   P   C   V   I   S   R   Q   L   R   V   S
238  CAC GGC TGC GTC TCC AAG ATC CTG TGC AGG TAC CAG GAG ACT GGC TCC ATA
 80   H   G   C   V   S   K   I   L   C   R   Y   Q   E   T   G   S   I
289  CGT CCT GGT GCC ATC GGC GGC AGC AAG CCC AAG gtgagcgggc gggccttgcc..
 97   R   P   G   A   I   G   G   S   K   P   K
```

For the following eight mutations, a short sequence is given, with the number of the first nucleotide shown. The changed nucleotide (or the first changed one if several change) is underlined. For each mutation, give the correct nomenclature (a) as a DNA change (b) (where appropriate) as a protein change.

c.15	CGGCGCTGTGGCCAGGATGATGC
c.43	GGCCCGGGGTAGAACTACCCGCG
c.78	GCTGGAAGTTAAGGGAGGGCCTC
c.86	TGTCCACTCCACTCGGCCAGGGC
c.121	CTCGGCGGCGTTTTATCAACGGC
c.130	GTTTTGATCAACGGCAGGCCGCT
c.248	TCTCCGAGATCCTGTGCAGGTAC
c.283	TCCATTCCTGGTGCCATCGGCGG

(3) Referring to the *PAX3* sequence in *Box 6.3*, write out the mutant sequence of each of the following, formatted as in Question 2:

p.N47H

c.247_248ins(C)

c.185_202del

p.E61X

c.85+6G>T

c.86–2A>G

p.V29M

(4) Referring to the *PAX3* sequence in *Box 6.3*, for each of the following mutations, select one of the following options:

(a) Synonymous

(b) Mis-sense

(c) Nonsense

(d) Frameshift

(e) Non-frameshifting insertion / deletion

(f) Splice-site mutation

(g) Initiator codon

(h) Terminator codon

(i) Intronic

(1) c.85+1G>A

(2) c.86T>A

(3) c.86–18T>G

(4) c.101insGCC

(5) c.118C>T

(6) c.172_173delAA

(7) c.216C>G

(8) c.270C>G

(5) The effects of a mutation can be studied at the protein level as well as by DNA sequencing. If a suitable antibody is available, mutations can be classified into CRM^+ and CRM^-. CRM means cross-reacting material. Classify each of the types of mutation in *Box 6.1* in this way, commenting on cases where the result is hard to predict.

(6) A student wrote the following answer to a question about the genetics of cystic fibrosis:

> 'The gene for cystic fibrosis is recessive. If you have two copies of the gene you have cystic fibrosis, but if you only have one copy you are just the same as somebody who doesn't have any copy'.

> Comment on this.

07 | What is epigenetics?

After working through this chapter you should be able to:

- Define epigenetic, imprinting, uniparental disomy, CpG island
- Explain how DNA is methylated, and how the methylation patterns can be heritable
- Describe two methods by which methylation patterns can be studied
- Explain the roles of CpG sequences in gene control and mutation
- Describe X-inactivation and its consequences for carriers of X-linked recessive conditions and balanced X-autosome translocations
- Give examples of pedigree patterns and sporadic syndromes dependent on imprinting

7.1. Case studies

CASE 16	Portillo family	**177**	188	216	389

- Sickly boy, Pablo
- Family history of similar symptoms
- Blood tests suggest X-linked severe combined immunodeficiency

Pilar and Pedro Portillo come from very close families and three generations live in the same part of town. When Pablo was born in 1989 Pilar and Pedro were happy that they had three children, but Pablo was a much more sickly baby than his siblings. He always seemed to have a cough, an ear infection or diarrhea and he failed to gain weight. Pilar's maternal grandmother encouraged Pilar to get an appointment for Pedro at the specialist children's hospital because Pablo's problems were very similar to those of her own two sons who had both died before they were one year old. She hoped there might be treatment available to stop Pablo deteriorating further. At the hospital Pablo was admitted immediately for investigations.

The blood tests showed that Pablo had a very low lymphocyte count. T cells and NK (natural killer) cells were absent; B cells were present but non-functional. *Box 7.1* gives some basic details about these cells. These findings, together with the family history, suggested a diagnosis of X-linked severe combined immunodeficiency (X-SCID). This was very bad news because without successful treatment the prognosis is very poor. The doctors suggested bone marrow transplantation was Pablo's best hope (see *Chapter 8*).

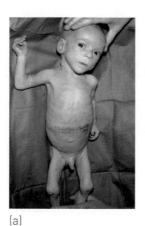
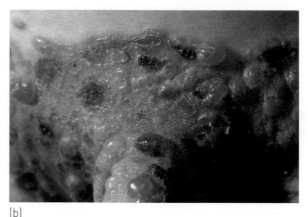

(a)   (b)

Figure 7.1 – Problems with immunodeficiency.
(a) Failure to thrive and skin problems. (b) Herpes simplex developing over an
area with eczema (Koebner phenomenon). Photo. (a) courtesy of Dept of Medical
Illustration, Manchester Royal Infirmary and (b) courtesy of Dr Andrew Will, Royal
Manchester Children's Hospital.

BOX 7.1

Types and functions of lymphocytes

All three types of lymphocyte are derived from bone marrow. B cells and NK cells mature in
the marrow but T cells undergo a process of maturation in the thymus gland. B cells give rise
to plasma cells that secrete immunoglobulins. NK cells are large granular lymphocytes with a
characteristic morphology; they account for up to 15% of blood lymphocytes and provide a first
line of defense against virally infected cells. **T lymphocytes** are involved in the regulation of the
immune response and in cell-mediated immunity, and they help B cells to produce antibody.
Mature T cells express antigen-specific T cell receptors plus the CD3 molecule. In addition,
mature T cells express either CD4 or CD8 cell surface molecules that enable them to play a role
in cell and antibody-mediated immunity (CD4+) or to become cytotoxic (CD8+).

| CASE 17 | Qian family | 178 | 190 | 389 |

- Girl, Kai, aged 2 years,
  showing slow development
- Seizure
- ? Angelman syndrome

Chu-Li and Chan are a hard working couple who have an import business. When
their first child Kai was born Chu-Li's mother moved from Hong Kong to help
look after the baby. She had looked after several grandchildren before but even
she found it hard to get Kai to feed well or to settle and sleep. Kai was slow
to gain weight and achieve her developmental milestones. She appeared very
jittery although she seemed happy and laughed a lot. By 2 years of age she wasn't
showing any signs of talking and an appointment was made with a pediatrician.
However, before this could happen she had a seizure and was admitted to the
children's ward.

It was clear to the pediatrician that there were major problems with Kai's
development. She noted that Kai, who had just learned to walk, did so with

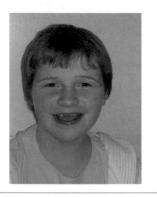

Figure 7.2 – A 10-year-old girl with Angelman syndrome.
She has a mutation in the *UBE3A* gene. Photo. courtesy of Dr Jill Clayton-Smith, St Mary's Hospital, Manchester.

rather stiff legs held well apart. She had lots of jerky movements especially with her arms. She laughed a lot and tended to protrude her tongue and dribble. Her records showed that her head circumference at birth was normal but it was now just below the 3rd centile. She arranged for Kai to have an EEG and the result confirmed her clinical suspicions. There were generalized EEG changes with runs of high-amplitude delta activity with intermittent spike and slow wave discharges. The pediatrician told the parents that she was sure Kai had a condition called Angelman syndrome. The family were shocked because they said no one else in the family had problems. They wanted to know what had caused the condition and if it might happen again. The pediatrician said that she needed to refer them to the genetics clinic because there were different ways that Angelman syndrome could occur and sometimes another child in a family could be affected.

| CASE 18 | Rogers family | **179** | 190 | 389 |

- Baby boy, Robert, born to older parents
- Floppy at birth; failed to suck
- Genetic tests in pregnancy showed normal male karyotype
- ? Prader–Willi syndrome

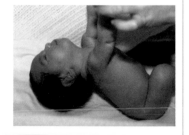

Figure 7.3 – A baby with Prader–Willi syndrome.
Note the marked hypotonia.

Ralph and Rowena Rogers had both been married before and each had a child by their first partners. Although Rowena was 38 years old when they married, they decided to try for a baby and were delighted when, after a few months, a pregnancy was confirmed. They wanted as many tests as possible to ensure a healthy baby. An amniocentesis test (see *Chapter 14*) showed a normal male karyotype and scans didn't show any problems. Rowena did mention that she didn't feel many fetal movements but put that down to the fact that she was very busy. Labor occurred on her due date and was a rather long affair but a baby boy was born weighing 3.2 kg. The family decided to call him Robert. When he was put to the breast he didn't try to suck at all and the doctor noticed he was very floppy. The doctor mentioned his concerns to Ralph and Rowena and said he was going to ask for an urgent chromosome test to rule out Down syndrome. Rowena reminded him that the amniocentesis test had shown a normal chromosome pattern and so the doctor decided to wait and see how Robert progressed. He needed feeding by tube because he couldn't suck well and had marked truncal hypotonia. The pediatrician talked to the geneticist on the telephone and described Robert's problems. Suspecting Prader–Willi syndrome, the geneticist said he would see the family urgently in his next clinic. In the genetics department the Rogers family were seen at the same clinic as the Qian family (Case 17), which was an informative coincidence, especially for the medical student who attended because he was doing a special module in genetics.

7.2. Science toolkit

Epigenetic effects are heritable changes in gene expression that depend on changes in the way DNA is packaged into chromatin, rather than on changes in the sequence. In *Disease box 2* we saw how the conformation of chromatin is determined by an interplay between modifications of histones, methylation of DNA and positioning of nucleosomes, and in *Section 3.4* we saw how gene expression depends on the local chromatin conformation. Chromatin conformation can be heritable because patterns of DNA methylation are heritable (see below), and when such effects are inherited they are called epigenetic. Normally the heritability is from cell to daughter cell, rather than from parent to child. Whether epigenetic changes in humans can ever be transmitted from parent to child is controversial, and is discussed further in *Section 7.4*.

Epigenetic controls are central to human development. As an embryo develops from a fertilized egg, cells become more and more specialized. Specialization involves manipulating the chromatin conformation along a chromosome so that only a specific subset of all the genes in the genome are expressed. The pattern of packaging along the chromosome has to be heritable in order that a differentiated cell can give rise to a clone of similarly differentiated daughter cells. There is intense interest in reversing this process in the laboratory, producing induced pluripotent stem cells by epigenetic reprogramming of differentiated cells. Cells from a patient might be induced to form new tissues or even whole organs to replace damaged or defective ones, without any of the problems of transplantation from a donor.

In clinical genetics, epigenetic effects are important in at least three contexts: X-inactivation, imprinting and cancer. Epigenetic reprogramming in cancer is discussed in *Chapter 12*; the three cases at the start of this chapter have been chosen to illustrate the other two effects.

X-inactivation

The fact that people can be entirely normal while having either one (46,XY) or two (46,XX) X chromosomes requires explanation. Having an extra or missing copy of an autosome that contained that many genes would be lethal. The explanation lies in a mechanism of dosage compensation called **X-inactivation** or **lyonization** (named after its discoverer, Dr Mary Lyon).

Early in the life of every human (and other mammalian) embryo, at the blastocyst stage, each cell somehow counts its number of X chromosomes. All Xs except one are then permanently inactivated. The inactivated chromosome remains intact but most of its genes are not expressed (some X-linked genes do escape the general inactivation; why and how they do so is the subject of current research). Which X remains active is a random choice in each cell. However, once the choice is made, it is remembered by all the daughters of that cell (*Figure 7.4*). X-inactivation is an epigenetic process, depending on a change in chromatin conformation that is heritable from cell to daughter cell. It is not heritable through a pedigree. In the female germ-line the inactive X is re-activated, and meiosis picks one X chromosome at random to go into the egg. Both X chromosomes in a 46,XX fertilized egg are active, and it is random which one will later be inactivated in any one daughter cell.

X-inactivation is controlled by a gene called *XIST* located on the proximal long arm of the X chromosome at Xq13. *XIST* is expressed only by the *inactive* X.

Figure 7.4 – X-inactivation is an epigenetic process.
Because of X-inactivation every female is a mosaic of cell lines with different active X chromosomes.

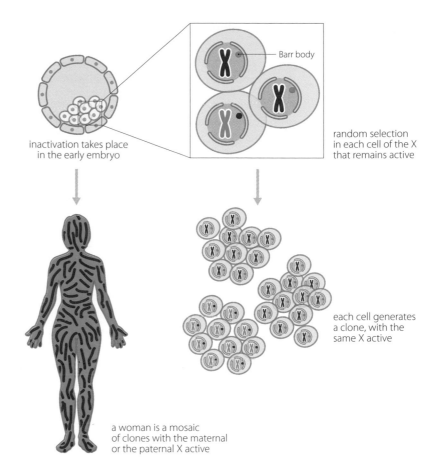

Barr body

inactivation takes place in the early embryo

random selection in each cell of the X that remains active

each cell generates a clone, with the same X active

a woman is a mosaic of clones with the maternal or the paternal X active

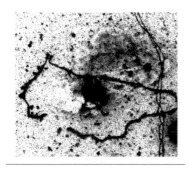

Figure 7.5 – Electron micrograph showing the X and Y chromosomes paired in prophase I of meiosis through the pseudoautosomal regions at the tips of their short arms. Reproduced from Connor and Ferguson Smith (1991) *Essential Medical Genetics*, 3rd edn, with permission from Blackwell Publishing, Oxford.

It produces a large non-coding RNA that physically coats the inactive X. This triggers a change in the chromatin conformation to make the chromosome heterochromatic and silence its genes. The XIST RNA spreads along the inactive X, moving outwards from Xq13 without ever jumping on to the active X. Heterochromatin has a tendency to spread along a chromosome, and this may be an extreme example of that general tendency. On a female karyotype such as *Figure 2.9* the two X chromosomes are indistinguishable – but this is because the chromosomes are being seen during mitosis when all chromosomes are highly condensed and largely inactive. On completion of cell division, while the other chromosomes of a female cell decondense, the inactive X remains condensed. In female cells it can be seen as a spot of densely staining chromatin at the edge of the nucleus, the Barr body. Counting Barr bodies was used in the past as a way of counting the number of X chromosomes (for sex tests on athletes, for example). Normal females and XXY males have one Barr body per cell; normal males and 45,X females have none, and 47,XXX females have two.

The 2.6 Mb of sequence immediately adjacent to the tip of the X chromosome short arm has special properties. A homologous sequence is present at the short arm tip of the Y chromosome; the two pair in meiosis (*Figure 7.5*) and have an obligatory crossover in this region. Genes in this region escape X-inactivation. Men and women each have two active copies of these genes, and the pattern of inheritance of variants appears autosomal. For this reason the region is called the **pseudoautosomal region**. There is another small pseudoautosomal region, 300 kb long, at the tip of the long arm – but this does not usually pair or cross-over with its counterpart on the Y chromosome in meiosis.

X-inactivation has implications for female carriers of X-linked diseases, as shown below in the cases of the Davies and Portillo families (Cases 4 and 16), and for female carriers of X:autosome translocations, as described in the final section of this chapter. See the case of the Ingram family (Case 9) in the next section for further discussion of X-inactivation.

Imprinting – why you need a mother and a father

For a heterozygous person, the parental origin of each allele is not normally relevant when thinking about their phenotype. However, some observations suggest that there are functional differences between the maternal and paternal components of somebody's genome. Occasional accidents produce 46,XX conceptuses that have either two maternal or two paternal genomes. Despite being ostensibly chromosomally normal, such conceptuses always develop very abnormally, and quite differently from each other (*Figure 7.6*). Experiments in mice demonstrate the same effects. Evidently there is some difference between maternal and paternal genomes, and normal development requires one of each.

Figure 7.6 – Conceptuses that have two maternal or two paternal genomes cannot develop normally.

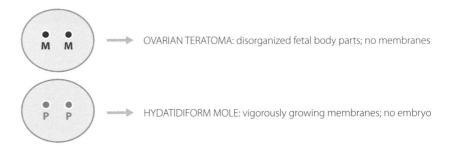

OVARIAN TERATOMA: disorganized fetal body parts; no membranes

HYDATIDIFORM MOLE: vigorously growing membranes; no embryo

More refined experiments in mice allowed the contribution of each individual chromosome to this effect to be studied. Ingenious manipulations allow mice to be generated that have correct chromosome numbers, but both homologs of one particular pair are derived from just one parent. This is called **uniparental disomy** (UPD). For some chromosomes the resulting mice are normal, but for others they are abnormal, and the particular abnormalities seen depend on whether the mice have two maternal or two paternal copies of the chromosome in question. Rare human cases of UPD were also discovered by chance. Later it became apparent that certain human syndromes could be caused by UPD, as described below.

These and other observations suggest that there are human (and mouse) genes that behave differently depending on their parental origin. They must carry some sort of *imprint* that marks their origin. It is important to remember that genes are not intrinsically paternal or maternal. If a man passes on to his child an imprinted gene that he inherited from his mother, he received it with a maternal imprint but

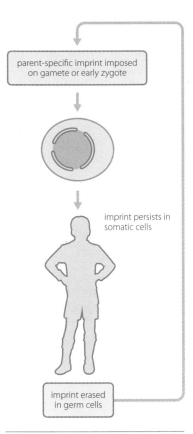

Figure 7.7 – Imprinting is epigenetic and reversible.

passes it on with a paternal imprint. Thus imprinting must be reversible, so that it can be erased and re-imposed with each generation (*Figure 7.7*). Imprinting is an epigenetic phenomenon: the expression of imprinted genes is modified, and the modification persists through all the cell divisions that lead from a fertilized egg to an adult person, but the DNA sequence is not changed. Our understanding of imprinting in humans has been greatly enhanced by the study of certain rare syndromes, in particular the two conditions described in Cases 17 and 18, Angelman and Prader-Willi syndromes.

DNA methylation and the heritability of chromatin conformation

DNA methylation plays an important role in determining the conformation of chromatin, and it also holds the key to the heritability of epigenetic changes. In humans and other mammals methylation takes the form of adding methyl groups to the 5-position of cytosines to form 5-methyl cytosine (5MeC). The methyl group of 5MeC lies in the major groove on the outside of the double helix, where it is accessible to DNA-binding proteins but does not interfere with the base-pairing in the interior (*Figure 7.8*).

Methylation is almost entirely restricted to cytosines that lie immediately 5′ of guanines in so-called CpG dinucleotides (the 'p' represents the phosphate group that links the two together). Each 5′-CpG-3′ in one strand of the double helix is partnered by a 5′-CpG-3′ in the opposite strand (remember, the strands are antiparallel). Not every CpG is methylated, but if a CpG in one strand is methylated, so is the CpG on the opposite strand, so that both strands carry the same pattern of methylated and unmethylated CpGs. This is the result of the action of a maintenance methyltransferase enzyme. When DNA is replicated, all CpG sequences on the newly synthesized strand are initially unmethylated. However, the maintenance methyltransferase subsequently methylates any CpG on the newly synthesized strand that lies opposite a methylated CpG on the parental strand (*Figure 7.9*). By this process the pattern of methylation is inherited from mother cell to daughter cell.

In addition to the maintenance methyltransferase, cells have two *de novo* DNA methyltransferases, so that the pattern of methylation, though heritable, is not fixed during the life of a cell. It differs according to the type of cell and its current

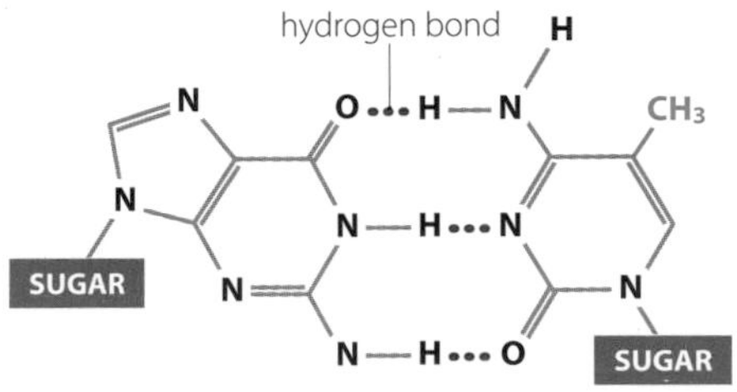

Figure 7.8 – 5-methyl cytosine base-pairs with guanine in exactly the same way as unmodified cytosine.

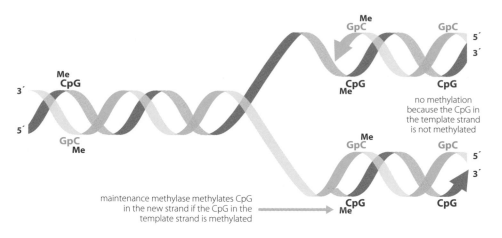

Figure 7.9 – The role of 5-methyl cytosine in epigenetics.
When the DNA is replicated a maintenance methylase specifically methylates CpG sequences in the newly synthesized strand whenever they occur opposite a methylated CpG in the template strand. As a result, patterns of CpG methylation are heritable.

metabolic state. *De novo* DNA methylation is part of the mechanism of dynamic regulation of gene expression that enables a cell to respond to external signals, adjusting its metabolism or differentiating. A combination of DNA methylation and histone modification converts the uniform chromatin fiber into a dynamic and highly differentiated structure (Hendrich and Bickmore, 2001).

The 'histone code' was described in *Disease box 2*. DNA methylation and histone modification are interdependent. Methylated DNA binds proteins that can modify histones, and modified histones in turn act as docking sites for DNA methyltransferases. When things go wrong, gene expression is dysregulated. Rett syndrome (see *Disease box 7*) is the result of loss of function of the *MECP2* gene which encodes a 5MeC-binding protein. MECP2 protein binds to methylated regions of DNA, where it represses gene activity, either directly or by recruiting histone deacetylases and other transcriptional repressors. Methylation of CpG dinucleotides upstream of a gene is a key signal for controlling gene expression. In general, methylation suppresses gene expression – for example the inactive X chromosome is heavily methylated compared to its active counterpart – but there are counter-examples. In imprinted regions of the genome there are sequences that are differentially methylated depending on the parental origin. Studies of DNA methylation are important both for understanding the mechanism of imprinting and for making diagnoses. The next section describes how this can be done.

Studying DNA methylation

Methylation patterns in DNA are much more difficult to study than sequence changes. As shown in *Figure 7.8*, 5MeC base-pairs with G indistinguishably from unmethylated cytosine, and so behaves identically to C in most laboratory tests. The hybridization properties of a DNA strand are unaffected by its methylation status, so hybridization-based tests cannot be used to investigate methylation. PCR and sequencing both depend on making copies of the sequence under investigation, and regardless of the state of methylation of the original DNA, the copies will be unmethylated. Thus none of the methods described in *Chapters 4* and *5* can be used to check the methylation pattern of a DNA sequence. Methylation studies mostly use three techniques:

- *Precipitation of methylated DNA by anti-5MeC antibodies.* This is a method of studying genome-wide patterns of methylation. Whole-genome DNA is fragmented and exposed to an antibody against methylated DNA. The precipitated fragments can be identified by sequencing or by hybridization to microarrays.

- *Digestion by methylation-sensitive restriction enzymes.* Certain restriction enzymes whose recognition site includes a CpG sequence, will cut the site only if it is unmethylated (for example, *Ecl*X1, see *Figure 4.12*); *Hpa*II cuts CCGG sequences, but will not cut C^{Me}CGG. Other enzymes are unaffected by methylation – for example *Msp*I cuts CCGG regardless of methylation. This difference can be exploited in various ways to reveal whether or not a particular CpG is methylated. In the investigation of Pablo Portillo (Case 16, see below) a sequence that included a CpG site was PCR amplified from DNA that had previously been digested with *Hpa*II. If the site was unmethylated, the template would have been cut in two, and no PCR product could be formed.

- *Bisulfite sequencing.* When DNA is treated with sodium bisulfite under carefully controlled conditions, cytosine is converted by deamination into uracil, but 5MeC is resistant to the reagent. Uracil is not a natural base in DNA, but it base-pairs with adenine in just the same way as thymine does. If a bisulfite-treated template is copied by PCR or used in a sequencing reaction, every unmethylated C in the original sequence appears as a T, while methylated Cs remain as C. Comparing the untreated and bisulfite-treated sequence reveals the pattern of methylation (*Figure 7.10*).

A variant of this method uses allele-specific PCR (*Figure 5.6*) to check the methylation status of one specific C. Primers are designed with 3′ terminal nucleotides G or A to match the C or U in the bisulfite-treated template. The G primer will amplify only the methylated template; the A primer amplifies only

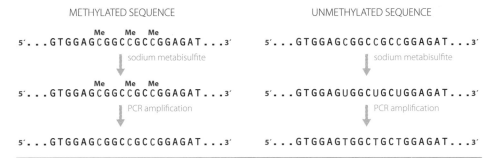

Figure 7.10 – The bisulfite method for analyzing DNA methylation.
Bisulfite treatment converts C to U. 5MeC remains unchanged. After PCR amplification, cytosines that were unmethylated are represented by thymines in the PCR product.

the unmethylated sequence. This method works best if the rest of the sequence to which the primer must hybridize is free of variably methylated cytosines, otherwise these too may be modified by the bisulfite treatment and prevent the primer hybridizing efficiently.

7.3. **Investigations of patients**

| CASE 4 | Davies family | 4 | 10 | 67 | 104 | 155 | **186** | 281 | 389 |

- Boy (Martin) aged 24 months, parents Judith and Robert
- Clumsy and slow to walk
- Family history of muscular dystrophy
- Pedigree shows X-linked recessive inheritance
- Order diagnostic DNA test
- Frameshift mutation in the dystrophin gene

Several of Martin's female relatives are obligate or possible carriers of this X-linked recessive disease. As a result of lyonization, a normal adult XX female is a mosaic of clones, some of which have the paternal X active while others have the maternal X active. A carrier of an X-linked disease is a mosaic of normal and abnormal clones. The consequence depends on what the affected gene does, and where the cells are.

- Where the gene product is diffusible, there is an averaging effect. Carriers of X-linked hemophilia have half the normal level of the affected clotting factor (subject to the usual individual variation). The clotting time is noticeably increased above normal, but the blood still clots sufficiently well to avoid disease.
- Where the gene product is fixed, there are patches of normal and affected tissue. These may be demonstrable, for example, in anhidrotic ectodermal dysplasia (OMIM 305100), where the affected skin lacks sweat glands. The size of the patches depends on whether the tissue consists of many small clones or a few large ones, and on how much cell mixing occurs during development of that particular tissue.
- In Duchenne muscular dystrophy the picture is complicated by the fact that muscle cells are multinucleate, being formed by fusion of myoblasts. Staining a muscle biopsy with a dystrophin antibody shows a patchy distribution of dystrophin in individual muscle cells of heterozygous females, reflecting the random nature of X-inactivation (*Figure 7.11*). Occasional carriers have significant muscle weakness, presumably because by bad luck they inactivated mainly the normal X in their muscle cells. They are known as **manifesting heterozygotes**. Most carriers show biochemical evidence of subclinical muscle damage in the form of elevated levels of creatine kinase in their serum. As mentioned in *Chapter 4* the CK level can be used to give an estimate of a woman's risk of being a carrier, but the estimate is rarely sufficiently close to 0% or 100% to be a useful guide for reproductive decisions. Only DNA analysis can do that.

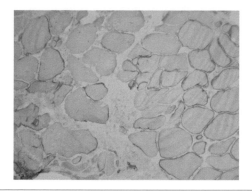

Figure 7.11 – A muscle biopsy from a female carrier of Duchenne muscular dystrophy stained with an antibody against dystrophin.
Note the patchy distribution of staining around the outer membranes of cells (compare with the sections from an affected boy and a normal control in *Figure 1.4*). Photo. courtesy of Dr Richard Charlton, Newcastle upon Tyne.

| CASE 9 | Ingram family | 26 | 41 | 69 | 104 | **187** | 389 |

- Isabel – first daughter of Irene and Ian
- Small stature despite tall parents
- ? Turner syndrome
- Diagnosis confirmed by karyotyping

Isabel Ingram has a single X chromosome, 45,X and has Turner syndrome. Given that the X-inactivation mechanism exists in order to allow normal development in people with differing numbers of X chromosomes, one might ask why there is anything wrong with her. The answer is probably that, even discounting the pseudoautosomal regions, not all genes on the X chromosome are subject to X-inactivation. An investigation of transcription levels (Carrel and Willard, 2005) showed surprising deviations from the conventional picture of blanket X-inactivation. Even outside the pseudoautosomal regions, about 15% of X-linked genes escaped inactivation partially or totally, and a further 10% showed differences between different inactive X chromosomes in the degree of inactivation.

Some X-linked genes that escape inactivation have counterparts on the Y chromosome, and these will have lower expression levels in women with Turner syndrome than in normal men or women. Those without functional Y-linked counterparts will have levels of expression in normal males similar to those in Turner females – but maybe the higher expression of these genes in XX females is responsible for some of the differences between males and females. Intriguingly, it has been claimed that Turner women whose X is of maternal origin may have behavioral problems of the sort that are mainly seen in boys (whose X chromosome, of course, is of maternal origin), while Turner women with a paternal X are free of such problems. If true, this would be evidence of imprinting.

- Sickly boy, Pablo
- Family history of similar symptoms
- Blood tests suggest X-linked severe combined immunodeficiency

Severe combined immunodeficiency can be either an autosomal recessive or an X-linked condition. At first it may seem surprising that an immunodeficiency should be X-linked – one might expect immunodeficiencies to be caused by mutations in the immunoglobulin genes, which are located on chromosomes 2, 14 and 22. But production of antibodies requires not only intact structural genes for those proteins, but also properly functioning B cells, whose successful development must require numerous other genetically controlled steps. In *Chapter 8* we will see some of the complicated processing that is needed to enable these cells to produce an effectively infinite repertoire of antibody molecules. Moreover, in combined immunodeficiency there is an absence of T cells as well as a functional defect in the B cells that produce antibodies. Its cause must be a failure of a much earlier stage of cell differentiation.

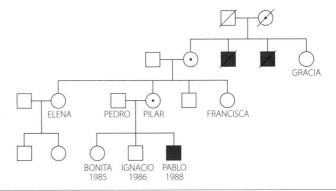

Figure 7.12 – Pedigree of severe combined immunodeficiency in the Portillo family.
The pattern shows that this is the X-linked form of this rare disease. The mother, grandmother and great-grandmother of the proband are obligate carriers. His sister, two aunts and cousin are at risk of being carriers.

When the pedigree (*Figure 7.12*) was taken it seemed clear that baby Pablo has the X-linked form of SCID. One immediate consequence for the family is to clarify the risks for relatives. Had the disease been the autosomal form, any relatives who were carriers would not be at risk of having affected children unless their partner was also a carrier. Because SCID is very rare, this risk is low provided they marry outside the family. However, now we know the condition is X-linked, Pilar's sisters, aunt and daughter are at substantial risk, although for her brother and normal son the risk is negligibly low.

At the time the family came to attention, it was not known what gene defect was responsible for X-SCID. However, it was possible to do carrier testing by looking at the pattern of X-inactivation in at-risk females. The X-SCID defect prevents development of B and T lymphocytes, therefore all lymphocytes in a carrier woman must be cells that happened to inactivate the defective X chromosome. Carriers will therefore show completely non-random inactivation in their lymphocytes, although in all their other tissues the normal random X-inactivation may be seen.

The methylation-sensitive restriction enzyme *Hpa*II was used to check the randomness of X-inactivation, as follows. The androgen receptor gene on the X chromosome contains a variable length $(CAG)_n$ trinucleotide repeat (see *Disease box 6*). The test will only work in women whose two X chromosomes have different sized repeats – but fortunately these are the majority of women because the repeat is highly polymorphic. Near the repeat are two CCGG sequences that are methylated in females on the inactive X, but unmethylated on the active X (and on the only X in males). A DNA segment containing both the $(CAG)_n$ repeat and the two CCGG sites is PCR-amplified from the person's DNA, with or without prior digestion with *Hpa*II (*Figure 7.13*).

(a)

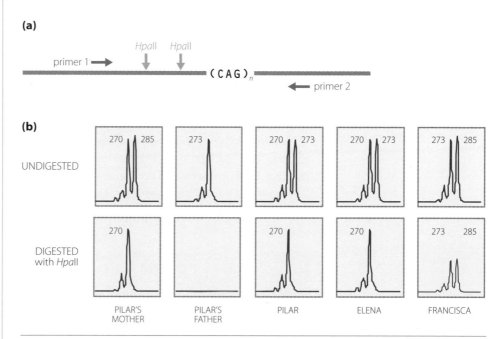

(b)

Figure 7.13 – A test for randomness of X-inactivation.
(a) The region of the androgen receptor gene on the X chromosome used in the test. The positions of the PCR primers, the trinucleotide repeat and the *Hpa*II sites are shown. (b) Results of the tests. The PCR products were sized and quantitated on a DNA sequencer.

- When the PCR is performed on a straightforward DNA sample from a woman, it amplifies the sequences from both the active and inactive X chromosomes. PCR is not affected in any way by methylation of the DNA. Assuming the woman is heterozygous for two different sized $(CAG)_n$ repeats, when the PCR product is run on a sequencer we see two equal sized peaks (*Figure 7.13b*).
- A second PCR reaction is performed on DNA that has been digested with *Hpa*II. All the PCR product will be derived from the inactive X chromosome. The unmethylated active X will have been cleaved by the *Hpa*II before the PCR procedure, preventing it from amplifying. A conventional DNA sample contains DNA from a large number of lymphocytes. If X-inactivation is random, about half the cells will have

had one X inactivated and about half will have had the other one inactivated. When the PCR product from the *Hpa*II-digested sample is run on a sequencer, we would see the same peaks as when we amplified undigested DNA, just each peak is about half size.

- If X-inactivation is non-random, one of the peaks will be selectively lost in the PCR product from the pre-digested DNA. The sequencer can quantitate the relative peak areas, and so give a precise figure for the proportion of cells that have each X active. Any female who is a carrier of X-SCID will show completely skewed X-inactivation in her lymphocytes.

This test showed that Pilar, her sister Elena and their mother had non-random X-inactivation in their lymphocytes. A chromosome giving a 270 bp PCR product was always inactivated. This was the one that Pilar and Elena had inherited from their mother. Pilar and Elena's other X gave a 273 bp PCR product (presumably the (CAG)$_n$ repeat had one more unit) and was fully digested by the *Hpa*II enzyme, showing that it was active in every lymphocyte. This came from their father. Francisca had the paternal 273 bp allele but she had inherited her mother's 285 bp allele. The *Hpa*II digest amplified both her chromosomes to approximately equal degrees, showing that in Francisca X-inactivation was random. Thus Pilar and Elena (and their mother) were carriers of the immunodeficiency, while Francisca was not. At the time this testing was done the defective gene had not been identified and though the gene had been mapped there was some uncertainty about the data. Their story is taken further in *Chapter 8*.

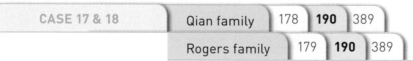

| CASE 17 & 18 | Qian family | 178 | **190** | 389 |
| | Rogers family | 179 | **190** | 389 |

Qian family
- Girl, Kai, aged 2 years, showing slow development
- Seizure
- ? Angelman syndrome
- Check for causative mutation with FISH

Rogers family
- Baby boy, Robert, born to older parents
- Floppy at birth; failed to suck
- Genetic tests in pregnancy showed normal male karyotype
- ? Prader–Willi syndrome
- Check for causative mutation with PCR

These two cases are considered together because although the symptoms of PWS and Angelman syndrome are completely different, the causes of both conditions have a great deal in common. Three-quarters of cases of each condition are caused by a deletion of chromosome 15q11–q13. It was natural to suppose that since the two syndromes are so different, the deletions causing them must also be different at the molecular level – but they are not. The deletions are caused by recombination between misaligned repeats – the same mechanism as we saw in Williams syndrome and the Di George–VCFS syndrome. The same 4 Mb stretch of DNA is normally deleted in each condition.

The breakthrough in understanding these conditions came when it was realized that the difference between them was due not to different sized deletions, but to different parental origins of the deleted chromosome. In PWS it is always the paternal chromosome 15 that is deleted, while in Angelman syndrome it is always the maternal copy. Thus imprinted genes at 15q11-q13 lie at the heart of the pathology. The cases of each syndrome that do not have a deletion have other disturbances affecting this chromosomal region (see below).

A FISH test for deletions. The deletion is sometimes just visible under the microscope (*Figure 7.14*) but it can readily be checked using FISH (see *Section 4.2*)

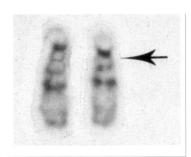

Figure 7.14 – The 15q11–q13 deletion in Prader–Willi or Angelman syndrome patients is sometimes just visible under the microscope in a standard cytogenetic preparation. In most cases a molecular test (FISH or MLPA) is needed to make the diagnosis.

or MLPA (*Section 5.2*). The array-CGH data shown in *Figure 4.8* are from a patient with PWS. This would be an expensive technique to use simply to check for the standard PWS deletion, but would be appropriate for an atypical case where there was doubt about the location or size of any deletion. In the present two cases a FISH probe for 15q11 identified a deletion in Kai Qian, confirming the diagnosis of Angelman syndrome. However, no deletion was seen in Robert Rogers, and so the provisional diagnosis of PWS still needed confirming.

A PCR test for the presence of maternal and paternal imprints. PWS is always caused by lack of a paternally imprinted copy of the 15q11–q13 region, but this can arise in various ways other than by deletion. A PCR test can be used to check directly for PWS arising through any of the possible causes (and similarly for Angelman syndrome). Certain CpG sequences within the critical region are differentially methylated on chromosomes carrying a paternal or a maternal imprint. This difference may constitute the actual functional imprint or may be a consequence of the imprints – either way it allows a reliable test for the imprinting status. DNA is treated with sodium bisulfite to convert unmethylated cytosines into uracil. The different methylation patterns in paternally and maternally imprinted DNA protect different cytosines from attack by the bisulfite. Thus the paternally and maternally imprinted copies of the same sequence are converted by the bisulfite reaction into different DNA sequences. These are then PCR-amplified using primers specific for the maternal or paternal bisulfited sequence. The two reactions give different sized products, and so can be run together in a single tube (*Figure 7.15*).

Using DNA polymorphisms to test for uniparental disomy. The PCR test showed that Robert Rogers only had the maternal imprint, which confirmed the diagnosis of PWS even though no deletion had been seen with FISH. Since FISH tests for the presence of only the one particular sequence within 15q11–q13 that was used as the probe, array-CGH could have been used for further investigation of Robert, to check sequences all across the PWS candidate region in case he had

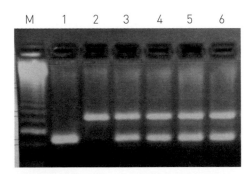

Figure 7.15 – **Using methylation-sensitive PCR to diagnose the state of imprinting of chromosome 15q11–q13.**
Chromosomes carrying a maternal imprint give a 313 bp product; those carrying a paternal imprint give a 221 bp product. Normal people show both bands (lanes 3–6); Angelman patients lack the 313 bp product (lane 1) and Prader–Willi patients lack the 221 bp product (lane 2). Lane M contains size markers. See Zeschnigk *et al.* (1997) for full details of the method. Photo. courtesy of Dr Simon Ramsden, St Mary's Hospital, Manchester.

an unusual deletion. In the present case, however, the next step was to check for uniparental disomy.

About 30% of PWS patients have two intact copies of chromosome 15, but both inherited from the mother. Uniparental disomy (UPD) can be detected by looking at the inheritance patterns of polymorphisms in the DNA of chromosome 15. Scattered in non-coding DNA all over the genome are short runs of tandemly repeated $(CA)_n$ nucleotides. The number of CA units present in one of these so-called microsatellites often varies between normal people. This number can be checked by PCR-amplifying a DNA fragment that includes the repeat and sizing it on a gel, in the same way as we checked the number of units in the $(CAG)_n$ repeat in the Huntington disease family (Ashton family, Case 1, see *Section 4.3*). The repeats used in the present investigation are not pathogenic, but serve as markers to identify the parental origin of the chromosomes. See *Chapter 9* for a fuller discussion of these DNA polymorphisms.

Figure 7.16 shows two possible results. In the first example (*Figure 7.16a*) it happens that the particular alleles in the three samples are such that we can't work out the parental origin of the marker alleles in the child. Remember that these are non-pathogenic polymorphisms that have no role in causing PWS or any other disease, so it is purely a chance matter which alleles a person happens to have. Such a result in Robert would show that he did have two copies of this particular sequence, and since this is a sequence from within the PWS critical region, it would confirm the FISH test showing that he did not have a deletion. In Robert's case the result (*Figure 7.16b*) was more informative. We see that Robert has no paternal alleles. He might be homozygous or hemizygous (having only a single copy) for the maternal allele; by itself this result is compatible with either a deletion or UPD. Because we already know there is no deletion, it demonstrates UPD. This is isodisomy, in which he has two copies of the same maternal chromosome. UPD could be confirmed by finding a similar pattern with a second chromosome 15 marker (microsatellite alleles occasionally mutate, so it is prudent to confirm any finding using a second independent microsatellite).

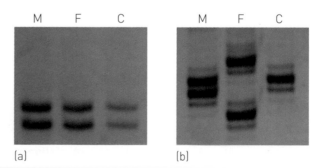

Figure 7.16 – Segregation of chromosome 15 markers in children with Prader–Willi syndrome.
M, mother; F, father; C, child. (a) In this case it is not possible to say which of the child's alleles are inherited from which parent. (b) In this example, the child does not inherit either of his father's alleles. Photo. courtesy of Dr Simon Ramsden, St Mary's Hospital, Manchester.

Robert has inherited no copy of chromosome 15 from his father. Under the microscope Robert's karyotype looks completely normal, but the microsatellite analysis shows that both his copies of chromosome 15 come from his mother. The phenotype of PWS is identical in patients with UPD or those with the more common paternal deletion, showing that PWS is caused by lack of a paternal copy of the 15q11–q13 sequence, and that lack of paternal copies of genes elsewhere on chromosome 15 has no additional effect. A few cases of non-deletion Angelman syndrome are also caused by UPD – in that case, having two paternal and no maternal copy of chromosome 15.

The origins of uniparental disomy. The UPD explains why Robert has PWS – but how does UPD arise? When the first example was reported (a child with cystic fibrosis in 1988) it was supposed that an egg that happened, through non-disjunction, to contain two copies of the relevant chromosome had, by extraordinary good luck, been fertilized by a sperm that happened, by non-disjunction, to lack any copy of that chromosome. If such a lucky coincidence were its sole cause, UPD would be vanishingly rare. In fact, though uncommon, it is seen far too frequently to be explained by such rare coincidences. A much more likely origin is through **trisomy rescue** (*Figure 7.17*). We know that every possible trisomy occurs at conception, but nearly all are incompatible with survival to term and miscarry spontaneously. But as *Figure 7.17* shows, a chance non-disjunction

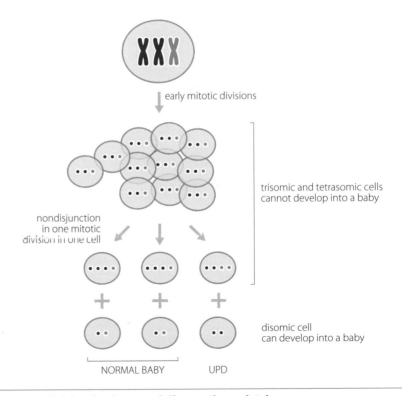

Figure 7.17 – Origin of uniparental disomy through trisomy rescue.
The initial conceptus is trisomic. A non-disjunction event in one mitotic division generates one disomic cell. If this happens very early in development that one cell is able to form the whole baby. By chance, one time in three the two copies will both be from the same parent.

in an early mitotic division of a trisomic conceptus might generate one cell with a normal chromosome count. If that happened early enough in embryogenesis, that one cell may be able to develop into a complete baby. Assuming the mitotic non-disjunction is random, one time in three the result would be UPD. Supporting this view, UPD accounts for 29% of PWS cases but only 1% of Angelman syndrome. We know that the non-disjunctions that produce trisomies usually occur in the maternal meiosis, so we would expect most trisomic conceptuses to have two maternal and one paternal contribution. Therefore trisomy rescue is far more likely to generate maternal UPD than paternal UPD. It may be significant that Robert's mother Rowena was 38 years old when Robert was conceived.

Other causes of PWS and Angelman syndrome. Deletion or UPD account for nearly all cases of PWS and most cases of Angelman syndrome (*Table 7.1*) but some have other causes. If either PWS or Angelman syndrome were the result of loss of function of one gene in the candidate region, then loss of function point mutations in the gene (on the appropriate parental chromosome) should have the same effect. The deleted region contains a number of genes, several of which show imprinted expression (*Figure 7.18*). As is usually the case with imprinted regions, some genes are expressed only from the paternal, and others only from the maternal chromosome. Checking each gene for mutations revealed point mutations in the *UBE3A* gene in around half of the non-deletion, non-UPD Angelman cases. Interestingly, this gene shows imprinted expression in brain but not in other tissues – thus imprinting can be tissue-specific.

Table 7.1 – **Causes of Prader–Willi syndrome and Angelman syndrome**

Cause	PWS	AS
Del15(q11–q13)	70% (paternal)	75% (maternal)
Uniparental disomy	29% (maternal)	1% (paternal)
Point mutation	–	10% (*UBE3A*)
Imprinting error	1%	3%

No point mutations of a single gene have been found in PWS, but studies of patients with rare small deletions have implicated the SNRPN transcript. This remarkable gene produces a huge paternal-specific transcript, at least 460 kb long that contains at least 140 exons. Only the first ten exons encode protein.

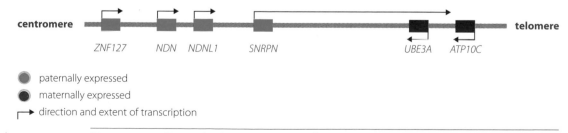

centromere   telomere

ZNF127   NDN   NDNL1   SNRPN   UBE3A   ATP10C

● paternally expressed
● maternally expressed
→ direction and extent of transcription

Figure 7.18 – **Genes in the Prader–Willi / Angelman syndrome region.**

The remaining exons are all non-coding. However, many small nucleolar RNAs (snoRNAs) are made from the RNA of *introns* from this region. These snoRNAs are required for modifying bases in ribosomal and other functional non-coding RNAs. It appears that PWS is caused by a deficiency of snoRNAs that, in turn, affects the functioning of the splicing machinery and so affects expression of other, unrelated, genes.

In a few otherwise unexplained cases of either syndrome, there seems to be a fault in the imprinting mechanism. Marker studies (as in *Figure 7.16*) show that chromosomes from both parents are present and complete, but methylation-specific PCR (as in *Figure 7.15*) shows that both carry the same parental imprint. Evidently something has gone wrong with the imprinting mechanism, so that either the paternal chromosome carries a maternal imprint, causing PWS, or vice versa, causing Angelman syndrome. These rare cases are examples of **epimutations** – mutations that change the epigenetics but not the DNA sequence. They provide valuable research material for scientists investigating the imprinting process.

7.4. **Going deeper ...**

CpG as a mutation hotspot

We have seen how sodium bisulfite converts cytosine to uracil by deamination (removal of the amino group). But cytosine in DNA also has a tendency to deaminate spontaneously. It is estimated that in every cell 100 cytosine bases lose their amino group every day. Cells have an enzyme that recognizes uracil in DNA and repairs the damage by replacing uracil with cytosine. 5-methyl cytosine also deaminates spontaneously. Deamination of 5-methyl cytosine produces thymine (*Figure 7.19*). This is a natural component of DNA, so the change is not obvious and is not always repaired. Thus CpG dinucleotides have a natural tendency to mutate to TpG. A review of the mutation databases that have been established for many diseases clearly shows that CpG sequences are hotspots for mutation.

The mutability of CpG sequences has had evolutionary consequences. Of the bases in the human genome 41% are C or G, so we might expect 4.2% (0.205×0.205) of all dinucleotides to be CpG. The observed frequency is one-fifth of this. Bulk human DNA is highly depleted of CpG sequences – they have been methylated

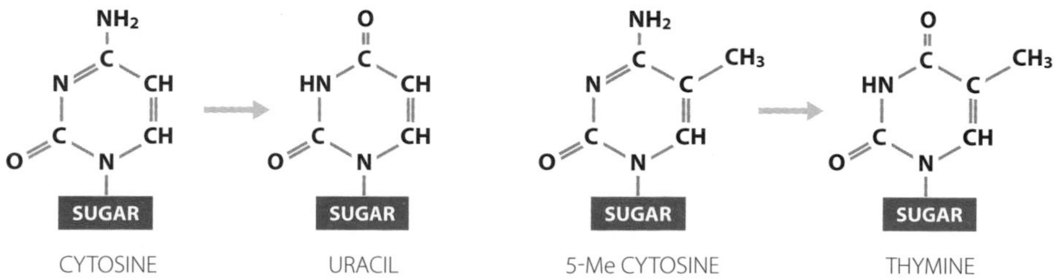

Figure 7.19 – Deamination of cytosine produces uracil, an unnatural base in DNA, but deamination of 5-methyl cytosine produces thymine.

and over evolutionary time converted to TpG by deamination. However, scattered around the genome are about 27 000 so-called **CpG islands** (the exact number depends on how an island is defined). These are stretches of DNA, normally 1 kb or less in length, where there has been no loss of CpG sequences. Presumably this is either because these sequences do not get methylated, or because they are functionally important and so natural selection ensures that they are not lost.

About 50% of human genes have a CpG island in or near the promoter region. The regulation of transcription may be different in genes that have CpG islands and those that do not. CpG islands normally remain unmethylated, regardless of whether the associated gene is active or not. They become abnormally methylated in some cancer cells, which silences the gene (see *Chapter 12*), but not in normal cells. Promoters that do not have CpG islands nevertheless do contain individual CpG dinucleotides, and reversible methylation of these is an important part of gene regulation.

X-inactivation has implications for women who carry an X:autosome translocation

Translocations can occur between the X chromosome and an autosome, just as between any two chromosomes. A woman who carries a balanced X:autosome translocation needs to inactivate one X chromosome, just like any other woman. As always, in each cell of the embryo one of the two X chromosomes is chosen at random for inactivation. If the structurally intact X is chosen for inactivation, everything goes normally. However, any cell that chooses to inactivate the translocated X runs into problems. The inactivation process starts at the X-inactivation center on the proximal long arm and moves outwards along the chromosome. It cannot reach the part of the X chromosome that has been separated by the translocation from the inactivation center. This detached portion therefore remains active. As a result, the cell will have two active copies of all X-chromosome genes distal to the translocation break. Moreover, as the wave of inactivation moves along the translocated chromosome it may not stop precisely at the X–autosome boundary. In some cases autosomal genes near the boundary are also inactivated. The overall result is to create genetic imbalances that are usually severe enough to prevent the cell contributing to further development (*Figure 7.20*). Thus as the embryo develops into a baby, all the tissues of the baby are formed by cells that happened to inactivate the structurally intact X.

A woman who carries an X:autosome translocation therefore shows completely biased X-inactivation. This may not matter, but in some cases it does. Any mutated gene on her translocated X chromosome will affect her phenotype just as it would affect a male, since this is the only active X chromosome in every cell of her body. Equally, if the translocation breakpoint happens to disrupt a gene, she will show the full phenotype associated in males with loss of function of that gene. For example, about two dozen unrelated women are known world-wide who have severe Duchenne muscular dystrophy despite having no family history of the disease. Each of these women has an X:autosome translocation. Each translocation involves a different autosomal breakpoint, but in each case the break on the X chromosome is at Xp21 and it disrupts the dystrophin gene.

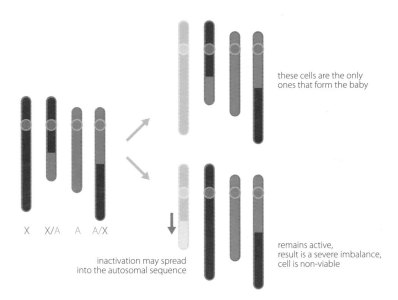

Figure 7.20 – Effect of X-inactivation in an embryo with a balanced X:autosome translocation.

these cells are the only ones that form the baby

inactivation may spread into the autosomal sequence

remains active, result is a severe imbalance, cell is non-viable

X   X/A   A   A/X

Other imprinting-related disorders

The study of imprinting-related disorders takes us into some of the most intricate and poorly understood areas of human genetics, and full accounts are well beyond the scope of this book. Apart from 15q11–q13, a number of other chromosomal regions are known to contain imprinted genes (*Table 7.2*). Like the Prader–Willi/Angelman region, these usually contain clusters of imprinted genes, some expressed only from the maternal and some only from the paternal chromosome. In PWS and Angelman syndrome loss of either the maternal or the paternal chromosome causes a specific syndrome, while having two copies of either seems to make no difference (UPD cases are phenotypically identical to deletion cases). Other imprinted regions may only show effects with loss from one parent, or may show specific dosage effects from having two copies of one parental chromosome. In all cases, various different events can cause the same disorder, as in *Table 7.1*.

Table 7.2 – Some diseases that may involve imprinting-related mechanisms

Syndrome	OMIM #	Chromosomal location	Affected gene
Prader–Willi syndrome	176270	15q11–q13	*SNRPN*
Angelman syndrome	105830	15q11–q13	*UBE3A*
Beckwith–Wiedemann syndrome	130650	11p15.5	*H19, IGF2, KCNQ1OT1*
Silver–Russell syndrome	180860	7p11.2 11p15.5	*GRB10*? *H19, IGF2*
Pseudohypoparathyroidism	103580	20q13.2	*GNAS1*
Transient neonatal diabetes mellitus	601410	6q24	*ZAC/HYMAI*

On chromosome 11p15, *hyper*methylation of the *H19–IGF2* region on the maternal chromosome causes Beckwith–Wiedemann syndrome, with fetal overgrowth, while *hypo*methylation of the same region on the paternal chromosome causes Silver–Russell syndrome, with intrauterine growth retardation.

What is the purpose of imprinting?

Several theories have been proposed to explain why imprinting should have evolved (see Wilkins and Haig, 2003). The conflict theory of imprinting suggests that, seen in 'selfish gene' terms, parents have conflicting interests. A father's genes are best propagated by his having plenty of children. If his partner dies from exhaustion, he can always grab another woman from the next cave. A woman's genes are best propagated if she takes care of herself and doesn't devote too many resources to any one child. Thus paternal genes promote fetal growth, even at the expense of the mother, while maternal genes limit the resources a fetus can take from her. This fits with the observations on hydatidiform moles and ovarian teratomas: the paternal genes promote proliferation of the placenta and membranes, which extract nutrients from the mother; maternal genes do the opposite. However, not every imprinted phenotype fits this theory – for example, we might expect babies with PWS to be small, and those with Angelman syndrome to be big, which is not the case.

How far do epigenetic effects determine individual differences?

Imprinting seems to be limited to a small number of genes – currently just a few dozen. However, epigenetic effects are essential to the everyday lives of cells. Dynamic changes in chromatin conformation allow a cell to respond to external signals, and heritable changes allow stable differentiation of tissues. Subtle changes in DNA methylation and histone modification can change the behavior of cells. As we will see in *Chapter 12*, epigenetic changes are widespread and important in cancer. How much of the many differences between individual people might also be due to epigenetic differences?

Problems in reproductive technology demonstrate that quite subtle influences early in development can have lasting epigenetic effects. There is an increased risk of Beckwith–Wiedemann syndrome and other imprinting defects among babies born by *in vitro* fertilization. The risk is not large (about 1 in 5000), but it is definitely larger than for babies conceived naturally. The abnormal circumstances of IVF conceptions are thought to somehow interfere with epigenetic programming. Imperfect epigenetic reprogramming of somatic cell nuclei is believed to be the reason why cloned mammals produced by somatic cell nuclear transfer (the technique that produced Dolly the sheep) are often abnormal (Horsthemke and Ludwig, 2005). When a cloned animal is born it is often oversized and there are high rates of neonatal death.

A controversial theory (the 'Barker hypothesis', see Barker, 1995) holds that the general balance of a person's metabolism (their tendency to obesity, hypertension, etc.) is largely determined by their nutritional status in intrauterine and early neonatal life. If true, this permanent adaptation would most probably depend on epigenetic mechanisms. The *IGF2* gene might be a key player in this process, as it has important roles in the regulation of metabolism and is known to be subject to subtle methylation effects. The Barker hypothesis has considerable implications for human genetics, because it implies that the search for susceptibility factors

Rett syndrome

Rett syndrome (OMIM 312750) is a childhood onset disorder, affecting almost exclusively females. Dr Andreas Rett, an Austrian physician, first described the disorder in 1966. Usually there is a period of normal early development followed, between 6 and 18 months, by apparent regression with loss of purposeful use of the hands and the onset of characteristic hand-wringing or other stereotypic movements. Head growth slows and over 50% develop seizures. Breathing irregularities including hyperventilation and apnea are common and eye contact is difficult to achieve. The course, severity and age of onset of the condition vary from child to child. Some girls never learn to walk or talk whilst others retain these skills to a certain extent. The condition can remain stationary for many years although complications like scoliosis occur. In later years further deterioration may lead to loss of muscle bulk, limitation of mobility and liability to chest infections.

The majority of cases of Rett syndrome are the only case in a family. However, there were a few reported cases of affected sisters, or half-sisters with the same mother, which supported the hypothesis that Rett syndrome was caused by a mutation in a gene on the X chromosome, and that it was likely to be lethal in males. Mutations in methyl-CpG-binding protein 2 gene (*MECP2*) were found in these rare families and in a large majority of girls with classic Rett syndrome. *MECP2* mutations were also found in some males with a severe neonatal encephalopathy, and indeed in occasional families with a girl with Rett syndrome, a male sibling with such a history of encephalopathy had been reported.

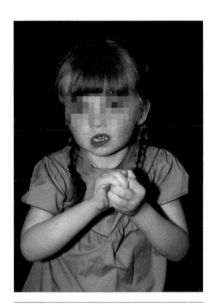

A girl with Rett syndrome, showing the characteristic hand-wringing.

The function of the MeCP2 protein in transcriptional silencing and epigenetic regulation of methylated DNA has been described above. There is a suggestion of genotype–phenotype correlation in that milder disease is observed in those with mis-sense mutations than in those with truncating mutations and in those with mutations that do not affect DNA binding. However, several individuals have been reported who have the same mutation but different phenotypes. Thus other factors such as X chromosome inactivation may influence severity. The genes regulated by MeCP2 activity are not yet all identified. It is also not understood why a period of normal development should occur.

Atypical phenotypes are described with earlier or later onset, or with milder or more severe effects and only a third of these carry an *MECP2* mutation. Some of those with early onset infantile spasms and severe phenotypes do not have *MECP2* mutations; instead they have *de novo* mis-sense mutations in another gene on the X chromosome, *CDKL5*. It has been speculated that the CDKL5 protein may be involved in regulating the phosphorylation of MeCP2. This is an example of using a phenotype to start unraveling a developmental pathway (see *Chapter 6*).

to conditions like obesity, hypertension and Type 2 diabetes should focus on epigenetic changes, rather than on DNA sequence variants, as described in *Chapter 13*.

Still more controversially, a number of epidemiological observations support the idea of *transgenerational* epigenetic effects. This is a difficult area to study. Understandably, the hypotheses being tested are novel and not very precise, and the datasets include large numbers of variables. This raises considerable problems of interpretation. Transgenerational effects down the female line are anyhow difficult to interpret because transmission of metabolic signals across the placenta could be the explanation. For effects transmitted down the male line, epigenetic transmission is a strong candidate. Examples of possible male-line transgenerational effects include:

- Historical studies from northern Sweden that show an association between the childhood food supply of the father and/or the paternal grandparents and the proband's longevity or risk of diabetic / cardiovascular mortality (Kaati *et al.*, 2002, Pembrey *et al.*, 2006).
- A contemporary UK cohort study that shows an association between paternal *onset* of smoking in mid-childhood and increased body mass index in their future sons at 9 years (Pembrey *et al.*, 2006).
- A contemporary population from Taiwan that shows an association between paternal betel nut chewing and early onset of the 'metabolic syndrome' in his offspring (Chen *et al.*, 2006). The 'metabolic syndrome' (see *Section 13.1*) includes obesity, insulin resistance, raised blood pressure and increased risk of diabetes and cardiovascular disease, so there is some overlap in the outcomes of these three transgenerational responses.

These are reasons to be skeptical. Primordial germ cells in embryos undergo extensive demethylation of their DNA, which would seem to limit their ability to transmit epigenetic marks to offspring – but the demethylation is unlikely to be complete. One has also to ask why, given that it is desirable to be adapted to one's environment, the proposed transgenerational epigenetic effects appear to adapt us to our grandparents' environment rather than our own. Supporters of epigenetic programming might reply that transgenerational effects are only a very small part of the general epigenetic programming, but because they are counter-intuitive they force us to take epigenetic explanations seriously.

7.5. References

Barker DJP (1995) Fetal origins of coronary heart disease. *Br. Med. J.* **311**: 171–174. For a hostile comment see Paneth N and Susser M (1995) Early origin of coronary heart disease (the 'Barker hypothesis') *Br. Med. J.* **310**: 411–412. *Full text of both articles is freely available at* http://bmj.bmjjournals.com.

Carrel L and Willard HF (2005) X-inactivation profile reveals extensive variability in X-linked gene expression in females. *Nature,* **434**: 400–404.

Chen TH-H, Chiu YH and Boucher BJ (2006) Transgenerational effects of betel-quid chewing on the development of the metabolic syndrome in the Keelung Community-based Integrated Screening Program. *Am. J. Clin. Nutr.* **83**: 688–692.

Hendrich D and Bickmore W (2001) Human diseases with underlying defects in chromatin structure and modification. *Hum. Mol. Genet.* **10**: 2233–2242.

Horsthemke B and Ludwig M (2005) Assisted reproduction: the epigenetic perspective. *Hum. Reprod. Update,* 11: 473–482

Jones PA and Baylin SB (2003) The fundamental role of epigenetic events in cancer. *Nature Rev. Cancer,* 3: 415–428. *This review is about cancer but the mechanisms they describe are general.*

Kaati G, Bygren LO and Edvinsson S (2002) Cardiovascular and diabetes mortality determined by nutrition during parents' and grandparents' slow growth period. *Eur. J. Hum. Genet.* **10**: 682–688.

Pembrey ME, Bygren LO, Kaati G, *et al.* (2006) Sex-specific male-line transgenerational responses in humans. *Eur. J. Hum. Genet.* **14**: 159–166.

Wilkins DF and Haig D (2003) What good is genomic imprinting: the function of parent-specific gene expression. *Nat. Rev. Genet.* 4: 359–368.

Zeschnigk M, Lich C, Buiting K, Doerfler W and Horsthemke B (1997) A single-tube PCR test for the diagnosis of Angelman and Prader-Willi syndrome based on allelic methylation differences at the *SNRPN* locus. *Eur. J. Hum. Genet.* 5: 94–98.

Useful websites

For an up-to-date source of information on imprinting and a list of imprinted genes see http://igc.otago.ac.nz

7.6. Self-assessment questions

(1) Suppose a gene on chromosome 6 is imprinted so that it is expressed only when it is inherited from the father. Complete absence of gene expression causes an unusual facial appearance. Draw a possible pedigree that you might see if a loss of function mutation in the gene is segregating in a large family.

(2) Repeat the exercise in SAQ1 assuming that imprinting is such that the gene is expressed only from the maternal chromosome.

(3) In the X-inactivation test, as performed on Pilar Portillo and her sisters (Case 16), after *Hpa*II digestion the product was boiled for 10 min so as to thoroughly destroy all traces of the restriction enzyme before adding the reagents for the PCR reaction. Why was this necessary?

(4) The diagram shows types for three DNA polymorphisms on chromosome 15 in the parents of a child. Marker A maps within the PWS / Angelman syndrome critical region; the other two markers map distal to this region. Write possible marker genotypes for their child if he has:

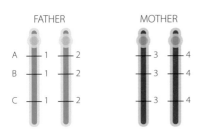

(a) PWS due to a deletion

(b) Angelman syndrome due to a deletion

(c) PWS due to uniparental disomy

(d) Angelman syndrome due to uniparental disomy

(e) PWS due to an imprinting error

(f) Angelman syndrome due to a mutation in the *UBE3A* gene

(5) Repeat exercise 4 assuming that in the paternal meiosis there was a crossover between the positions of markers A and B, and in the maternal meiosis between the positions of markers B and C. (NB this is not unrealistic – there is normally at least one crossover in each chromosome arm in each meiotic division.)

(6) Part of a DNA sequence is as follows:

```
          m                        m        m  m     m
5′   CACTGCGGCAAACAAGCACGCCTGCGCGGCCGCAGAGGCAG   3′
```

The cytosines indicated are either all methylated or all unmethylated, depending on the parental origin. The DNA is treated with sodium bisulfite and then a PCR primer is used to make a complementary strand. The primer used is off the diagram to the right. Design 10-nucleotide primers to specifically amplify the methylated and unmethylated versions of this sequence in conjunction with the downstream primer, and write out the sequence of this part of the PCR product. (Real primers would be 20–40 nucleotides long – they might need to be longer than normal PCR primers because it might be impossible to avoid some mismatches depending on which cytosines were methylated).

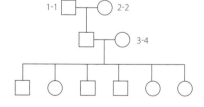

(7) The pedigree shows genotypes for a polymorphic DNA marker that is located in the Xp–Yp pseudoautosomal region. Mark in possible genotypes for all the people in the pedigree.

CHAPTER 08

How do our genes affect our metabolism, drug responses and immune system?

Learning points for this chapter

After working through this chapter you should be able to:

- Describe the basic principles of inborn errors of metabolism and give examples of diseases caused by metabolic blocks
- Give examples of individual variations in response to drugs, explaining their importance
- Discuss critically the prospects for personalized medicine based on genetic testing
- Describe the general nature and function of the major histocompatibility complex and the role of HLA matching in transplantation
- Describe in outline the genetic mechanisms underpinning our ability to mount a specific immune response against virtually any foreign antigen

8.1. Case studies

| CASE 19 | Stott family | **203** | 214 | 389 |

- Second pregnancy; scan suggests baby boy
- Baby born with ambiguous genitalia
- FISH to chromosomes
- ? Congenital adrenal hyperplasia

Sarah and Steven Stott had already had a daughter and were pleased when the scan in their second pregnancy seemed to indicate the baby was a boy. However, when the new baby was examined by the nurse soon after birth she was worried and the pediatrician was called. She explained to Sarah and Steven that the baby had ambiguous genitalia and might be a little boy with an abnormality called hypospadias, or a little girl who was virilized by an underlying hormone problem. Otherwise the baby was well, but the pediatrician arranged for urgent tests for sodium and potassium, and for chromosome analysis. Using FISH studies the cytogenetics lab. was soon able to report that the baby was chromosomally a girl, and the biochemical tests were normal. The pediatrician asked her pediatric endocrinology colleague to become involved and samples were sent off for 17-hydroxy progesterone and testosterone levels to be assessed. Samples were also sent to the molecular genetics lab. for genetic testing for congenital adrenal hyperplasia. When the results came back they indicated that this was the diagnosis, and the baby, who by then had been called Susie, had the less severe type where salt is not lost. Her levels of 17-hydroxy progesterone and testosterone

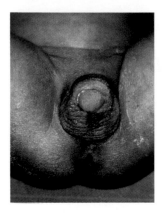

were raised and mutations had been found in both copies of Susie's *CYP21* genes. Hydrocortisone treatment was started and surgery was planned for later that year. When Sarah and Steven looked back at Susie's first week they recalled how difficult it was for them because they were very worried about the baby, couldn't tell their friends and relations whether they had had a girl or boy, and couldn't choose a name for the baby.

Figure 8.1 – Ambiguous genitalia of a baby girl with the simple virilizing form of congenital adrenal hyperplasia.

| CASE 20 | Tierney family | **204** | 215 | 312 | 389 |

- 4-year-old boy, Jason
- Pale with extensive bruising and tachycardia
- ? Acute lymphocytic leukemia

Jason is a previously fit and well 4 year old boy who presented with a two-week history of extensive bruising and a pain in his back. His mother took him to the family doctor who noted that he was pale and tachycardic (a fast heart rate) without obvious fever. Blood tests revealed a low hemoglobin level (anemia), a raised white blood cell count (90×10^9/ l, normal range $4-11 \times 10^9$/ l) and low platelet level. Analysis of the blood count showed a high level of lymphocytes. These results raised the possibility of a diagnosis of childhood acute lymphocytic leukemia.

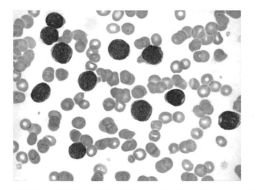

Figure 8.2 – Typical appearance of acute lymphocytic leukemia.
Small blasts with high nuclear–cytoplasmic ratio, some with prominent nucleoli.
Photo. courtesy of Dr John Yin, Manchester Royal Infirmary.

8.2. Science toolkit

In this chapter we cover three areas of genetics, all of which concern causes of genetic differences between people:

- inborn errors of metabolism
- common variation in drug responses (**pharmacogenetics**)

- the systems that enable us to mount an immune response against virtually any foreign antigen, but that also lead to transplant rejection (**immunogenetics**)

The present section and *Section 8.4* are each divided into three parts, covering these three areas.

Inborn errors of metabolism

The concept of inborn errors of metabolism was developed at the very dawn of clinical genetics (see *Box 8.1*). If a metabolic pathway requires the sequential action of several enzymes, a loss of function mutation in any one of the genes encoding those enzymes will lead to a metabolic block (*Figure 8.3*). Substrate accumulates before the block, and there is a lack of product downstream of the block.

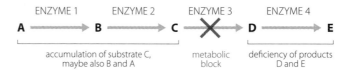

Figure 8.3 – **Effects of a metabolic block in a simple pathway.**

- In a biosynthetic pathway the most noticeable effect is likely to be the absence of the end product. For example, tyrosinase is the key enzyme for biosynthesis of melanin, and homozygous loss of function of tyrosinase causes albinism (*Figure 8.4*).
- In a degradative pathway, it is usually the accumulation of the blocked substrate that causes problems. The lysosomal storage diseases are typical examples. Lysosomes are vesicles that contain a collection of around 40 different hydrolytic enzymes that are required to degrade a variety of large molecules. Lysosomes import high molecular weight material, but can only export the low molecular weight products of degradative reactions. A deficiency of one or other of the lysosomal enzymes therefore causes undegraded or partially degraded high molecular weight material to accumulate within the lysosome. This can lead eventually to the death of the cell. Patients with lysosomal storage diseases are normal at birth, but there is a progressive deterioration as undegraded material builds up in the lysosomes. For instance, in mucopolysaccharidoses like Hunter syndrome (OMIM 309900) and Hurler syndrome (OMIM 607014), lack of one or another enzyme required for the breakdown of glycosaminoglycans (mucopolysaccharides) leads to accumulation of undegradable and unexportable high molecular weight material. *Figure 10.1* illustrates the consequences in one lysosomal storage disease, Tay–Sachs disease.
- The high concentration of substrate upstream of a block in a degradative or synthetic pathway can also lead to the production of abnormal metabolites. For example, in phenylketonuria (see **Vlasi family, Case 22** in *Chapter 11*) a block in the normal catabolic pathway for phenylalanine

leads to an accumulation of phenylalanine in the blood and tissues (*Figure 8.4*). This eventually spills over into production of phenylketones. The porphyrias are caused by accumulation of pathogenic intermediates in a blocked synthetic pathway.

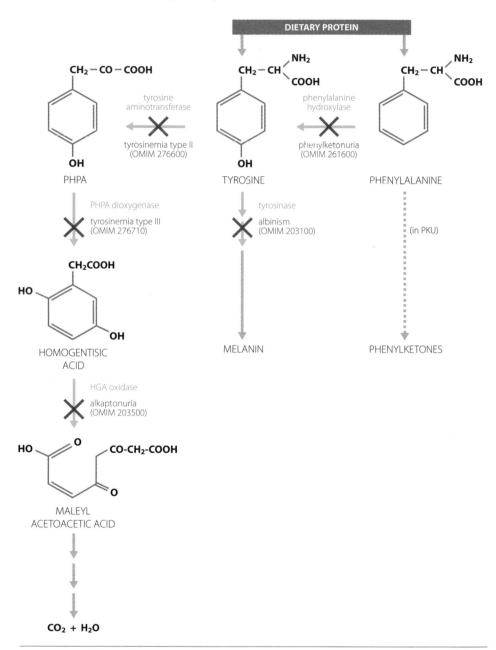

Figure 8.4 – Metabolism of the amino acids phenylalanine and tyrosine.
Consequences of a metabolic block can include absence of product (albinism), excretion of the material immediately upstream of the block (alkaptonuria), or excretion of alternative metabolites of a blocked substrate (phenylketonuria). PHPA = *p*-hydroxy phenylalanine.

BOX 8.1

Some history

The concept of *inborn errors of metabolism* goes back to the very early days of human genetics: in 1902 Archibald Garrod published a paper entitled 'The incidence of alkaptonuria: a study in chemical individuality'. Alkaptonuria (OMIM 203500 – see *Figure 8.4*) is a rare recessive condition in which affected individuals lack homogentisate 1,2-dioxygenase (also called homogentisic acid oxidase) and accordingly excrete in their urine large amounts of homogentisic acid, an intermediate in the catabolism of phenylalanine and tyrosine. This readily darkens on exposure to air, hence the name. Garrod noted that parents of patients were often first cousins, and that brothers and sisters were sometimes affected. He speculated that alkaptonuria might be a mendelian recessive condition – a remarkable insight, given that Mendel's work had only been rediscovered two years previously. In a series of lectures in 1908, Garrod coined the term 'inborn error of metabolism' and suggested cystinuria and pentosuria as further examples.

Rather like Mendel, Garrod was perhaps ahead of his time. Geneticists at the time were more concerned with understanding the basic mechanisms of heredity, and biochemists with understanding basic biological chemistry. Patients with exceedingly rare diseases were not amenable to experimental investigation. It was over 30 years later that Beadle and Tatum developed a suitable experimental system, X-ray mutagenesis and biochemical analysis of the fungus *Neurospora crassa*. Their 1941 paper 'Genetic control of biochemical reactions in *Neurospora*' does not contain the phrase associated with their names, 'one gene – one enzyme' but does say:

> It should be possible, by finding a number of mutants unable to carry out a particular step in a given synthesis, to determine whether only one gene is ordinarily concerned with the immediate regulation of a given specific chemical reaction.

Within five years, Beadle had clearly enunciated the one gene – one enzyme hypothesis and placed it at the centre of contemporary understanding of gene action. At that time neither the structure of proteins nor that of genes was known. A further seminal development was the demonstration by Ingram in 1956 of the difference between normal hemoglobin and hemoglobin S. By the early 1960s all the basic concepts of biochemical genetics were in place.

Biochemical genetics is defined more by its methods and practitioners than by anything else. During the period 1960–1990, before PCR became routine, possibilities for clinical genetic testing by DNA analysis were limited. Biochemists, however, had a sophisticated knowledge of metabolic pathways and enzymology, and they applied this to any suitable genetic condition. They used specialized tools, such as gas chromatography coupled to mass spectrometry (GC–MS), to identify abnormal metabolites in blood or urine. They ran large-scale newborn screening programs, and were closely involved in managing children in whom they diagnosed inborn errors. All this set them a little apart from mainstream clinical genetics. Nowadays the two have very much come together. The biochemists have not abandoned their GC–MS and other special technologies, but the use of DNA methods and of concepts from biochemistry and cell biology is now universal across all of clinical genetics.

Congenital adrenal hyperplasia (CAH), the condition affecting Susie Stott (Case 19), illustrates a rather more complex situation. CAH is a result of a metabolic block that prevents the production of the glucocorticoid and mineralocorticoid hormones. *Figure 8.5* shows the main synthetic pathways. All steroid synthesis starts from cholesterol. The enzymes involved are mostly members of the cytochrome P450 family of oxidative enzymes. P450 enzymes are also involved in the metabolism of many drugs, as we shall see below. Several of the enzymes act on multiple, closely related substrates and some of them catalyze more than

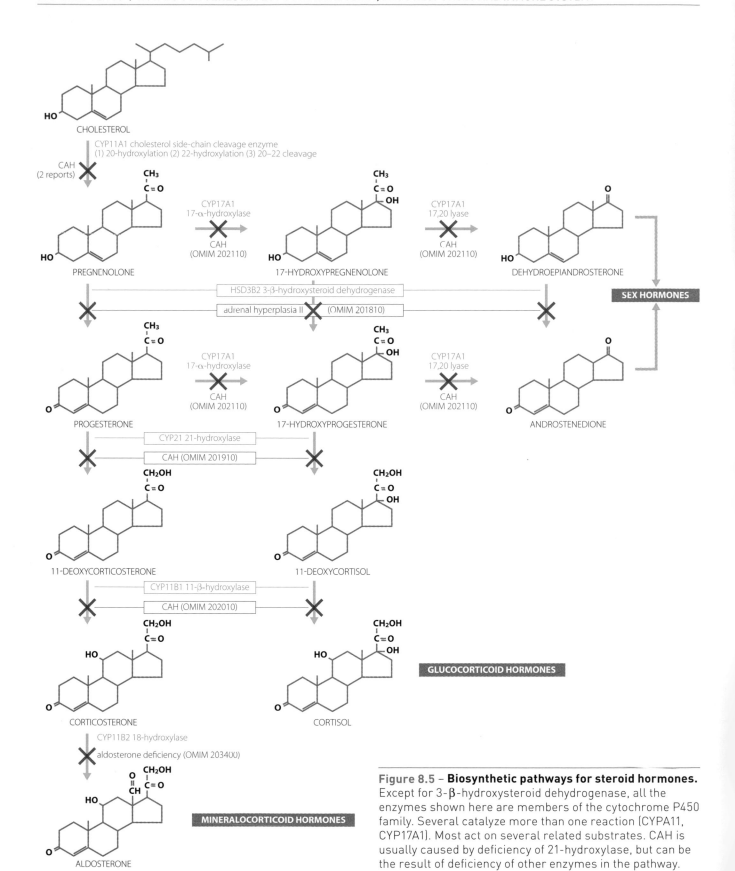

Figure 8.5 – Biosynthetic pathways for steroid hormones. Except for 3-β-hydroxysteroid dehydrogenase, all the enzymes shown here are members of the cytochrome P450 family. Several catalyze more than one reaction (CYPA11, CYP17A1). Most act on several related substrates. CAH is usually caused by deficiency of 21-hydroxylase, but can be the result of deficiency of other enzymes in the pathway.

one reaction. The result is more of a meshwork than the simple linear pathway of *Figure 8.3*.

CAH could result from failure of any of five enzymes highlighted in the figure, although 95% of cases are due to deficiency of 21-hydroxylase. In the most severe form (salt-wasting CAH) the lack of aldosterone causes episodes of life-threatening loss of salt through the kidneys. Susie is an example of the milder 'simple virilizing' form. The absence of the glucocorticoid and mineralocorticoid hormones causes increased secretion of adrenocorticotrophic hormone (ACTH) via a feedback loop, and this in turn leads to increased production of androgens. Females are virilized *in utero* to varying degrees by the excess androgens. The internal anatomy is normal female, but the external genitalia may be ambiguous, requiring plastic surgery soon after birth. A mild or attenuated form of CAH is a cause of infertility in adult females. The different pathologies are partly due to different mutations in the 21-hydroxylase gene (gene deletion or truncating mutations causing complete loss of function versus mis-sense mutations causing partial loss), or to different numbers of gene copies (see below).

As described in *Box 8.2*, mutations at the 21-hydroxylase locus often occur through interaction with an adjacent pseudogene. A practical consequence of this interesting genetic mechanism is that the mutations it produces are limited to those already present in the pseudogene. Around 75% of all mutations can be found by checking for a few specific variants already present in the pseudogene, without having to sequence all 10 exons of the gene. This was the procedure followed in the case of the Stott family (Case 19).

Deletions and gene conversions in 21-hydroxylase deficiency

BOX 8.2

Research into the genetics of 21-hydroxylase deficiency has revealed an interesting mutational mechanism. The *CYP21* gene is part of a tandemly duplicated sequence lying within the major histocompatibility complex (MHC) on chromosome 6p21. We will consider the primary functions of the MHC below, when discussing immunogenetics. Here we note that there is a 30 kb tandem duplication (see *Box figure 8.1*). The *C4A* and *C4B* genes both encode complement factor 4, but only one of the duplicated *CYP21* genes is functional. *CYP21A1P* is an inactive pseudogene. Compared to its functional counterpart *CYP21A2* it has acquired several mis-sense mutations plus splicing, frameshifting and nonsense mutations, any one of which would make it non-functional. As mentioned in *Chapter 3*, duplicate copies of genes often degenerate into pseudogenes because there is no selection against random mutations.

We have already seen how such repeated sequences are hotspots for duplication and deletion mutations through recombination between misaligned repeats (*Disease box 3*). The non-functional product has a 30 kb deletion of one C4–21OH unit. This mechanism is responsible for about 20–25% of 21-hydroxylase mutations, and also for the existence of a complex range of haplotypes in the general population, containing one or three copies of the repeat, with varying numbers of functional genes and pseudogenes. In the majority of CAH patients, however, the normal duplicated structure is still present, but the functional gene has acquired inactivating mutations identical to one or more of those present in the pseudogene. Analysis of flanking sequence variants showed that they are not recombinant. This is evidence of **gene conversion**, a process in which a short DNA sequence is replaced by one copied from, in the vast majority of cases, a highly homologous sequence in the immediate vicinity, but without recombination. Analysis of 21-hydroxylase mutations provided the first evidence that gene conversion, a mechanism well known in fungi, also occurred in mammals.

BOX 8.2 – continued

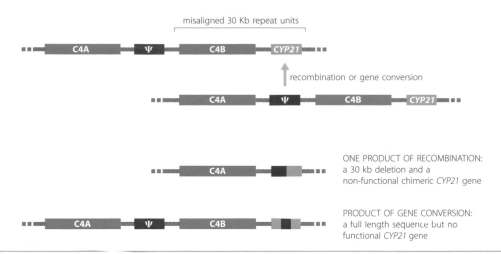

Box figure 8.1 – Most 21-hydroxylase mutations are the result of actual or abortive recombination between misaligned C4-21OH repeats. Actual recombination produces deletions and duplications; 20–25% of mutant alleles have the 30 kb deletion. Aborted recombination results in gene conversion in which part of the functional gene sequence is replaced by sequence from the pseudogene (ψ).

Although the end result is different, gene conversion is in fact a product of the recombination mechanism. As explained in *Chapter 2*, recombination does not involve two clean cuts being made in the recombining chromosomes at precisely identical places. Rather, a loose strand from the first cut invades the other partner. Subsequent events can lead either to full recombination or to replacement of a short stretch of the invaded receptor sequence by the invading donor sequence. Mismatch repair enzymes may then 'correct' any mismatches in the recipient sequence to match the donor sequence; alternatively the heteroduplex may persist until the next round of DNA replication produces one daughter cell with the full duplex donor sequence. Gene conversion is difficult to prove. It usually replaces only a very short stretch of sequence, 100 bp or so. If all the products of the conversion can be recovered and characterized, as in some fungi, the non-reciprocal nature of the exchange is apparent; otherwise the effect cannot be distinguished from close double recombination.

Pharmacogenetics

It has been known for years that many drugs work in only a proportion of the people taking them, and some may produce unwanted or dangerous effects in some people (*Table 8.1*). Adverse reactions to drugs are a serious clinical problem. It has been estimated that they are responsible for around 100 000 deaths each year in the US, while in the UK 1 in 15 hospital admissions have been attributed to this cause. Much of this individual variation in response is genetically determined. Genetic factors affect both the pharmacokinetics (the absorption, distribution, metabolism and excretion of the drug – in other words, what the body does to a drug) and the pharmacodynamics (the actual effect of the drug on its target organ, or what a drug does to the body).

Many of the most striking individual differences in response are due to large individual variations in the rate of metabolism of drugs. For a substantial proportion of all prescription drugs (maybe 25–30%) their elimination starts with an enzymic oxidation catalyzed by one of three enzymes, CYP2C9, CYP2C19 and CYP2D6. These are members of the large P450 family of enzymes that we

Table 8.1 – **Examples of drugs that produce serious side effects in some people**

Drug	Effect
Azathioprine	Life-threatening bone marrow suppression from normal dose in people with low activity thiopurine methyl transferase
Fluorouracil	Fatal nervous system toxicity from standard doses in people with deficiency of dihydropyrimidine dehydrogenase (1%)
Hydralazine	Risk of systemic lupus erythematosus in slow acetylators
Isoniazid	Risk of polyneuropathy in slow acetylators
Succinylcholine	Prolonged apnea in people with butyrylcholinesterase deficiency
Warfarin	Excessive bleeding in people with low-activity *CYP2C9* or *VKORC1*

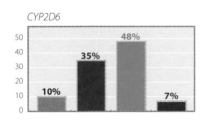

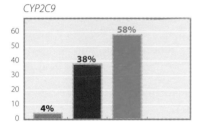

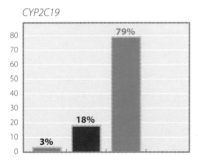

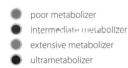

● poor metabolizer
● intermediate metabolizer
● extensive metabolizer
● ultrametabolizer

Figure 8.6 – Polymorphisms in the *CYP2D6*, *CYP2C9* and *CYP2C19* genes cause common variations in enzyme activity.
Variation is present in all populations but at different frequencies; these figures are for white people of Northern European origin and are redrawn from the data of Service (2005).

encountered when considering steroid biosynthesis. For each of these enzymes, common polymorphisms affect their activity. People can be classified as poor, intermediate, extensive and ultra-rapid metabolizers (*Figure 8.6*). The clinical effect of a given dose of drug is greater in a poor metabolizer, and much less in an ultra-rapid metabolizer because of the different rates of elimination of the drug. If a standard dose is used, ultra-rapid metabolizers may get no benefit from the drug, while poor metabolizers may suffer effects of an overdose.

Some drugs require P450 action to convert them into their active form. Codeine is converted by CYP2D6 to its active form, morphine. Poor metabolizers get no pain relief from standard doses of codeine, while ultra-rapid metabolizers are at increased risk of adverse effects such as breathing problems and sedation.

Many other enzyme systems are involved in pharmacokinetic variations. A long-standing example is the surgical muscle relaxant suxamethonium (succinylcholine). Normally its effect is short-lived because it is rapidly broken down by butyrylcholinesterase, but individuals who are homozygous for a low activity variant of the enzyme (see OMIM 177400) are unable to eliminate the drug in this way and suffer dangerously prolonged apnea. Other drugs are metabolized via acetylation, and people can be divided into fast and slow acetylators depending on the activity of *N*-acetyl transferase.

The case of the Tierney family (Case 20) concerns a variant of thiopurine methyl transferase (TPMT). This enzyme catalyzes the first step in the breakdown of the immunosuppressant drugs azathioprine and 6-mercaptopurine. These are widely used in transplantation, for treating inflammatory bowel disease and inflammatory arthritis, and for acute lymphocytic leukemia. In 1980, cases were first described of TPMT deficiency in red blood cells, and subsequent studies established that reduced red blood cell TPMT activity was associated with adverse effects of thiopurine drugs, including azathioprine and 6-mercaptopurine. About

10% of the UK population are heterozygous for a low activity allele, and 0.3% are homozygous. These people are much more sensitive than normal homozygotes to the effects of these powerful drugs. In low-activity homozygotes, normal doses can cause life-threatening bone marrow toxicity and collapse of the hemopoietic system. TPMT status can be tested either by measuring the enzyme activity or by DNA analysis of the gene.

TPMT tests do not predict all cases of neutropenia or the other side effects associated with use of these drugs. However, for the 1 in 300 individuals who are deficient in TPMT there is a very high risk of profound early onset neutropenia if treated with standard doses of thiopurine drugs. Therefore, in 2004, the US Food and Drug Administration (FDA) directed that 6-mercaptopurine should include labeling information outlining the availability of genetic and phenotypic tests to determine TPMT status. See McLeod and Siva (2002) for further discussion.

The examples above all concern pharmacokinetics, but there are also clinically significant variations in pharmacodynamics, the actual response of the target molecule or cell to the drug. Some drugs are now being deliberately designed to act only on one specific genotype, as described in *Section 8.4*. That section discusses the scope for personalized prescribing, where a drug is offered in conjunction with a genetic test.

For further discussion of genetic effects on drug performance, see the reviews by Evans and McLeod (2003), and Weinshilboum (2003).

Immunogenetics

Immunogenetics involves two main aspects:

- understanding how we can produce an apparently infinite number of different specific antibodies, in a clear exception to the one gene – one polypeptide hypothesis
- understanding how we can distinguish self from non-self, and mount an immune response against almost any foreign cell or antigen

Here we outline the genetics behind the recognition problem; the mechanisms for generating antibody diversity are outlined in *Section 8.4*. Immunogenetics is a large subject, and the treatment here is necessarily introductory. Any recent immunology textbook will go much more deeply into this fascinating area of genetics. For background and much further detail on the recognition problem as described below, a good source is Chapter 5 of *Immunobiology* by Janeway *et al.* (2001), which is available on the NCBI Bookshelf (see *References*).

As is well known, transplanted organs are rejected unless they are tissue-matched. This will turn out to be a problem for Pablo Portillo (Case 16) who needs a bone marrow transplant (see *Section 8.3*). The major determinants of rejection are antigens encoded by genes in the MHC on chromosome 6p21.3. Transplants that are fully matched at the MHC will not normally be rejected. Unfortunately, full MHC matching is seldom achievable, except between identical twins, because the MHC is the most polymorphic and variable region in the human genome.

Genes are densely packed within the MHC – the 'classical MHC' contains around 200 genes in a 4.1 Mb region; the 'extended MHC' (*Figure 8.7*) is 7.6 Mb long and contains over 400 genes – though nearly half of these are non-expressed pseudogenes. Unusually, many of the genes are functionally related. In higher organisms functionally related genes are usually scattered apparently randomly over the genome, except for some clusters of recently duplicated and diverged genes. In the MHC, however, most of the genes play some part in the immune process – although there are exceptions, such as the 21-hydroxylase gene mentioned above. Within the MHC, the key determinants of self versus non-self recognition are cell surface molecules encoded by a series of structurally related genes, the Human Leukocyte Antigen (HLA) genes.

HLA molecules are divided into Class I and Class II.

- Class I molecules are present on the surface of most nucleated cells. They consist of a heavy chain, encoded by an HLA gene, and a constant light chain, β2-microglobulin, encoded on chromosome 15. There are 26 Class I genes in the MHC, but only nine are functional. The HLA-A and HLA-B molecules are the most important Class I antigens for tissue matching. Both loci are highly polymorphic: with 511 recorded alleles, the HLA-B locus is the most polymorphic in the human genome.
- Class II antigens are found mainly on B-lymphocytes and macrophages. They consist of alpha and beta chains, both encoded within the MHC. Of the 24 Class II loci, 15 are functional. The main Class II molecules are DR, DP and DQ, and again these are highly polymorphic (in 2001 a World Health Organization committee listed 323 DRβ alleles).

Clearly there has been selection in favor of this very extensive variability. Alleles frequently differ by substantial blocks of amino acid residues, suggesting that recombination and gene conversion have both been important in generating the diversity.

HLA molecules present peptides derived from foreign proteins to T-lymphocytes. Class I molecules present endogenous antigens to CD8$^+$ T cells, while Class II

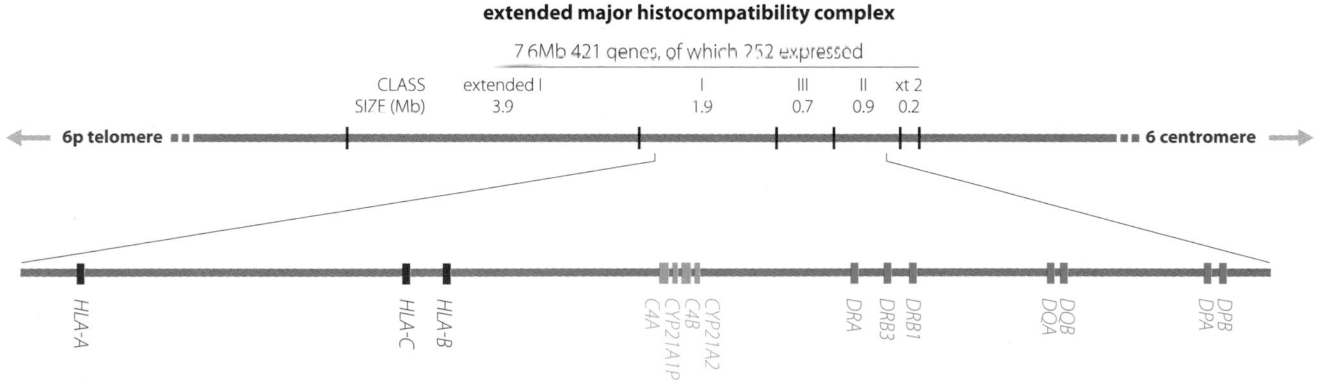

Figure 8.7 – The human MHC locus at 6p21.3 is conventionally divided into Class I, II and III regions, with extensions at either end.
The figure shows the most important genes for tissue matching, together with the C4 / 21-hydroxylase cluster. Data from Horton *et al.* (2004).

molecules present exogenous antigens to CD4$^+$ T cells. T cells initiate an immune response to either non-self peptides presented by self-HLA molecules, or cells carrying non-self-HLA molecules. T cells that respond to self peptides presented by self-HLA molecules occur but are eliminated during early development ('clonal deletion'). The response to cells carrying non-self-HLA molecules is the cause of transplant rejection. Ideally a transplant donor and recipient should be matched for both alleles at the HLA-A, -B and -DR loci (i.e. six matches). With modern immunosuppressive treatments, transplantation across mismatches is often successful, but immunosuppression brings problems of its own.

8.3 Investigations of patients

CASE 19	Stott family	203	**214**	389

- Second pregnancy; scan suggests baby boy
- Baby born with ambiguous genitalia
- FISH to chromosomes
- ? Congenital adrenal hyperplasia
- PCR testing for mutations

Molecular investigation of CAH is quite challenging. The analysis has to focus on the functional gene, *CYP21A2*, and distinguish it from the highly homologous pseudogene, *CYP21A1P*. As described in *Box 8.2*, most pathogenic changes are due to small parts of the functional gene being replaced by nearly identical sequence from the pseudogene. The analysis must also be able to identify deletions of the functional gene against a background of variable copy numbers of both the functional gene and the pseudogene in the normal population. Because the numbers of gene and pseudogene copies vary between healthy people, it is important to compare results from the patient with those from both parents, bearing in mind that a parent might have a deletion on one chromosome masked by a duplication on the other.

The functional and pseudogenes are distinguished by locus-specific PCR. A PCR primer will only work if the 3′ end nucleotide is correctly base-paired to the template sequence (see *Figure 5.6*). Thus the known sequence differences between the functional gene and the pseudogene can be exploited to design PCR assays that specifically test the functional gene for particular short sequences derived from the pseudogene. Large deletions can be characterized by Southern blotting, normally by comparing the positions and intensities of hybridizing bands in each parent and in the affected child, or MLPA (see *Section 5.2*) can be used to quantify the copy number specifically of the functional gene.

The results (*Figure 8.8*) showed that Susie Stott was a compound heterozygote for two sequence changes, both of which are characteristic of the pseudogene and must have been introduced into the functional gene by gene conversion. The *CYP21A2* gene she inherited from her father contains an 8 bp deletion in exon 3, c.332_339del. This creates a frameshift and as a result the gene is completely non-functional. From her mother Susie inherited a gene containing a single variant nucleotide in exon 4, c.518T>A. This causes the mis-sense amino acid change p.I173V. This mutant allele retains a low level of residual 21-hydroxylase activity and, because of this, Susie probably had enough residual 21-hydroxylase activity to escape the severe salt-wasting phenotype, but not enough to avoid *in utero* virilization.

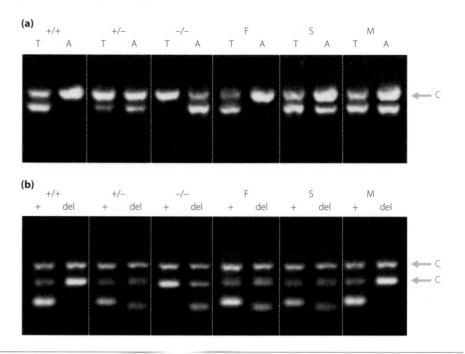

Figure 8.8 – Using locus- and allele-specific PCR to identify the 21-hydroxylase genotype.
The gels test for two variants, c.332_339del and c.518T>A, that are specific to the pseudogene, but which may be introduced into the functional gene by gene conversion. (a) Testing the functional gene for the c.518T>A mutation by allele-specific amplification of the T (left track) or A (right track) allele. (b) Testing for the c.332_339 deletion. The left track of each pair amplifies only the non-deleted allele (+); the right track amplifies only the deleted allele (del), which runs a little faster because it is smaller. In each gel the lanes marked +/+, +/– and –/– are control samples homozygous for the normal allele, heterozygous, and homozygous for the mutant allele, respectively. The lanes marked F (father), S (Susie) and M (mother) show the analysis of the Stott family. We see that Susie inherited the c.518T>A mutation from her mother and the c.332_339del mutation from her father. All bands marked C are PCR controls. Photos courtesy of Dr Simon Tobi, St Mary's Hospital, Manchester.

| CASE 20 | Tierney family | 204 | **215** | 312 | 389 |

- 4 year old boy, Jason
- Pale with extensive bruising and tachycardia
- ? Acute lymphocytic leukemia
- Bone marrow test and check diagnosis
- TPMT enzyme analysis prior to 6-mercaptopurine treatment

The blood counts on Jason raised the possibility of a diagnosis of childhood acute lymphocytic leukemia (ALL). The diagnosis of ALL was confirmed by the pediatrician at the local hospital who performed a bone marrow test, which revealed a large number of blast cells (immature lymphocytes, see *Figure 8.2*). Jason was admitted to hospital and treated with induction chemotherapy including prednisolone, vincristine, daunomycin and L-asparaginase. He responded well to this treatment and progressed to consolidation treatment with methotrexate. He was then started on maintenance treatment of 6-mercaptopurine and methotrexate, which was planned to continue for 3 years.

Prior to treatment with 6-mercaptopurine a blood sample was taken for TPMT enzyme analysis. As mentioned above, this drug causes severe adverse effects in people with low TPMT activity. Three variant alleles account for 80–95% of intermediate or low activity cases (*Table 8.2* and *Figure 8.9*).

Table 8.2 – Common low-activity thiopurine S-methyl transferase alleles

Allele	Frequency in Caucasians
TPMT*2	0.5%
TPMT*3A	5%
TPMT*3C	0.5%

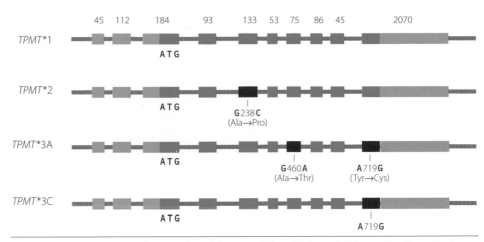

Figure 8.9 – Sequence of normal and low-activity alleles of thiopurine S-methyl transferase.
Note that the TPMT*3A sequence includes two mis-sense changes. Numbers show the size of exons in bp. Sequences in green are non-coding.

The TPMT test on Jason revealed a normal level of enzyme activity. However, after treatment started Jason suffered severe neutropenic sepsis, an infection associated with a very low neutrophil count. He was given intravenous antibiotics and supportive treatment and recovered well. The doctors noted that before he had the TPMT test he had been given a blood transfusion to correct his anemia. Because the TPMT enzyme test is performed on red blood cells, this may have provided an inaccurate measure of his TPMT status. A blood sample was therefore sent for TPMT genotyping. This revealed that Jason was homozygous for the TPMT*3A allele, predicting absent TPMT activity. He was recommended on the maintenance treatment with a reduced dose of 6-mercaptopurine and remained disease free.

| CASE 16 | Portillo family | 177 | 188 | **216** | 389 |

- Sickly boy, Pablo
- Family history of similar symptoms
- Blood tests suggest X-linked severe combined immunodeficiency
- Check that bone marrow transplantation is appropriate

In the previous chapter we saw the pedigree of this family (*Figure 7.12*). Baby Pablo has been diagnosed with SCIDX1. Bone marrow transplantation is the treatment of choice for severe immunodeficiencies such as Pablo has. At first sight an immunodeficient patient would seem an ideal choice as a transplant recipient. Pablo lacks all T-cell function and therefore cannot reject a graft. However, a problem with bone marrow transplants is graft-versus-host (GvH) disease. If the grafted bone marrow successfully reconstitutes an immune system it will recognize the host tissue as foreign and initiate an immune response that could be fatal. Good matching should reduce the risk of this. Pablo and other family members were typed for HLA-A, -B and -DR with the results shown in *Figure 8.10*.

Sibs have a 1 in 4 chance of sharing both MHC haplotypes. Unfortunately neither of Pablo's sibs Ignacio or Bonita turned out to be a perfect match. His parents, of course, each shared one haplotype with him. Transplant donor registries were searched in the hope of finding a well-matched unrelated donor, but not

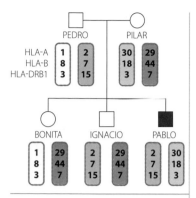

Figure 8.10 – Results of HLA typing in the Portillo family. Because the *HLA-A*, *-B* and *-DR* loci are close together on chromosome 6, they are normally inherited as a block (haplotype).

Table 8.3 – Frequencies of Portillo family alleles and haplotypes in a Spanish population

Locus	Allele	Frequency
HLA-A	1	0.095
	2	0.230
	29	0.083
	30	0.107
HLA-B	7	0.056
	8	0.052
	18	0.071
	44	0.179
HLA-DRB1	3	0.123
	7	0.179
	15	0.052

Haplotype	Observed frequency	Calculated frequency
A1-B8-DR3	0.023	0.00011
A2-B7-DR15	0.019	0.00067
A29-B44-DR7	0.051	0.00266
A30-B18-DR3	0.035	0.00093

Note that HLA genes tend to occur in particular combinations. The observed frequency of each haplotype is much greater than the product of the individual allele frequencies (shown in the Calculated frequency column). This is an example of linkage disequilibrium. See *Chapter 13* for more discussion. Data from www.allelefrequencies.net; note that the nomenclature has been simplified.

surprisingly no perfect or even good match could be found. *Table 8.3* shows the frequencies in Spaniards from Murcia of each of the alleles and of the whole haplotypes carried by Portillo family members. Even though these are among the commonest haplotypes in that population, the chance a randomly selected member of the population would have the same two haplotypes as Pablo is 1 in 1500.

Time passed, and eventually it was decided to act on his mother Pilar's offer to donate some of her own marrow. A new technique gave hope that GvH disease could be minimized. The problem is caused by T cells in the donor marrow, and in the 1980s techniques were developed to deplete human marrow of T cells. This made it, in principle, possible to restore immune function by bone marrow transplantation in patients with any form of SCID. Some T cells are inevitably present, so it is still preferable to match the transplant as well as possible, but mismatches are no longer a major problem. The method had recently become available in her regional transplant center, and so bone marrow was taken from Pilar, depleted of T cells, and infused into Pablo. However, the results were disappointing. The child acquired only low levels of T-cell function. Evidently the marrow had engrafted poorly. Despite receiving a booster transplant, again from his mother, he succumbed to a cytomegalovirus infection and died at the age of 14 months. Experience suggests that the success rate is much lower in transplants performed after about 3.5 months of age. Buckley (2004) gives an authoritative and readable review of bone marrow transplantation in SCID.

Pablo died in 1989. At that time the gene causing the family disease had not been identified. The options open to his parents, if they wanted more children and wished for prenatal testing, were limited. They could opt for fetal sexing and terminate any pregnancy where the fetus was male. Given that in half those cases the fetus would have been unaffected, this was not acceptable to Pilar or Pedro. The geneticists could use genetic markers to try to identify whether a male fetus had inherited Pilar's normal or abnormal X chromosome, as described in *Chapter 9*. A DNA sample had been banked from Pablo to help with this, or with mutation analysis once the gene had been identified. The problem was that genetic mapping of X-SCID at that time had not provided an unambiguous localization. Probably the defective gene mapped to the proximal long arm, at Xq12-q13, but there was some question over whether this was true of all cases. Thus there was a risk that an inappropriate genetic marker would be used, and a false negative result obtained. Pedro and Pilar were unwilling to take this risk, and in any case they already had two healthy children and decided not to have more; Pedro had a vasectomy.

In 1993 the faulty gene in X-SCID was identified as *IL2RG*. This encodes the gamma subunit that is part of the receptors for several different cytokines (interleukins 2, 4, 7, 9 and 15). Lack of cytokine signaling prevents development of T cells and NK cells; B cells are present but do not produce antibodies. The gene is quite small, consisting of eight exons covering 4.2 kb at location Xq13. A variety of loss of function mutations have now been described in affected males.

The DNA sample from Pablo Portillo was retrieved from the freezer and tested. A C>T substitution was found in exon 7 that converted a CGA codon for arginine 293 into a TGA stop codon (*Figure 8.11*). Note that this mutation is of a CpG sequence and is probably a result of deamination of a 5-methyl cytosine. It has been reported several times in unrelated cases, confirming that this particular CpG sequence is a mutational hotspot. Previously Pilar's sisters Francisca and Elena had been carrier-tested by checking for non-random X-inactivation (*Chapter 7*). Now they were re-contacted and offered a definitive mutation test. Both accepted. PCR-amplifying and sequencing exon 7 of the gene confirmed the X-inactivation pattern, showing that Elena was a carrier but Francisca was not. A note was made to contact Pilar's daughter Bonita and Elena's daughter when they were about 16 and could make an informed decision about carrier testing.

```
NORMAL SEQUENCE      C G G A C G A T G C C C C G A A T T C C C A C C C T G A A G
                      R   T   M   P   R   I   P   T   L   K
MUTANT SEQUENCE      C G G A C G A T G C C C T G A A T T C C C A C C C T G A A G
                      R   T   M   P   X
```

Figure 8.11 – The mutation in the *IL2RG* gene that produced X-SCID in Pablo Portillo.
X in the mutant sequence means a stop codon.

Years later another affected baby was born in a different branch of the family, and by that time there were more possibilities for treatment. This story will be taken up again in *Chapter 14*.

8.4. **Going deeper ...**

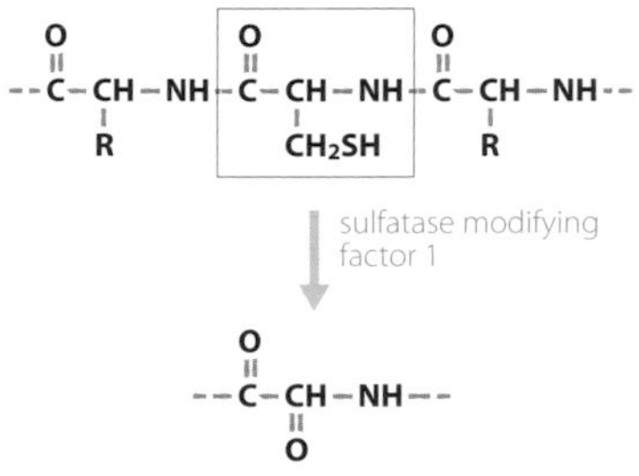

Inborn errors of metabolism

One gene – many enzymes?

The one gene – one enzyme hypothesis, though not true in all circumstances, is the essential guiding idea in biochemical genetics. How then can we explain diseases where a single gene defect results in defects in multiple enzymes? Two examples illustrate how defects in post-translational modification can cause loss of activity of multiple enzymes:

- Mucolipidosis II (OMIM 252500) patients have disproportionate dwarfism, a coarse face and mental retardation, similar to those with Hurler syndrome (OMIM 607014). Both diseases involve lysosomal enzyme defects, but whereas Hurler syndrome is caused by loss of function of one specific lysosomal enzyme, α-L-iduronidase, lysosomes in patients with ML II (also known as I-cell disease) have deficiencies of a whole range of enzymes. ML II is one of the family of carbohydrate-deficient glycoprotein diseases. Lysosomal enzymes require a specific attached carbohydrate as a signal that they should be transported to lysosomes after they are synthesized in the cell cytoplasm. In ML II this signal is defective. There is almost complete absence of lysosomal targeting, and instead most lysosomal enzymes are secreted into the bloodstream. The signal consists of *N*-acetylglucosamine-1-phosphate attached to mannose sugars that are in turn attached to the polypeptide chains of many lysosomal enzymes. The underlying defect in ML II is in a single enzyme, the transferase needed to produce the signal molecule (*GNPTAB* gene).

- Multiple sulfatase deficiency (OMIM 272200) combines the features of six mendelian diseases that are each caused by deficiency of one specific sulfatase enzyme. mRNAs for each individual enzyme appear to be produced normally. This is again a defect in post-translational processing. All the affected enzymes have an unusual amino acid, formylglycine, as part of their active site. This is produced by modifying a cysteine residue in the protein after it has been synthesized (*Figure 8.12*). Multiple sulfatase deficiency is the result of loss of function mutations in the gene encoding sulfatase-modifying factor (SUMF) I, the enzyme responsible for the modification.

Figure 8.12 – The active site of several sulfatases requires post-translational modification of cysteine to formylglycine by the SUMF enzyme. Loss of SUMF function produces multiple sulfatase deficiency.

One enzyme – one disease?

There is no neat one-to-one correspondence between enzymes and diseases. You cannot take a metabolic pathways chart and write in beside each reaction the disease that results from an inborn error in that step. To begin with, any disease that is the result of failure of a multi-step pathway could be produced by a block at any step in the pathway. Thus several inborn errors might produce the same disease. This is similar to the way that defects in many different genes can produce inherited hearing loss. Also, many enzymes are dispensable – perhaps lack of the reaction product has no obvious adverse effect, or maybe there are other ways of achieving the same function. Thus some enzyme defects would not produce a disease. Vitamin C biosynthesis provides an interesting example of this – an inborn error that all humans have, and that only manifests as disease in exceptional environments (*Box 8.3*). In other cases the result is a distinct phenotype, but one that we would not classify as a disease. Lactose intolerance is an example (*Box 8.4*). Finally, different degrees of deficiency in one enzyme may produce phenotypes that are sufficiently different to be classed as different diseases – see the example of DTDST deficiency below.

Genotype–phenotype correlations

Most inborn errors involve loss of function mutations, and as is usually the case with loss of function mutations, there is often extensive allelic heterogeneity (see *Chapter 6*). Because biochemists can measure enzyme activity quantitatively, inborn errors are a promising field for establishing genotype–phenotype correlations. We might expect a mutation that causes a partial loss of activity of an enzyme to cause a milder disease than one causing total loss.

In many cases this expectation is fulfilled. CAH illustrates this. In one study (see OMIM 201910) a complete lack of enzyme activity usually produced the salt-wasting form; a 2% residual activity produced the simple virilizing form, and 10–20% activity produced the non-classical forms. However, as in many other examples, the correlation between enzyme activity and phenotype was far from perfect. Mutations in a sulfate transporter enzyme provide another example. High molecular weight sulfated polysaccharides are important components of connective tissue, and loss of function mutations in the Diastrophic Dystrophy Sulfate Transporter (DTDST) enzyme cause skeletal dysplasias. Four different autosomal recessive skeletal dysplasia syndromes, which were distinguished on clinical grounds, turned out all to be caused by defects in DTDST. In ascending order of severity they are:

BOX 8.3

Inability to make vitamin C – a universal inborn error in humans

If you lived on the diet that your dog or cat eats, you would develop scurvy because of lack of vitamin C. How do they stay healthy despite never eating lemons? It turns out that almost all animals have the enzymes necessary to synthesize ascorbic acid, and so are not dependent on an external supply. Exceptions to this include humans and other higher primates, guinea pigs, fruit-eating bats and the red-vented bulbul bird. All these species lack the enzyme L-gulono-gamma-lactone oxidase (GULO), which catalyzes the last step of ascorbic acid biosynthesis. The human version of this gene, on chromosome 8p21, is a defective pseudogene with missing exons and other mutations, relative to the functional mouse *gulo* gene. Human cells transfected with the mouse *gulo* gene make their own ascorbic acid. Presumably the defective species all had such a fruit-rich diet that there was no selective pressure against *GULO* loss of function mutations.

D-glucuronic acid → L-gulonic acid → L-gulonolactone —**X**→ 2-keto L-gulonoloactone → L-ascorbic acid

---

Box figure 8.2 – Biosynthesis of ascorbic acid.
The final reaction is non-enzymic and occurs spontaneously. **X** indicates the metabolic block in humans.

Lactose intolerance – a common metabolic polymorphism

Most adults of Northern European origin have a dominant trait: hereditary persistence of intestinal lactase. This makes them able to tolerate a diet rich in milk. Conversely, most people in East Asia and in tropical and subtropical regions of the world shut off production of intestinal lactase in early childhood. It is quite common for people who lack intestinal lactase to suffer abdominal distension, pain, and diarrhea if they drink fresh milk. Dairy products such as cheese and yoghurt contain less lactose and cause fewer problems. Across the world the correlation with milk drinking is close – for example, certain nomadic tribes in Africa (e.g. the Bedouin, and the Beja people of Sudan) who drink fresh milk have high levels of persistence of intestinal lactase, whereas most African populations are non-persistent.

Persistence or non-persistence of lactase is not an inborn error but a common polymorphism: both states are common among normal people. The ancestral state is undoubtedly non-persistence, as found in most mammals. Evidently there has been powerful selection for the persistence variant among populations who have taken up dairy farming. This must all have happened within the last 9000 years, making it one of the strongest selective changes in recent human history.

The causative DNA variant has proved hard to identify. Recent data point to a C/T polymorphism 14 kb upstream of the start codon of the lactase gene on chromosome 2q21. In a survey of 236 individuals from four populations (Finnish, French, European American and African–American), every individual with one or more T alleles had persistent lactase, while every individual homozygous for the C allele had non-persistence. This variant is typical of the sort of variants that are likely to surface as susceptibility factors for common diseases (*Chapter 13*). Mendelian diseases are usually the result of mutations that cause major loss or gain of function of a gene, but here we have an example of a change that modifies the timing of expression of a gene without affecting the integrity of the gene product.

- multiple epiphyseal dysplasia 4 (MED4, OMIM 226900),
- diastrophic dysplasia (DTD, OMIM 222600).
- atelosteogenesis type II (AOII, OMIM 256050)
- achondrogenesis type 1B (ACG1B, OMIM 600972).

Many different mutations have been reported in the *DTDST* gene. An interesting paper by Karniski (2001) explores the relationship between enzyme activity and clinical phenotype.

Enzyme activity was measured for a series of reported mutant alleles (*Figure 8.13*). Most patients are compound heterozygotes, and it is important to remember that what matters in physiology is the overall level of activity provided by the two alleles of the gene. Grouping the mutations into zero (0), low (L) and medium (M) activity, Karniski reported the following genotypes in patients:

Disease	Observed genotypes of individual cases
MED, DTD	M/M, L/L, L/L, M/0
AOII	L/0, L/0, L/0, M/0
ACG1B	0/0, 0/0, L/L, M/0

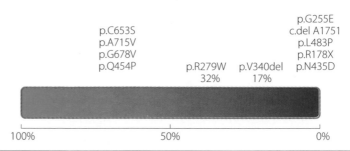

Figure 8.13 – Enzyme activity, as percentage of normal, of products of mutant *DTDST* alleles.
Data from Karniski (2001).

The general conclusion is that genotype–phenotype correlations exist, but they are usually rather loose. A paper by Scriver and Waters (1999) describes why this might be so.

Phenylketonuria (PKU, OMIM 261600) is an inborn error caused by lack of phenylalanine hydroxylase (we will meet an example in *Chapter 11*, Case 22). Phenylalanine accumulates upstream of the block, and high levels of phenylalanine damage the developing brain. Thus the major clinical problem of PKU is mental retardation. Many different mutations have been described, leading to varying degrees of loss of function. The question Scriver and Waters ask is how far a patient's IQ can be predicted from a knowledge of the mutation. The answer is, not very far, and *Figure 8.14* summarizes their arguments why this is so (their paper is recommended reading).

Pharmacogenetics

Many genetically determined differences in pharmacokinetics and pharmaco-dynamics have been known for decades, but until recently personalized prescribing has been a topic for talk rather than action. There are several reasons for this slow uptake.

A cynic might argue that drug companies would not wish to develop a genetic test for drug efficacy if its only effect was to reduce the size of the market for their drug. They would be much keener to identify the genotypes responsible for rare idiosyncratic adverse reactions – but that is an exceedingly difficult task. Pharmaceutical companies now try to design drugs so that they are not metabolized by the P450 system or other highly variable enzymes. Thus the main targets for pharmacogenetic testing would be established drugs, most of which are now out of patent protection. The industry has little incentive to develop and market tests for drugs that are not bringing in much money.

One obstacle to personalized medicine concerns the logistics of incorporating genetic testing into routine clinical practice. It puts a delay between seeing the patient and prescribing a treatment. Personalized prescribing might really take off if there were a bedside dipstick test that allowed instant genotyping. An alternative in countries with integrated healthcare systems and electronic patient records might be to perform a single once-in-a-lifetime microarray analysis of all the genes associated with major pharmacogenetic variation. Data from the analysis

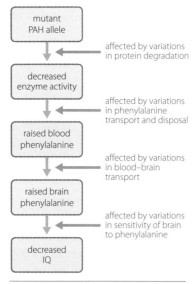

Figure 8.14 – In phenylketonuria many factors weaken the correlation between genotype and phenotype.
PAH: phenylalanine hydroxylase; This figure summarizes the arguments of Scriver and Waters (1999).

would become part of a person's standard medical record, available whenever there was a need to prescribe any drug. For some situations, for example with psychiatric drugs and cancer chemotherapy, a delay of a few days would be a price worth paying if the result was much more effective treatment. Microarray-based expression profiling of tumors is finding some application in guiding cancer treatment (see *Chapter 12*), but the core problem is the often poor genotype–phenotype correlation. Even when there is reasonable understanding of the genetics, genotypes may not be sufficiently predictive of the optimum drug and dosage to be clinically useful. The anti-coagulant warfarin is an interesting case.

Warfarin is widely prescribed to people who have coronary artery disease or venous thrombosis, especially after surgery. The therapeutic window – the range of doses that are effective and not harmful – is narrow. Too little, and the patient gets no benefit; too much and there is a risk of serious, even fatal, bleeding. The safe but effective dose varies 20-fold between individuals, and adverse effects of inadequate or excessive doses are a major cause of emergency hospital admissions, second only to those caused by problems with insulin. Warfarin targets vitamin K epoxide reductase (VKOR), an enzyme that helps maintain the level of vitamin K, an essential clotting co-factor. Breakdown of the drug depends on several P450 enzymes, especially CYP2C9. Individuals with low-activity variants of CYP2C9 and/or some variants of VKOR are at risk of serious bleeding episodes when given a standard dose of warfarin. However, many other factors also affect a person's response. These include the age of the patient, the presence of other illnesses, the concurrent use of other drugs, and variation in other genes involved in handling the drug. The right dose for a given individual is found by trial and error, with careful monitoring. Genotyping can shorten the trial and error period, but does not make accurate enough predictions to obviate the process.

This rather negative picture is changing with the development of anticancer drugs that are specifically designed to target certain tumor genotypes. Typical of these is imatinib (Gleevec® / Glivec®). As described in *Chapter 12*, tumors carry mutant genes whose action is central to the ability of the cells to evade the normal controls on proliferation. One of these, the Bcr–Abl tyrosine kinase, is characteristic of chronic myeloid leukemia (CML). It is part of the intracellular signal transduction cascades described in *Disease box 8* that relay external growth signals to the cell nucleus, but the mutant kinase stimulates the cell to grow even in the absence of the appropriate signal. Imatinib is a small molecule designed specifically to inhibit the mutant kinase, and it has revolutionized treatment of CML, being extremely effective at inducing remission.

Other drugs target different specific tumor genotypes. Trastuzumab (Herceptin®) is a monoclonal antibody against the ERBB2 receptor – it targets breast cancers that have multiple copies of the *ERBB2* gene. Gefitinib (Iressa®) and erlotinib (Tarceva®) target tumors with certain specific mutations in the *EGFR* (epidermal growth factor receptor) gene, and so on. These drugs are highly effective against tumors having the specific target genotype, and completely ineffective against similar tumors that lack the relevant variant. They are also extremely expensive. Thus in oncology, for certain tumors it is becoming routine to genotype a biopsy before deciding which drug to prescribe. If similarly targeted drugs are developed for other areas of medicine, personalized prescribing will become more common.

Immunogenetics

In *Section 8.2* we mentioned two challenging aspects of immunogenetics: how antigens are recognized as self or non-self, and how the effectively infinite diversity of antibody molecules is produced. The role of the MHC in recognition was described above; here we discuss the remarkable genetic mechanisms that underlie antibody diversity.

Antibodies are proteins (immunoglobulins, Ig) composed of heavy and light polypeptide chains. These can be assembled in various ways to produce the different classes of antibody – IgA, IgD, IgE, IgG and IgM. Each class has a specific heavy chain and a choice of κ or λ light chains. The five types of heavy chain are all encoded at the *IGH* locus on chromosome 14, and the light chains at the *IGK* or *IGL* loci on chromosomes 2 and 22, respectively. Each of these loci, however, contains a large pool of possible coding sequences (*Figure 8.15*). The C-terminal part of each Ig chain of a given class is constant, but the N-terminal part, that carries the antigen binding site, is highly variable. Mature immunoglobulin genes have a conventional multi-exon structure, with a single exon encoding the N-terminal variable region and several exons encoding the constant region. However, the exon encoding the variable region is the product of highly variable DNA rearrangements during B cell maturation.

As explained in the caption to *Figure 8.15*, the sequence encoding each variable region is made by joining a V (variable), J (joining) and (for heavy chains) D (diversity) segment, each chosen from a range of alternatives. Do not confuse this process with the splicing of exons and introns. Exons and introns are spliced in the RNA transcript by the spliceosome (*Chapter 3*). Ig genes are spliced at the DNA level specifically in B lymphocytes. The product is a multi-exon gene whose primary transcript is spliced in the usual way.

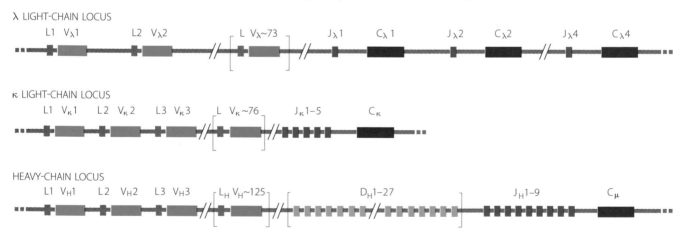

Figure 8.15 – Each type of immunoglobulin gene is assembled by DNA rearrangements that occur specifically in B lymphocytes.
In light chains one of 73 (λ) or 76 (κ) V regions is joined to one of 5–11 J regions, giving 365–836 combinations. In heavy chains one of 27 D regions is joined to one of nine J regions, and the new sequence is then joined to one of about 125 V regions, giving about 30 000 combinations. This combinatorial diversity is only one of the ways in which B cells are enabled to produce an almost infinite diversity of immunoglobulins. Redrawn from Janeway *et al.* (2001) with permission from Garland Science.

The total diversity of antibodies depends on several additional mechanisms.

- Unlike conventional genetic recombination, the specialized mechanism joining V, D and J segments adds or removes random small numbers of nucleotides at the junctions. Where the result produces a frameshift, the rearranged gene is non-functional, but in the one-third of cases where the reading frame is conserved, a whole extra layer of diversity is created.
- After gene rearrangement is complete, a process of somatic hypermutation introduces random point mutations at high frequency into the variable region of the genes in activated B cells.
- The different classes of heavy chain in IgA, IgD, IgE, IgG and IgM are made by yet another specialized recombination mechanism. Each rearranged IgH gene has at its 3′ end sequences encoding each of the five types of constant region (only the C_μ is shown in *Figure 8.15*; the others are downstream of this). Only the C sequence closest to the VDJ exon is used. Class switching occurs by an intramolecular recombination event that physically excises one or more C sequences, so that a different one lies adjacent to the VDJ sequence.
- Finally, the combination of a heavy chain and a light chain in an antibody molecule provides yet another source of combinatorial diversity.

It remains only to add that a similar generator of diversity operates on the T cell receptor genes. For more detail of all of these processes, consult an immunology textbook, such as Janeway *et al.* (2001).

RAS–MAPK syndromes

Figure 8.4 illustrated the spectrum of inborn errors of metabolism that result from blocks in phenylalanine metabolism. This *Disease box* illustrates an analogous situation in a cell signaling pathway. The RAS–MAPK (mitogen-activated protein kinase) pathway is involved in control of cell proliferation and differentiation. Errors in different components of the pathway produce a series of dysmorphic syndromes – inborn errors of development, so to speak.

The RAS–MAPK pathway (see *Box figure 8.2*) relays signals from cell surface receptors to the nucleus. Receptors for several different signals trigger conversion of proteins of the RAS family from inactive GDP-bound forms to the active RAS–GTP. Accessory proteins assist the conversion (SHP2 encoded by *PTPN11* and guanine exchange factors such as SOS1) or reverse it (GTPase

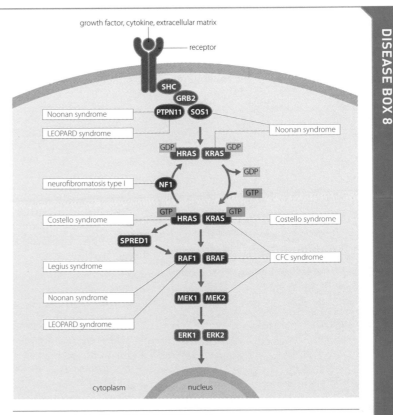

DISEASE BOX 8

Box figure 8.2 – **The RAS–MAPK pathway.**

activating proteins such as neurofibromin, the product of the *NF1* gene). The RAS–GTP proteins trigger phosphorylation and activation of BRAF. BRAF then phosphorylates MEK1 and MEK2, activating them to phosphorylate and activate ERK1 and ERK2. These latter proteins are members of the MAPK family of protein kinases that can affect gene transcription so as to promote cell proliferation or differentiation.

Excessive RAS–MAPK signaling causes hyperproliferation. Strong gain of function mutations, especially of the three Ras genes (*HRAS*, *KRAS* and *NRAS*) and of *BRAF*, are very common in tumors (see *Chapter 12*). These are always somatic mutations. Inherited mutations are usually less strongly activating and cause a spectrum of disturbances of development (see *Box table 8.1* and *Box figure 8.3*). These conditions are dominant, and are commonly the result of *de novo* mutations of paternal origin. Cells in the male germ-line that acquire such mutations may enjoy a proliferative advantage, leading to an expanded clone of mutation-bearing gametes. This effect has been well documented for gain of function mutations in fibroblast growth factor receptors, which signal through the RAS–MAPK pathway. Several of the syndromes can be caused by mutations in any one of several genes, while different mutations in the same gene can cause different syndromes.

Thinking in terms of pathways, rather than individual genes, has enabled geneticists to make sense of a previously confusing set of overlapping syndromes.

Box table 8.1 – Syndromes caused by disturbances to the RAS–MAPK signaling pathway

Syndrome	OMIM number	Genes involved	Molecular pathology and features
CFC	115150	*BRAF* *KRAS* *MEK1* *MEK2*	Mild gain of function mutations, resulting in increased RAS–MAPK signaling. Coarse facial features, heart defects, developmental disability
Costello	218040*	*HRAS*	Gain of function mutations resulting in increased RAS–MAPK signaling. Coarse facial features, severe feeding problems, failure to thrive, short stature, heart defects, developmental disability, papillomata. Increased risk of tumors
Noonan	163950	*PTPN11* *SOS1* *KRAS* *NRAS* *RAF1* *CBL*	Mild gain of function mutations resulting in increased RAS–MAPK signaling. Short stature, pectus excavatum, heart defects, downslanting palpebral fissures and ptosis. Mild learning disability
NF1	162200	*NF1*	Loss of function mutations in an inhibitor of RAS action resulting in increased RAS–MAPK signaling. Café-au-lait patches, neurofibromas of skin and nerves, Lisch nodules in the eye. Macrocephaly. May have similar facies to Noonan syndrome
Legius	611431	*SPRED1*	Loss of function mutations in a negative regulator of RAS–BRAF interaction, resulting in increased RAS–MAPK signaling. Café-au-lait patches without the other complications of NF1
LEOPARD	151100	*PTPN11* *RAF1*	Loss of function mutations, resulting in reduced RAS–MAPK signaling; the name is an acronym for the clinical features: Lentigenes, EKG conduction abnormalities, Ocular hypertelorism, Pulmonary stenosis, Abnormal genitalia, Retardation of growth, and Deafness

*Costello syndrome is dominant, despite having an OMIM number starting with 2, which would normally denote a recessive condition. Some early reports interpreted the mode of inheritance wrongly.

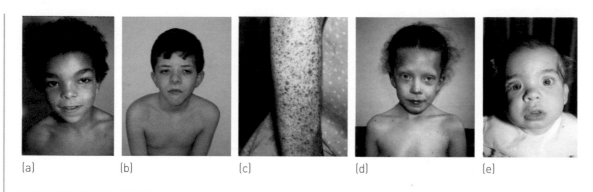

(a)　　　　(b)　　　　(c)　　　　(d)　　　　(e)

Box figure 8.3 – **Syndromes due to mutations in genes encoding proteins involved in RAS–MAPK pathway.**
(a) NF1; note café-au-lait patches and wide-spaced eyes. (b) Noonan syndrome patient with *PTPN11* mutation; note downward slanting palpebral fissures and pectus excavatum. (c) LEOPARD syndrome; arm demonstrating multiple lentigenes; patient also had deafness and EKG abnormalities. (d) CFC syndrome patient with *MEK2* mutation; note coarse hair and facial features and lentigenes. (e) Costello syndrome patient with *HRAS* mutation; note hypotonic face with coarse features and epicanthic folds. Also note bright blue eyes that are striking in many patients with syndromes of RAS–MAPK pathway.

8.5. References

Buckley RH (2004) Molecular defects in human severe combined immunodeficiency disease and approaches to immune reconstitution. *Ann. Rev. Immunol.* **22**: 625–655.

Evans WE and McLeod HL (2003) Pharmacogenomics: drug disposition, drug targets and side effects. *New Engl. J. Med.* **348**: 538–549.

Horton R, Wilming L, Rand V, *et al.* (2004) Gene map of the extended human MHC. *Nat. Rev. Genet.* **5**: 889–899.

Janeway CA, Travers P, Walport M and Shlomchik M (2001) *Immunobiology*, 5th edn. Garland Science, New York. *Available on the NCBI Bookshelf* www.ncbi.nlm.nih.gov/books.

Karniski LP (2001) Mutations in the diastrophic dysplasia sulfate transporter (DTDST) gene: correlation between sulfate transport activity and chondrodysplasia phenotype. *Hum. Molec. Genet.* **10**: 1485–1490.

McLeod HL and Siva C (2002) The thiopurine S-methyltransferase gene locus – implications for clinical pharmacogenomics. *Pharmacogenomics*, **3**: 89–98.

Scriver C and Waters PJ (1999) Monogenic traits are not simple: lessons from phenylketonuria. *Trends Genet.* **15**: 267–272. *Highly recommended reading.*

Service RF (2005) Going from genome to pill. *Science*, **308**: 1858–1860.

Weinshilboum R (2003) Inheritance and drug response. *New Engl. J. Med.* **348**: 529–537.

Useful website

Personalised medicines: hopes and realities – a report by the Royal Society 2005: www.royalsoc.ac.uk/displaypagedoc.asp?id=17570

8.6 Self-assessment questions

(1) The diagram shows the biosynthetic pathways leading from precursor A to products E and G. Enzymes E1-E5 catalyze the reactions. E1 converts 90% of A to B and 10% to

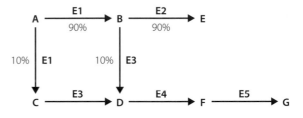

C. 90% of B is normally converted to E by E2, but 10% is converted to D by E3. Which enzyme(s) might be deficient in a condition marked by (a) deficiency of E and G, (b) deficiency of G only, and (c) deficiency of E together with a raised amount of G?

(2) Describe ways in which a mendelian condition might be the result of loss of function of several enzymes if, (a) each of several unrelated patients shows a loss of function of just one of the enzymes, different in each patient and, (b) if each patient shows loss of function of all of the enzymes.

(3) Acute intermittent porphyria is a dominant condition, yet it is estimated that 80% of people heterozygous for a pathogenic *PBGD* mutation go through their lives completely unaware of the fact, and never suffer an episode of the disease. Discuss possible reasons for this low penetrance.

(4) Discuss the case for regarding scurvy as a genetic disease. Can similar arguments be applied to other examples?

(5) Arthur, Bridget and their three children Charles, Daniel and Eliza were typed for the HLA-A, -B and -DR loci. The results (using a simplified nomenclature) were:

Arthur	A3,23;	B7,27;	DR3,4
Bridget	A2,23;	B15,27;	DR3,4
Charles	A3,23;	B15,27;	DR3,4
Daniel	A2,23;	B7,27;	DR3,4
Eliza	A2,3;	B27;	DR4

Assuming there is no recombination, so that a person's A, B and DR alleles are passed on as an unbroken haplotype, work out the haplotypes in this family.

(6) What features of the gene locus or mutational spectrum in a disease would lead you to suspect that gene conversion might be a major mutational mechanism?

09 | How do researchers identify genes for mendelian diseases?

After working through this chapter you should be able to:

- Describe the principle of genetic mapping in humans
- Identify recombinants and non-recombinants in a simple pedigree
- Describe the use of microsatellites and SNPs as genetic markers
- Describe in outline different routes by which human disease genes have been identified
- Describe the potential of whole exome or whole genome sequencing to identify disease genes
- Show how the Human Genome Project databases can be used to address clinical problems
- Show how linked markers can be used to track a disease gene through a pedigree

9.1. **Case studies**

| Dyschromatosis symmetrica hereditaria | **229** | 238 |

Although this condition (OMIM 127400) is rare and is not particularly troublesome clinically, we chose it because all the steps in the standard route for gene identification are described in a single paper in a source that is likely to be accessible to most readers (Miyamura *et al.*, 2003). Because these are real families, we have not tried to invent a clinical story.

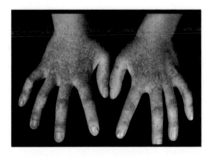 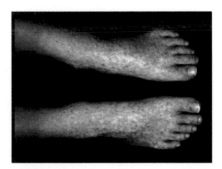

Figure 9.1 – Dyschromatosis symmetrica hereditaria
Patients with DSH have small hyperpigmented and hypopigmented macules on the backs of their hands and the dorsal surface of their feet. The abnormalities are otherwise asymptomatic and do not affect the general health of the person. The condition is autosomal dominant. Photos courtesy of Drs Tamio Suzuki and Yasushi Tomita, Nagoya University.

9.2. **Science toolkit**

Genes can be defined in two very different ways:

- as determinants of mendelian characters ('the Huntington disease gene', etc.)
- as functional units of DNA

Ultimately the two must correspond, and in this chapter we will see how corresponding pairs are identified. The Human Genome Project and related initiatives have given us a good catalog of genes as functional DNA units. For each gene we know its exact physical location, measured in base pairs of DNA from the end of a chromosome. The catalog is not perfect – genes whose product is a non-translated RNA are harder to define, and details of many protein-coding genes are incomplete. Nevertheless the current list and the associated physical map are a tremendous resource, at least for protein-coding genes.

However, knowing the human genome sequence does not in itself tell us anything about the Huntington disease gene – neither its DNA sequence nor its chromosomal location. Genes that are defined through phenotypes have to be identified using different methods. Once identified, they will almost always nowadays turn out to be genes that have already been defined as DNA units – but it is usually impossible to say in advance which functional DNA unit will be the right one. The major achievement of clinical genetics during the years 1985–2000 has been to identify the genes underlying the great majority of mendelian diseases and to make the connection between characters and DNA sequences.

There are several possible ways to identify the gene responsible for a mendelian character, including the following.

- If the amino acid sequence of the protein product is known, a cDNA sequence can be worked out by reading the genetic code table. An oligonucleotide probe can be synthesized corresponding to the sequence, and used to screen a cDNA library to isolate a clone containing the cDNA (see *Box 9.1*).
- If one member of a gene family has been shown to cause a certain disease, other members of the same family are candidates for related diseases. For example, after the fibrillin gene was shown to be mutated in Marfan syndrome (see Case 10, Johnson family) a related gene, fibrillin 2, was a good candidate for a related condition, congenital contractural arachnodactyly (OMIM 121050).
- If a gene causes a phenotype in an animal, its human homolog is a candidate for a similar human condition. *Sox10* was shown to cause the *Dominant megacolon* mutation in mice. Its human homolog *SOX10* therefore became a candidate for the similar Type IV Waardenburg syndrome (OMIM 277580) in humans.
- If a gene product is part of a developmental, regulatory or metabolic pathway, and that gene is mutated in some but not all people with a certain disease, other genes in the same pathway are candidates for the remaining cases. The RAS–MAPK pathway described in *Disease box 8*, provides several examples.

- If a disease shows genuine anticipation (that is, it becomes more severe or has earlier onset in each succeeding generation – see *Disease box 4*) then it may well be caused by an unstable expanding DNA repeat. There are techniques for checking a patient's DNA directly for such repeat expansions. If an expansion in a particular gene is found, DNA from other patients can be checked for the same expansion.

However, none of these methods is generally applicable to *any* mendelian condition. In any case, because genotype–phenotype correlations are generally poor and hard to predict, the chance of phenotype-based predictions hitting on the correct gene is not high. Before investing much effort in mutation screening, most researchers would want some extra confirmation that they are looking in the right place. This confirmation comes from mapping the character.

Thus the standard route, by which the great majority of genes underlying mendelian characters have been identified, starts with mapping the character to reveal its chromosomal location. In pre-genomic days, once the location was known it was then necessary to clone all the DNA from the candidate region, identify every gene in the region, and screen each for mutations in affected people. That approach is called **positional cloning** and was an heroic undertaking. Nowadays, in the post-genome era, everything is much easier. Having mapped the gene, a list of genes at that location is downloaded from the databases, and suitable candidates picked for mutation screening. This is often called the **positional candidate** approach.

Identifying genes through their protein product

This was the route used in some early successes at identifying disease genes. Until the late 1970s, techniques for isolating and characterizing proteins outstripped those for isolating and characterizing human DNA. Examples include:

- *The α- and β-globin genes* – these were among the earliest human genes to be cloned, based on the knowledge that most of the protein synthesis in red cell precursors was of the two globin chains. RNA isolated from these cells therefore constituted an impure preparation of globin mRNA, and could be used to screen libraries to identify matching DNA clones.

- *Factor VIII* – this gene was identified in 1984 from information about the protein it encoded. It was known that hemophilia A was caused by a lack of blood clotting Factor VIII. A sufficient quantity of Factor VIII protein was isolated from pig blood to allow a partial amino acid sequence to be obtained. This was used to predict the sequence of the mRNA encoding those parts of the protein, by reading the genetic code table in reverse. The prediction contained many ambiguities – for example, the amino acid serine could be encoded by any of six codons. At the other extreme, tryptophan and methionine each have only a single codon. A run of 15 amino acids was chosen that minimized the ambiguities, and a mix of oligonucleotides was synthesized, including all possible sequences encoding the 15 amino acids. This mix was used as a probe to find a matching sequence in a pig genomic DNA library. Having isolated the pig *F8* gene, a pig clone was used to identify the human *F8* gene by screening a human library.

Modern techniques of proteomics may once again make it practicable to identify the gene defect underlying a disease through the study of changes in the protein repertoire.

Below we consider how the genes causing human phenotypes can be mapped, and then how the correct gene can be identified within the candidate region. In *Section 9.3* we go through the stages of a real example of the positional candidate method: the identification of the gene causing DSH. But technology moves on, and the new massively parallel DNA sequencing methods (described in *Chapter 5*) are making a radically new approach possible. Rather than first mapping the gene through family studies, and then sequencing genes in the candidate region to search for mutations, it is now possible simply to sequence every exon of every gene ('whole exome sequencing'), or even the whole genome, and search directly for the causative sequence change. In this new paradigm the critical step is the data analysis, to identify which of the innumerable sequence variants present in every person's genome is the pathogenic change. This approach is discussed in *Section 9.4* and illustrated in *Disease box 9*.

Fundamentals of gene mapping

All genetic mapping depends on the behavior of chromosomes at meiosis (*Figure 2.7*). Non-homologous chromosomes assort independently. This means that alleles at loci on different chromosomes have a 50% chance of ending up in the same gamete (non-recombinant) and a 50% chance of ending up in different gametes (recombinant). Loci that are on the same chromosome will travel together unless a crossover between the paired homologous chromosomes separates them (*Figure 9.2*). They will be separated if a crossover occurs at a position between the two loci. This will happen often to widely separated loci, but only rarely to those close together. Thus the chance of recombination between two loci is a measure of the distance between them. Loci that are separated by recombination in 1% of meioses are defined as being 1 centiMorgan (cM) apart.

Genetic distances, defined in this way and measured in centiMorgans, are not the same as physical distances, measured in bp, kb or Mb of DNA. The two would correspond exactly only if the chance of a crossover were identical in every stretch of a chromosome. In fact, some regions have a higher frequency of crossovers than others. The order of loci should still be the same on genetic and physical

Figure 9.2 – Crossing over between paired homologous chromosomes in the first division of meiosis produces recombination between genetic loci.
This example shows the effects on three loci, A, B and C, of two crossovers that happen to involve three of the four chromatids. Double crossovers can involve two, three or all four strands. NR, non-recombinant for this pair of loci; R, recombinant for this pair of loci.

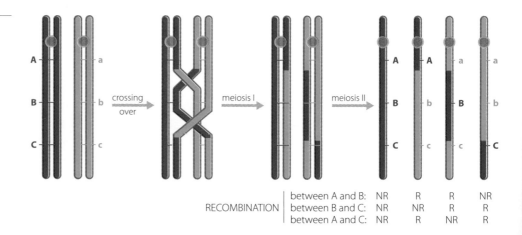

RECOMBINATION				
between A and B:	NR	R	R	NR
between B and C:	NR	NR	R	R
between A and C:	NR	R	NR	R

maps, but the spacing may be different. As a rule of thumb, 1 cM corresponds to 1 Mb – but there are considerable local variations.

Genetic mapping depends on studying two (or more) loci in a set of independent meioses and estimating the proportion of meioses where there was recombination between them. If the recombination fraction is significantly below 50%, the loci are said to be linked, and must be on the same chromosome. Unlinked loci may be on different chromosomes or may be on the same chromosome but distant from each other. Studying a series of linked loci and estimating the pairwise recombination fractions allows the loci to be arranged in order along a genetic map (*Figure 9.3*). The figure shows a breeding experiment in fruit flies, the organism in which the concepts of genetic mapping were developed by TH Morgan around 1910–

Three recessive characters were studied:

Vermilion (v)	vs. normal (red, v^+) eyes
Crossveinless (cv)	vs. normal (cv^+) wings
Cut (ct)	vs. normal (ct^+) wing border

The available fly stocks were:
red eyes, crossveinless and cut wings (v^+/v^+, cv/cv, ct/ct)
vermilion eyes, normal wings (v/v, cv^+cv^+, ct^+/ct^+)

(a) *Two lines were produced for the mapping experiment*
Triply recessive v/v, cv/cv, ct/ct with vermilion eyes, crossveinless and cut wings
Triply heterozygous, v/v^+, cv/cv^+, ct/ct^+ with an all normal phenotype

(b) *Triple heterozygotes are crossed with flies homozygous for all three recessive characters and the offspring phenotyped*
The male parent contributed the three recessive alleles, so the phenotype of each progeny fly gives a direct readout of the genotype of the maternal gamete that produced it.

(c) *For each pair of loci recombinants are identified and the recombination fraction calculated*
Gametes are recombinant if they contain a combination of alleles different from the parental combinations (v^+, cv, ct) and (v, cv^+, ct^+) – see the way the triply heterozygous females were obtained. Results were:

v	cv^+	ct^+	580	non-recombinant (*n* = 1172)
v^+	cv	ct	592	
v	cv	ct^+	45	recombinant between (v, ct) and cv loci (*n* = 85)
v^+	cv^+	ct	40	
v	cv	ct	89	recombinant between v and (cv, ct) loci (*n* = 183)
v^+	cv^+	ct^+	94	
v	cv^+	ct	3	recombinant between (v, cv) and ct loci (*n* = 8)
v^+	cv	ct^+	5	
			1448	

Note that only 276 of the 1448 gametes (19%) are recombinant. Clearly the three loci are linked.

(d) *Combining the data establishes the order and genetic distances of the loci*
The rarest class must be those that require a double recombination to produce them. This establishes that the gene order must be v – ct – cv.

Next, we count recombinants in each interval:

Between v and ct:	183 + 8	= 191/1448 = 13.2%
Between ct and cv:	85 + 8	= 93/1448 = 6.4%
Between v and cv:	183 + 85 + (2 × 8)	= 284/1448 = 19.6%

The map established by this experiment is: v – 13.2 cM – ct – 6.4 cM – cv.

Figure 9.3 – Genetic mapping in the *Drosophila* fruit fly.
Distances are genetic distances, measured in centimorgans (cM). Data from Griffiths *et al.* (1999)

1920. Experiments such as this established the methodology of genetic mapping; applying similar concepts to humans requires elaborate statistical methods.

Special problems of genetic mapping in humans

The need to use genetic markers

Human genetic mapping asks exactly the same questions as mapping in fruit flies, but the methods used have to be adapted to handle typical human families. Mapping always looks at pairs (or larger numbers) of loci. Although any meiosis may in fact involve a crossover between the two loci, we can only tell whether or not that has occurred if the person in whom the meiosis takes place is heterozygous at both loci. With the flies in *Figure 9.3* the experimenter could set up an appropriate cross. With humans we have to take families as we find them. The chance of finding families in which two diseases are segregating, so that there are double heterozygotes, is very low. Instead, we look for families in which the disease of interest is segregating, and then type them for genetic markers. Markers, for these purposes, need to have four properties:

- they must be inherited in a clean mendelian manner
- they must be sufficiently polymorphic that there is a good chance that a person, picked because they are heterozygous for the disease we are studying, is also heterozygous for the marker
- they must be reasonably easy to type, using material that family members are reasonably likely to be willing to provide
- markers must be available across the whole genome at reasonably close intervals. How close 'reasonably close' is depends on the family material available. If very large numbers of meioses can be studied, the whole genome could be tested using markers 40 cM apart. Realistic pedigree collections require markers no more than 10 cM apart. That translates to 300–500 markers, spread across the genome.

In the past, attempts were made to use blood groups, protein electrophoretic variants and tissue types as markers, but each failed one or more of the criteria listed. Only DNA polymorphisms can satisfy the requirements. Two types of polymorphisms are generally used (*Figure 9.4*).

- **Microsatellites** are short tandem repeats (for example, $(CA)_n$ sequences) that are present in everybody at the same specific chromosomal locations, but where the number of repeat units varies from person to person.

Figure 9.4 – Common types of DNA polymorphism.
(a) A $(CA)_n$ microsatellite, (b) an A/C SNP, (c) a C/T SNP that causes an RFLP (in this case loss of an *Eco*RI site by a CpG→TpG change). *Eco*RI recognizes the sequence GAATTC.

(a)
```
ctctcacagt agccacacac acaccgctgc acagcggcct                    n=5
ctctcacagt agccacacac acacaccgct gcacagcggc ct                 n=6
ctctcacagt agccacacac acacacaccg ctgcacagcg gcct               n=7
```

(b)
```
tttttttg tttcccttcc atgggtgata ttgcttcttg aaatacggac           A
tttttttg tttcccttcc atgggtgatc ttgcttcttg aaatacggac           C
```

(c)
```
tgcacagtga tgtggaattc gaaagctgac tgca                  EcoRI site present
tgcacagtga tgtggaattt gaaagctgac tgca                  EcoRI site absent
```

The early phases of the Human Genome Project were largely devoted to identifying and mapping suitable microsatellites from among 150 000 present in the human genome. They are genotyped by PCR-amplifying a segment of DNA containing the microsatellite and determining its size by gel electrophoresis (often using fluorescent labeling and a DNA sequencing machine). They have the advantage of having many possible alleles (that is, people might have 5, 6, 7 ..., etc. repeats), increasing the likelihood that a meiosis will be informative.

- **Single nucleotide polymorphisms** are less informative, because there are almost always only two alternative nucleotides at a polymorphic site. However, they are abundant (almost 15 million are cataloged in the dbSNP database, see *References*) and they can be typed by techniques that avoid gel electrophoresis. This is important because it allows various very high throughput techniques to be used, such as microarrays ('SNP-chips'). Some SNPs create or abolish a recognition site for a restriction enzyme, thus creating a **restriction fragment length polymorphism (RFLP)**. RFLPs were the original DNA markers, superseded by microsatellites for general mapping, but still useful because they are easy and convenient to type in a small laboratory.

All DNA polymorphisms have one big advantage as genetic markers: they can easily be located to a specific chromosomal region. Originally this was done by FISH (see *Section 4.2*) or related methods; now it can be done simply by searching the genome database for the location of adjacent unique sequences. Thus genetic mapping now has available a dense framework of markers, all mapped relative to one another and in defined chromosomal locations.

Recognizing recombinants

Figure 9.5 shows a pedigree where recombinants and non-recombinants can be counted unambiguously. A dominant disease is segregating in this family, and individuals have been typed for a DNA polymorphism that has alleles 1, 2, 3 and 4. Recombination between the disease and marker loci might have occurred in any meiosis in the pedigree, but we can only detect it in the offspring of the doubly heterozygous individual II–2. She received marker allele 2 with the disease gene from her mother and marker allele 4 with the normal allele at the disease locus from her father. Offspring who inherit either of those combinations are non-recombinant; those who inherit disease + 4, or normal + 2, are recombinant. There are two recombinants in ten meioses.

If we had DNA from only the lower two generations of the family in *Figure 9.5* (the grandparents were dead, or declined to give DNA) we could not tell which of

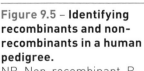

Figure 9.5 – Identifying recombinants and non-recombinants in a human pedigree.
NR, Non-recombinant. R, recombinant. See text for full details.

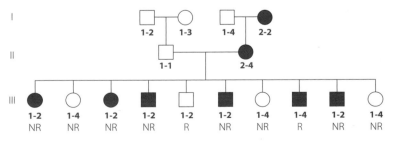

the offspring in the bottom generation were recombinant and which were non-recombinant. We would know there were two of one type and eight of the other, and we might guess that the two were probably recombinant, but we would not know. Individual II–2 might have inherited marker allele 4 with the disease, in which case there would be eight recombinants and only two non-recombinants. If we are collecting families with an uncommon genetic disease, we cannot restrict ourselves to families with the ideal structure of *Figure 9.5*. We will probably end up relying on families whose structure does not allow recombinants to be identified unambiguously.

To get round this problem, human gene mapping relies on computer programs that don't try to identify individual recombinants, but instead calculate the likelihood of the overall pedigree data, on the alternative assumptions that the two loci are linked (with a specified recombination fraction) or not linked. The ratio of the two likelihoods provides evidence for or against linkage. If the likelihood ratio supports linkage, the most likely recombination fraction is the one that gives the most favorable likelihood ratio. The output statistic from this analysis is the logarithm of the likelihood ratio, which is known as the **lod score**. The reasons for using this statistic, and its properties, are explained briefly in Strachan and Read (2010), or in detail in Ott (1999).

Getting enough meioses

Even in the most favorable circumstances – an ideally structured pedigree with no recombinants – a minimum of ten meioses is needed to provide statistically significant evidence of linkage. If we want to map a disease, we have to take the families as we find them. The structure is seldom ideal; vital people may be homozygous for the marker (remember we can only score doubly heterozygous meioses) and there will probably be some recombinants. Because of these factors, linkage analysis will seldom be successful with fewer than 20 meioses. This usually means that several families must be combined. It is then very important to be sure that they really do all have the same disease, caused by mutation at the same locus. Locus heterogeneity is a serious obstacle.

Protocol for a linkage trawl

A typical mapping project would start with collecting families where the disease of interest is segregating. Excellent clinical input at this stage is crucial to success. It is imperative to get the diagnosis right, to be confident that all the families really do have the same disease and that people are correctly classified as affected or unaffected. When diseases show variable expression (see *Disease box 1*), this can be a demanding task. Having ascertained the families, affected and unaffected family members must be persuaded to give a sample, usually blood, for the research. Fortunately, many people in families where a genetic disease is segregating are keen to help research, but there is no place for compulsion. Unlike fruit flies, individuals have every right to refuse.

DNA is extracted in the laboratory, and then the samples are genotyped for markers spaced across the genome. Over the years this has become much easier. Once it was a massive undertaking using Southern blots and taking years; in the project described in *Section 9.3* it was completed in a few weeks using a panel of microsatellite markers; now each sample can be genotyped for 500 000 or more SNPs in a single operation using a high-density microarray (a SNP chip). For each marker, the genotypes must be aligned to the pedigrees and checked for co-segregation with the disease under study. This is done using computer programs to calculate the lod scores. *Table 9.1* shows a real example.

As mentioned above, the statistical test of linkage is the lod score. This is the *log*arithm of the *odd*s of linkage (at a stated recombination fraction) compared to non-linkage. The essential points about lod scores are:

- each lod score refers to a specific recombination fraction; for each marker it is usual for the computer to calculate a table of lod scores for a series of possible recombination fractions (see *Table 9.1*)
- a lod score of +3 is the threshold of statistical significance ($P=0.05$).
- higher lod scores are stronger evidence of linkage; the lod score is logarithmic, so a lod score of 4 is ten times as good as a lod score of 3
- a lod score below –2 is significant evidence against linkage at the stated recombination fraction

The endgame: testing candidate genes for mutations

Once a reasonably small candidate region has been defined by linkage analysis, a list is drawn up of all the genes within the region. Once, this meant several years of work by a team of skilled postdoctoral researchers to discover the genes; now a suitable list can be downloaded from the Human Genome Project database (though it must be borne in mind that the list may be incomplete). Genes are prioritized for mutation testing on several criteria.

- **Function** – does available information on the gene function make it seem a likely candidate for this particular disease? Bear in mind, though, that the relation between biochemical function and disease symptoms is often very far from obvious. For example, the *FMR1* gene encodes an RNA-binding protein; loss of function mutations cause Fragile-X syndrome (OMIM 309550, see *Case 12*, the Lipton family in *Chapter 4*), the main features of which are mental retardation, a characteristic face and macro-orchidism.
- **Pattern of expression** – is the gene expressed in the tissues that are affected by the disease? Data on expression are available from analyses of cDNA libraries. A cDNA library prepared from a given tissue will contain only cDNAs of genes that are expressed in that tissue.
- **Other related genes** – are there related genes elsewhere in the genome, and if so, are any of them known to be mutated in a similar disease?
- **Animal models** – is there an animal mutant known for this gene, and if so is the phenotype appropriate? We would not look for an exact correspondence, but there should at least be points of resemblance.
- **Size and complexity** – all other things being equal, it is much easier to test a gene with two exons than one with 67.

Having established a prioritized list, each gene in turn is scanned for mutations in a panel of unrelated affected individuals – preferably those whose disease is known to map to the candidate location. Any of the techniques described in *Section 5.2* (*Methods for scanning a gene for any sequence change*) could be used, but the usual approach would be to sequence every exon. This is still not a completely routine task – not every exon of every gene is correctly represented in the databases, and some mutations are deep within introns, or otherwise hard to spot. However, barring ill luck, the whole process might take one scientist a few months. Nowadays collecting the necessary families and samples is the most difficult part of the work.

For loss of function diseases, it is reasonable to hope to find a diversity of nonsense, splicing and frameshift mutations in different unrelated people. Such a finding would unambiguously identify the gene as the correct one. If only one change is found, but in several unrelated affected people (as often happens with gain of function diseases), it will be important to check that this is not a common non-pathogenic polymorphism. That is done by typing a suitably large number of healthy controls from the same ethnic background. Final confirmation that the correct gene has been identified might come from constructing an animal model, using the techniques of targeted knockouts or RNA interference (Bantounas *et al.*, 2004; Iredale, 1999).

9.3 Investigations of patients

Dyschromatosis symmetrica hereditaria | 229 | **238**

Several Japanese families were ascertained in which this condition was segregating, and many family members donated blood for DNA extraction (*Figure 9.6*). DNA samples from three families were typed for 343 microsatellite markers spaced across the genome and lod scores were calculated. Most of the markers gave negative lod scores, but a series of adjacent markers on chromosome 1 gave the lod scores shown in *Table 9.1*.

Things to note about this table include:

*   Some of the lod scores are well above 3, showing strong evidence of linkage.
*   The fact that the lod score at zero recombination is minus infinity for every marker, means that with every marker there are some recombinants between the marker and the disease. In other words, none of the markers is extremely close to the disease locus.
*   The markers are shown in chromosomal order. The lod scores are much stronger for markers in the center of the table than those at the top and bottom. This implies that the disease locus is somewhere in the middle part of the region covered by these markers.
*   Don't try to read too much into the exact value of a strongly positive lod score. The lod score for one marker may be lower than that for an adjacent marker because one or two individuals happened to be homozygous for one marker and not for the other. Homozygous individuals contribute no information to the mapping process, so the lod score is lower. But the overall pattern shows strong support for linkage to markers in the central part of the region covered.

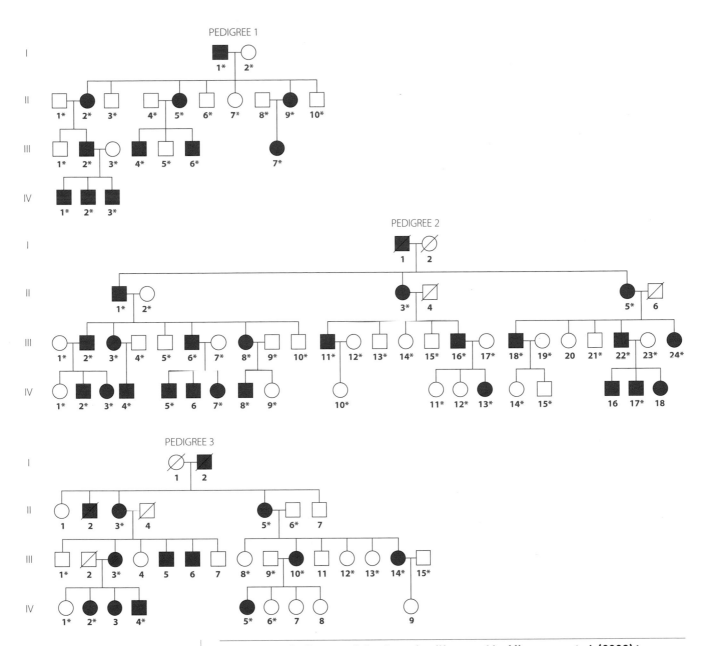

Figure 9.6 – Pedigrees of the three families used by Miyamura *et al.* (2003) to map the dyschromatosis gene.
Individuals marked with asterisks provided DNA samples. Adapted from Miyamura *et al.* (2003) with permission from Elsevier.

The markers shown in *Table 9.1* span a genetic distance of just over 60 cM on the long arm of chromosome 1. To narrow this down, the families were genotyped for a new set of closely spaced microsatellites across the candidate region. *Figure 9.7* shows the crucial parts of the data for *D1S498* and 11 new microsatellites that map in the 13 cM gap between *D1S498* and *D1S484*. For the 12 microsatellite markers in the figure, the different alleles are given arbitrary numbers, and the genotypes of seven individuals are shown, each as two haplotypes. The haplotypes are deduced by typing the parents. Rather than calculate lod scores (irrelevant

Table 9.1 – Linkage analysis in the families shown in *Figure 9.6*

Marker	LOD at θ =:						
	0	**0.05**	**0.1**	**0.15**	**0.2**	**0.3**	**0.4**
D1S424	–inf.	0.17	1.15	1.51	1.59	1.30	0.66
D1S206	–inf.	–1.21	0.56	1.29	1.59	1.51	0.90
D1S502	–inf.	3.81	4.88	5.02	4.75	3.51	1.68
D1S252	–inf.	5.46	5.96	5.78	5.29	3.77	1.79
D1S498	–inf.	4.49	4.43	4.09	3.62	2.42	1.06
D1S484	–inf.	1.80	2.99	3.34	3.31	2.62	1.42
D1S196	–inf.	–0.76	0.46	0.99	1.21	1.17	0.72
D1S218	–inf.	–7.17	–4.03	–2.40	–1.41	–0.36	0.02

The table shows lod scores calculated by computer for a series of microsatellite markers from the long arm of chromosome 1. θ symbolizes the recombination fraction. See text for discussion.

The microsatellites are named according to a standard scheme (D = DNA segment, 1 = on chromosome 1; S = single copy; the number just records the order in which each marker was first described).

Adapted from Miyamura *et al.* (2003) with permission from Elsevier.

since at this stage they knew that this region was linked to the disease locus), the researchers used the haplotypes to pinpoint individual recombinations.

In a given family, most affected people had inherited the same complete haplotype of markers with the disease gene – that is, in the meiosis in the parent who transmitted the disease gene to that individual, that region of chromosome had not been disrupted by any crossover. Most affected people in Family 1 had the haplotype shown in green in individual 1-I1 on his disease-related chromosome (*Figure 9.7*). Similarly in Family 2 most had the blue haplotype, and in Family 3 most had the yellow haplotype on their disease–bearing chromosome. However, several individuals had recombinant haplotypes, indicated in *Figure 9.7* by the part-colored boxes. Because these individuals were affected, they must have inherited the disease gene. This therefore had to be located within the colored segment of their recombinant haplotype, or in the immediately adjacent gap. Thus individual IV–3 in Family 1 tells us that the disease locus must lie above marker *D1S2777*. (Although *D1S2715* is the lowermost marker in the colored part of the haplotype, the disease gene might lie between this and the next marker down – but not at or below *D1S2777*.) Individual IV–4 in Family 3 tells us it must lie below marker *D1S2715* (in the yellow segment of the chromosome). Therefore it must actually lie between these two markers. The other recombinant individuals are consistent with this localization.

This analysis narrowed down the candidate region to just 500 kb at chromosomal location 1q21.3. A genome browser program was used to check this region in

INDIVIDUAL	family 1				family 2						family 3			
	1-I1		1-IV3		2-II1		2-IV4		2-IV5		3-III3		3-IV4	
D1S498	5	2	5	4	2	3	2	2	2	5	3	2	2	4
D1S2347	1	4	1	1	4	1	4	1	4	1	1	3	3	1
D1S2345	4	4	4	8	7	2	7	1	2	1	2	2	2	1
D1S2858	2	1	2	2	1	1	1	2	1	2	2	2	2	2
D1S305	6	6	6	7	6	5	6	1	6	6	6	8	8	2
D1S2715	5	6	5	5	1	1	1	5	1	3	6	3	3	1
D1S2777	1	4	4	3	3	3	3	3	3	3	5	3	5	3
D1S2624	3	3	3	3	5	1	4	3	5	1	4	2	4	4
D1S506	6	6	5	4	5	5	5	4	5	5	5	2	5	5
D1S2635	7	8	8	8	7	8	8	7	7	7	7	7	7	8
D1S2771	3	1	1	1	1	1	1	3	1	1	1	1	1	3
D1S2707	6	2	2	6	4	6	2	6	4	6	5	6	5	2

Figure 9.7 – Haplotypes of seven individuals from the three pedigrees in *Figure 9.6*.
See text for discussion. Reproduced from Miyamura *et al.* (2003) with permission from Elsevier.

the Human Genome Project database. Only seven genes were listed in the region. DNA from affected individuals in each pedigree (and another unrelated individual with the same disease) was then scanned for mutations in each gene. Single strand conformation polymorphisms (SSCP, see *Figures 5.8b* and *5.12*) were used to check each exon of each gene. Changes were found in each sample in one of the genes, *DSRAD* (double-stranded RNA-specific adenosine deaminase). Within a family, each affected person had the same change, but they were different between families, and not all in the same exon (exons 2, 10, 10 and 15 in the four unrelated cases).

It remained to be proven that the changes detected were the true pathogenic mutations. Pointers to this were as follows.

- Two of the four mutations were nonsense mutations, which are unlikely to be common polymorphic variants.
- The other two mutations were both mis-sense mutations involving amino acids that were completely conserved in the corresponding protein in 11 different animal species surveyed. Such conservation implies that these amino acids have important functions, so the mutations are unlikely to be common polymorphisms.
- DNA from 116 unrelated normally pigmented Japanese adults was tested for each mutation; none was found. Again, this argues against them being non-pathogenic polymorphisms.

Surprisingly, when the *DSRAD* gene was knocked out in mice, the result was an embryonic lethal, even in heterozygotes. Although unexpected, this does not disprove the identification of *DSRAD* as the dyschromatosis gene. Although the similarities between mice and humans greatly outweigh the differences, there are differences. These are especially likely to be seen where an effect is due to haploinsufficiency (where a 50% level of gene activity is not enough for normal function), as here. Note also that none of the research described shows why a 50% reduction in the activity of this gene should cause pigmentary abnormalities of the skin of just the hands and feet. Often identifying the gene is just the start of research into what it does.

| CASE 3 | Choudhary family | 3 | 9 | 66 | **242** | 262 | 389 |

- Girl (Nasreen) aged 8 months, parents Aadnan and Mumtaz
- Deaf
- Parents are first cousins
- Pedigree suggests autosomal recessive deafness

When we last met this family (*Chapter 3*), it was still only a hypothesis that Nasreen's deafness was autosomal recessive, or even that it was genetic at all, since there are so many different causes of hearing impairment. The fact that she had two affected uncles, and that all were offspring of consanguineous marriages, strengthened the case for it being autosomal recessive, but the only way to prove it would be to demonstrate a mutation. As described in *Chapter 3*, this is difficult because mutations in at least 50 different genes can cause autosomal recessive hearing impairment.

Although any one of over 50 genes might be responsible, in most populations mutations in one gene, *GJB2*, are by far the most common cause. This gene encodes the connexin 26 protein that forms gap junctions between cells in the inner ear. These are important for recycling potassium ions, which enter the hair cells when they fire in response to sound. *GJB2* is a very simple gene, having just two exons, and all the coding sequence is in exon 2. In specific populations particular mutations are common, for example, c.35delG in Europeans (see *Figure 6.2*) and c.235delC in Chinese. It is simple to test for the commonest mutations in the patient's ethnic group, and reasonably simple to sequence the whole small gene, so this test is often performed. It provides a definite answer in up to half of all cases. However, a negative result leaves the investigation no further forward.

The whole *GJB2* coding sequence was sequenced in Nasreen's DNA, but no mutation was found in either copy. Normally this would be the end of the story, but in this case the geneticist decided to try harder. Partly this was because the family were particularly keen to know the cause of Nasreen's hearing loss. Partly it was because she wanted to be able to give better recurrence risks to Nasreen's uncle Waleed and aunt Benazir (see *Figure 1.9* for the pedigree) who, as explained in *Chapter 1*, were planning to marry. Partly it was because the family structure allowed further investigation.

On the assumption that Nasreen, Waleed and his brother Mohammed all had the same autosomal recessive hearing loss, it was likely that one or other of Nasreen's great-great-grandparents had carried a mutation in heterozygous form, and that the three deaf individuals had each inherited two copies of that original mutant gene as a result of the consanguinity in the family. If they did indeed all have two copies of that ancestral chromosome segment, they should all be homozygous for the same set of marker alleles on the chromosomal region immediately surrounding the mutant gene. That would be something quite unlikely to happen just by chance. Searching for such shared regions of homozygosity in inbred families is known as **autozygosity mapping** (autozygosity means homozygosity by descent from a defined common ancestor). High resolution SNP chips provide a convenient tool for autozygosity mapping. As shown in *Figure 9.8*, samples from Nasreen, Waleed, Mohammed and two unaffected sibs were genotyped on SNP arrays, revealing a shared region of autozygosity at chromosome 3p21. The Hereditary Hearing Loss Homepage (see *Section 9.5*) provides lists of the locations of all known genes causing hearing loss. This showed that the *DFNB6* locus (OMIM 600971) mapped to the appropriate location.

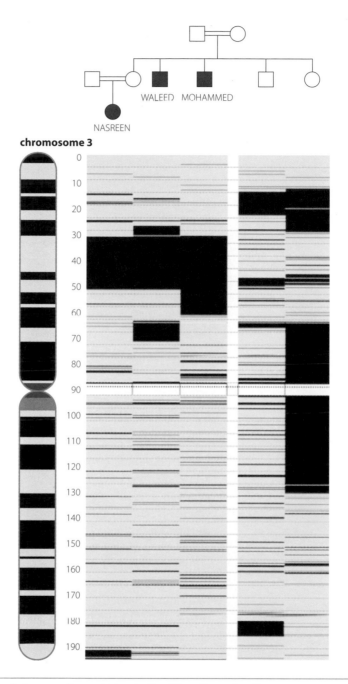

Figure 9.8 – Autozygosity mapping in the Choudhary family.
The three blacked-in individuals have profound hearing loss, presumed to be autosomal recessive (see *Figure 1.9*). DNA from these three and two unaffected sibs was genotyped on high-density SNP arrays. The graphic shows the results for chromosome 3. SNPs are represented by horizontal lines at the appropriate chromosomal location. Heterozygous SNPs are shown in green, homozygous ones in black. The white area marks the centromere. The three affected individuals are all homozygous for a contiguous set of SNPs across the 3p21 region, while the unaffected sibs are heterozygous for most of these SNPs. No other region of shared homozygosity was seen on other chromosomes. It is likely that this region contains the gene responsible for their hearing loss. Figure courtesy of Jill Urquhart, St Mary's Hospital, Manchester.

The gene responsible for *DFNB6* hearing loss had been identified as *TMIE* (transmembrane inner ear-expressed gene; OMIM 607237). Few families had been described with deafness caused by *TMIE* mutations, and without the evidence from the autozygosity mapping, *TMIE* would have been low on the list of candidate genes to test. The four exons of this gene were sequenced in Nasreen's DNA. She was homozygous for a frameshifting mutation, an insertion of four nucleotides in exon 2. Having identified the family mutation, the geneticist was now in a position to offer definitive carrier testing to any family members who wished it. As an alternative to autozygosity mapping, whole exome sequencing, as described in *Disease box 9*, would have been a good way of identifying the causative mutation in this family.

Interestingly, the five families previously shown to have *TMIE* mutations were all from the Indian subcontinent, and one of them had the same sequence change as Nasreen. If DNA could be obtained from an affected member of the Indian family, it would be possible to work out whether both families had inherited the mutation from an unknown common ancestor. If they had the same ancestral chromosome segment, they would have the same haplotype of SNPs immediately surrounding the mutation.

9.4. Going deeper ...

Using chromosomal abnormalities to suggest a candidate region or candidate gene

Rare individuals with a disease and a chromosome abnormality can sometimes allow an investigator to circumvent linkage analysis and go directly to testing genes in a candidate region. This is especially important for a dominant disease where affected people seldom reproduce. As mentioned in *Chapter 2*, occasionally the breakpoint of a chromosomal translocation or inversion disrupts a gene. If loss of one copy of that gene causes a disease, the person will have that disease. Thus clinicians should always keep an eye open for people who have both a mendelian disease and a chromosomal abnormality, especially if both occur *de novo* in one individual. Sometimes it will just be coincidence, but several such cases have provided the vital clue to identifying a disease gene. Rubinstein–Taybi syndrome (see *Disease box 2*) is a good example. Other examples are given in *Table 9.2*.

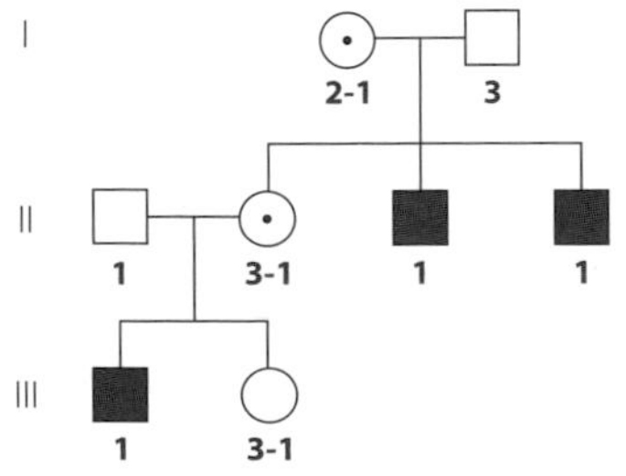

Gene tracking: using linked markers to predict genetic risks in a pedigree

In the dyschromatosis families, the investigators knew which individuals were affected or unaffected, and they tested many markers to find one that co-segregated with the disease. However, once research has identified a marker that reliably co-segregates with a disease, it is sometimes possible to use the marker to predict who in a family has or has not inherited the disease gene. This is known as **gene tracking**. *Figure 9.9* shows a hypothetical example. The pedigree shows an X-linked recessive disease and genotypes for a polymorphic marker that is known to be closely linked to the disease locus. Evidently the disease-bearing

Figure 9.9 – Using gene tracking to predict genetic risk. See text for discussion. NB, males have only one allele of any X chromosome marker.

Table 9.2 – Cases where an alert clinician provided a vital clue to identify a disease gene

Disease	Chromosomal location	Crucial clinical observation
Duchenne muscular dystrophy	Xp21.3	(a) a boy with DMD and a visible deletion at Xp21.3 (b) a woman with DMD and a balanced reciprocal X;21 translocation Both these cases pointed to Xp21.3 and gave researchers a handle on DNA from the disease region in the pioneering days of positional cloning
Type I Waardenburg syndrome	2q35	A boy with *de novo* disease and a *de novo* inversion of 2q35–q37.3 directed linkage analysis to those locations in the days when testing each marker required a week's work or more
Williams–Beuren syndrome	7q11.23	A family in which supravalvular aortic stenosis co-segregated with a balanced reciprocal translocation, t(6;7)(p21.1;q11.23) – see *Disease box 3*
Sotos syndrome	5q35	A patient with the disease and a balanced reciprocal translocation t(5;8)(q35;q24.1). The breakpoint was shown to disrupt the *NSD1* gene, which was then shown to be mutated or deleted in other cases of the syndrome

chromosome carries allele 1 of the marker. Individual III–2 inherited allele 3 from her carrier mother, and is therefore at very low risk of being a carrier. Her risk is not zero, because it is possible that there was a recombination between the disease and marker loci in the meiosis that produced the egg from which she developed. Note that you cannot deduce risk simply by looking at the individual marker genotypes (e.g. III–2 has the same marker genotype as her carrier mother, but in her case this means that she is not a carrier). You have to follow the segregation of a chromosome through the pedigree.

In the days when the loci for major diseases had been mapped, so that linked markers were known, but the disease gene had not yet been identified, gene tracking was an important part of clinical genetics. Once a disease gene has been identified it is usually preferable to check directly for mutations. Gene tracking is still sometimes used for some large genes with many exons, where scanning the whole gene for mutations is not cost-effective. A special application is the **fetal exclusion test**. In *Figure 9.10*, II–1 is at 50% risk of developing Huntington disease because his mother is affected. He has opted against having a predictive test for himself, but he and his wife do not want any child of theirs to suffer the same life-long anxiety. A direct prenatal test for the Huntington disease mutation (expansion of a $(CAG)_n$ repeat, see *Figure 4.18*) would say definitively whether or not a fetus carried it; but if it was positive, II–1 would know that he too carried the Huntington disease mutation, and he does not wish to know this. Instead, a linked marker is used. Fetus III–1 has inherited the chromosome that II–1 received from his unaffected father. It is therefore free of risk (barring recombination in the paternal meiosis). Fetus III–2 has inherited the chromosome that came from its affected grandmother. It is at 50% risk of having inherited the Huntington disease mutation. The parents had decided that they would terminate any such

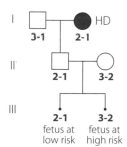

Figure 9.10 – A fetal exclusion test in Huntington disease.
Numbers are alleles of a marker closely linked to the HD locus. See text for further explanation.

pregnancy. That way, they were assured of having only unaffected children, without finding out whether or not II–1 carried the mutation. The downside is that any aborted fetus had a 50% chance of being entirely normal.

As mentioned above, the marker genotype of an individual tells us nothing in itself. What matters is the pattern of segregation of the disease and marker in the family. In *Figure 9.10*, the marker genotype 2–1 that is present in the affected grandparent, indicates a low risk when it is found in the fetus, while the fact that II–1 also types 2–1 tells us nothing about his disease status. The marker is not the disease gene; it is a non-pathogenic variant that just happens to lie on the same region of a chromosome as the disease gene.

Next generation sequencing and the coming revolution

The massively parallel DNA sequencing techniques discussed in *Chapter 5* are changing genetics in many ways, one of which is the search for disease genes. No longer is it always necessary to identify a candidate region for mutation hunting by linkage, autozygosity mapping or through a chromosomal abnormality. Instead, it is entirely feasible to sequence every exon of every gene (whole exome sequencing) or even the whole genome. The question then becomes, how easy will it be to identify the pathogenic change, given that the genome of every individual, healthy or diseased, will show several million differences from the reference human genome sequence, including probably 100 or so *de novo* changes that will not have been present in the DNA of either parent?

Disease box 9 shows that it can be done, at least for a recessive condition (where each patient will have two mutations in the same gene), and provided you have several unrelated affected individuals. Shortly after that work was published, the Nijmegen group showed they could do the same with a dominant condition, where each patient had only a single mutation (Hoischen *et al.*, 2010). An essential step in that work was to look for a gene that had different mutations in different unrelated patients. Clearly this is not a foolproof method for identifying novel disease genes. The exon capture methods work better with some exons than others. It might eventually be better to skip this step and sequence the whole genome. At each stage in the data analysis there is a risk of throwing out the baby with the bathwater. Time will tell how often it will be possible to identify a novel disease gene by sequencing the DNA of a single isolated patient. With the new technologies, sequences of individual human genomes are rapidly accumulating, and as we know more and more about the spectrum of rare variants that can be found in healthy individuals, it will become less of a challenge to pick out candidate pathogenic changes in the genomes of patients. Evolutionary conservation is an important criterion for selecting potentially significant mis-sense changes, while for dominant conditions the pathogenic change should be *de novo* – that is, not present in either parent.

It is worth noting that these new methods bring some potential ethical problems. As long as researchers sequenced only predetermined small segments of a subject's DNA it was unlikely that they would coincidentally discover some unrelated but important variant. Whole exome or whole genome sequencing changes this. In fact, this already happened in the Miller syndrome work described in *Disease box 9*: the affected sibs also turned out to be homozygous for a ciliary disorder. In this case the discovery simply explained an atypical aspect of their phenotype, but it is easy to imagine uncovering less welcome information. On the other hand, other techniques that look at the whole genome – conventional karyotyping or array-CGH for example – have always carried this risk, and it is familiar to clinicians in many other branches of medicine. It does mean that researchers in molecular genetics need to be careful in future to define in advance just what their subjects have consented to, and to be sure that they are in a position to refer subjects for proper counseling if necessary.

DISEASE BOX 9

Miller syndrome: identifying a disease gene by large-scale sequencing.

Miller syndrome (OMIM 263750) is characterized (see *Box figure 9.1*) by abnormalities of the face (micrognathia, cleft lip and/or palate, coloboma of the eyelids) and limbs (missing or hypoplastic fingers or toes). Only a few dozen cases have been described and in the only three reported multiplex families the parents were unrelated. Thus there was uncertainty whether the condition was recessive or dominant, with the multiplex families being due to germinal mosaicism in one parent.

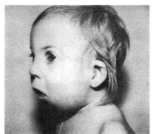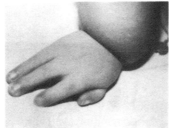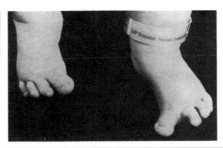

Box figure 9.1 – Clinical features of a patient with Miller syndrome.
Photos reproduced from Donnai, Hughes and Winter (1987) with permission from the BMJ Publishing Group.

This rare condition was chosen as a test-bed for a new approach to identifying disease genes (Ng *et al.*, 2010). The new massively parallel sequencing technology was used to sequence every exon of every gene ('whole exome sequencing') in just four affected individuals – two affected sibs and two unrelated cases.

This new approach to identifying disease genes rests on three key abilities:

* the ability to separate the *c.* 1% of protein-coding sequence in a person's genomic DNA (the 'exome') from the 99% of non-coding DNA

* the ability to sequence the 30 Mb exome with sufficient accuracy to identify all single base and larger variants, even when these are present in heterozygous form

* the ability to identify the pathogenic variant against the background of all the other variants revealed by the sequencing

For the first step, whole genomic DNA from the subject was fragmented and then hybridized to an immense cocktail of probes which, between them, covered the entire exome. Various companies have recently developed methods for massively parallel and flexible oligonucleotide synthesis that allow such whole exome probe cocktails to be prepared at manageable cost. These 'capture probes' may be anchored on a microarray or used in solution. In the latter case they are tagged with biotin, so that they and the genomic fragments hybridized to them can be recovered by binding them to streptavidin-coated magnetic beads. After hybridization, the unwanted DNA is washed away and the hybridized fragments are then released.

In sequencing, each individual stretch of the DNA must be sequenced many times to achieve the necessary overall accuracy – in the Miller syndrome study (Ng *et al.*, 2010), an average of 40 times. Unlike Sanger sequencing, where one specific piece of DNA is sequenced, the next generation technologies pick templates at random from a huge pool. Inevitably some fragments are missed. To be confident of including every fragment, especially both alleles in heterozygotes, each individual fragment must be given many opportunities to be picked up for sequencing. Even with 40-fold coverage, only 97% of bases were reliably identified.

After a computer has assembled the many millions of overlapping short sequence reads into an overall exome sequence, the next challenge is to identify the pathogenic change. A series of filters are applied.

1. The first stage of filtering has already happened: only coding sequences have been selected for study. Thus one assumption is that the pathogenic change is in an exon, not in a distant regulatory sequence or in a sequence encoding a functional RNA.

2. Next, sequence changes predicted not to affect coding or splicing are discarded. Sometimes this will be a mistake, because the computer programs that predict splicing effects are not infallible.

3. Next, any changes that are already present in databases such as dbSNP and previously reported genome sequences of healthy individuals are rejected. Again, there is a risk of rejecting the desired causative change because some variants that are listed in these datasets may cause a recessive or incompletely penetrant dominant condition.

4. Finally, remaining mis-sense changes are rejected if a computer program predicts that they would not affect the function of the gene product.

Box table 9.1 shows how the filters operated in this study.

Box table 9.1 – Numbers of genes containing sequence variants in Miller syndrome patients

Filter	Present in both affected sibs		Present in both sibs + 2 unrelated cases	
Model	Dominant	Recessive	Dominant	Recessive
NS/SS/I*	3940	2362	2654	1525
Not in previous datasets	228	9	8	1
Predicted damaging	83	1	2	0

Data are shown for genes present in both of two affected sibs and also in both these sibs and in two additional unrelated patients. On the dominant model, a gene is reported if it contains at least one variant; on the recessive model both alleles must contain a variant (but not necessarily the same one).
*NS/SS/I: non-synonymous/splice site/insertion-deletion variant.

The final filter gave a false prediction: in the only gene (*DHODH*, dihydroorotate dehydrogenase) that carried variants in both alleles in every patient, one of the two variants in the affected sibs was wrongly classified as not damaging. *DHODH* was definitively proven to be the Miller syndrome gene by identifying mutations in a further four cases.

9.5. **References**

Bantounas I, Phylactou LA and Uney JB (2004) RNA interference and the use of small interfering RNA to study gene function in mammalian systems. *J. Mol. Endocrin.* **33**: 545–557. *Free full text at* http://jme.endocrinology-journals.org/cgi/content/full/33/3/545

dbSNP public database: www.ncbi.nlm.nih.gov/SNP/

Donnai D, Hughes H and Winter RM (1987) Postaxial acrofacial dysostosis (Miller) syndrome. *J. Med. Genet.* **24**: 422–425.

Griffiths AJF, Gelbart WH, Lewontin RC and Miller JH (1999) *Modern Genetic Analysis.* WH Freeman, New York.

Hereditary Hearing Loss Homepage http://hereditaryhearingloss.org

Hoischen A, van Bon BW, Gilissen C, *et al.* (2010) *De novo* mutations of *SETBP1* cause Schinzel–Giedion syndrome. *Nat. Genet.* **42**: 483–485.

Iredale JP (1999) Demystified … gene knockouts. *Mol. Pathol.* **52**: 111–116. *Free full text at* http://mp.bmjjournals.com/cgi/reprint/52/3/111

Miyamura Y, Suzuki T, Kono M, *et al.* (2003) Mutations of the RNA-specific adenosine deaminase (DSRAD) gene are involved in dyschromatosis symmetrica hereditaria. *Am. J. Hum. Genet.* **73**: 693–699.

Ng SB, Buckingham KJ, Bigham AW, *et al.* (2010) Exome sequencing identifies the cause of a mendelian disorder. *Nat. Genet.* **42**: 30–35.

General background

Ott J (1999) *Analysis of Human Genetic Linkage*, 3rd edn. Johns Hopkins University Press, Baltimore. *A highly authoritative exposition of the basis of human genetic mapping.*

Strachan T and Read AP (2010) *Human Molecular Genetics*, 4th edn. Garland Science, New York. *This covers the material of this chapter in somewhat greater depth.*

9.6. **Self-assessment questions**

(1) The pedigree shows a family with a fully penetrant autosomal dominant disease. Genotypes are shown for a DNA polymorphism that has alleles 1 and 2.

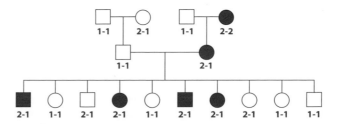

(a) Mark each meiosis as definitely non-recombinant, definitely recombinant, probably non-recombinant, probably recombinant or uninformative.

(b) What is the best estimate of the recombination rate?

(c) Test the significance of the deviation from the null hypothesis of 50% recombinants (no linkage) using χ^2. Is the result significant?

(d) In what proportion of such pedigrees would you expect to see the observed pattern of markers in generation III if there were no linkage between the marker and the disease? Call this L1.

(e) In what proportion of such pedigrees would you expect to see the observed pattern of markers in generation III if there were linkage (recombination fraction θ) between the marker and the disease? Call this L2 (L2 is a function of θ, of course).

(f) Tabulate the values of L1, L2, L2/L1 and $\log_{10}$(L2/L1) for $\theta = 0$, 0.05, 0.1, 0.15, 0.2....0.5.

(g) $\log_{10}$(L2/L1) is the lod score. What is the maximum lod score? Is this significant? Comment.

(2) In the family below, a fully penetrant autosomal dominant disease is segregating. The disease has been mapped to chromosome 2q35 in previous studies. The pedigree shows genotypes for four DNA polymorphisms from within the candidate region, arranged in chromosomal order. Can you narrow down the disease locus using these data?

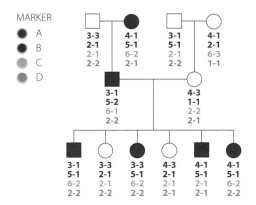

(3) Janet was pregnant with their second child when her husband John and 14 year old son Ben were killed in a car crash. Ben had cystic fibrosis. Janet desperately wants to have the baby, but feels she cannot cope with a second tragedy in the form of another child with cystic fibrosis. It was only after the double funeral that she raised the issue with her physician. He pointed out that prenatal diagnosis required DNA samples from Ben and John, who had been cremated. John's elderly parents were contacted and they agreed to give small mouthwash samples for mutation testing. A week later the laboratory requested blood samples so that they could do extensive sequencing, because the initial multiplex OLA test had not revealed any mutation in the parents' samples. However, by this time they were uncontactable, having embarked on a world cruise to forget their grief. A search through old files hit on a Guthrie blood spot card that

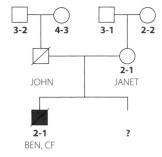

had been used for Ben's routine neonatal screening. The sample was too degraded to be used for mutation screening, but the laboratory was able to type it for a DNA polymorphism known to be tightly linked to the cystic fibrosis locus. All available DNA samples were typed for the marker, with the results shown. What are the possible genotypes and implications for the fetus if a prenatal test is carried out?

(4) Linkage studies have mapped the gene causing a mendelian disease to a 2 Mb region. Database searching shows this region contains the following genes:
- an enzyme involved in detoxification reactions in the liver
- a phosphate transporter
- a component of the large ribosomal subunit
- a nuclear-encoded component of the mitochondrial electron transport chain
- a ubiquitously expressed protein of unknown function containing a variable length run of glutamines
- an enzyme catalyzing one step in the tricarboxylic acid cycle
- a protein of unknown function expressed in the adult central nervous system and retina
- a transcription factor expressed only in restricted regions of early embryos
- a ubiquitously expressed transcription factor
- a component of the DNA damage repair pathway

What would be your first candidate for mutation testing if the disease in question was
- (a) an adult-onset neurodegenerative disease showing anticipation
- (b) a rickets-like skeletal malformation
- (c) absence of the pituitary gland
- (d) an accelerated aging syndrome
- (e) a combination of deafness and diabetes

CHAPTER 10 | Why are some conditions common and others rare?

Learning points for this chapter

After working through this chapter you should be able to:

- Define gene frequency, inbreeding, founder effect, coefficient of relationship
- Use the Hardy–Weinberg formula to calculate carrier frequencies for autosomal and X-linked recessive conditions
- Describe qualitatively the effects of inbreeding and use Sewall Wright's path coefficient method to calculate gene sharing by relatives
- Describe the consequences of heterozygote advantage and give examples
- Explain why it is difficult to change population gene frequencies by medical interventions

10.1. Case studies

CASE 21	Ulmer family	**253**	261	284	389

- Hannah, a 6-month-old baby girl
- Ashkenazi Jewish origin
- Tay–Sachs disease

Rachel and Uzi Ulmer's families originally came from Eastern Europe and are of Ashkenazi Jewish origin, though neither family was religious, and Rachel and Uzi didn't attend Jewish schools or the synagogue. Hannah was their third child; they had two healthy children, aged 5 and 3 when Hannah was born. Hannah seemed very well as a young baby and smiled and held her head up at the normal time. However, at her 6 month check, the doctor noted her head control was not good and arranged a further appointment 4 weeks later. He was more concerned then because her head control was even worse and she seemed less responsive. He undertook a full neurological examination and found that she had cherry red spots in the maculae of both eyes. He felt fairly sure that Hannah had Tay–Sachs disease (OMIM 272800) and arranged for blood samples to be sent to measure levels of hexosaminidase A. Sadly the levels were extremely low and the diagnosis was confirmed. Rachel and Uzi and their families were devastated at the poor prognosis they were given for Hannah, but resolved to try to make her life as comfortable as possible. Over the next 3 years Hannah deteriorated further; her limbs became spastic and she lost her vision and hearing. She died at the age of four and a half years.

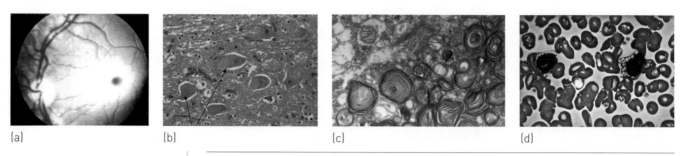

(a)   (b)   (c)   (d)

Figure 10.1 – (a) The characteristic cherry red spot on the retina of a child with Tay–Sachs disease. (b) Ballooned neurons in the central nervous system (arrows). (c) Abnormal cell bodies seen under the electron microscope. (d) Vacuolated lymphocytes. These are typical features of lysosomal storage diseases. Photos courtesy of Drs Ed Wraith and Guy Besley, Royal Manchester Children's Hospital.

10.2. **Science toolkit**

This chapter is about **gene frequencies**: what determines them, how they can change, and the way gene frequencies can be used to work out genetic risks in a variety of situations. Note that the term 'gene frequency' is a misnomer – we really mean *allele frequency* – but 'gene frequency' is too thoroughly established in genetic parlance to change now. Gene frequencies are numbers that lie between 0 and 1; traditionally they are symbolized as p and/or q.

Gene frequencies depend on the concept of a **gene pool**. This would consist of all the alleles at a particular locus in some defined population. The population might be anything from a small community to the whole of humanity. Within the gene pool, the gene frequency of allele $\underline{A}$ is the proportion of all the alleles that are $\underline{A}$. It is also the probability that a gene, picked at random from the pool, would be $\underline{A}$. Alleles can be defined in various ways for different purposes. Most discussion of gene frequencies in relation to disease classifies all alleles at a locus into just two categories, normal alleles and disease alleles. If you sequenced the DNA, you would probably find that each included quite a range of variants, and for some purposes you might wish to count each sequence variant as a separate allele. Whatever scheme you use to classify alleles, the frequencies of all the alleles in a population must add up to 1.

Clinicians are usually more interested in frequencies of genotypes than frequencies of alleles. They want to know the probability that a randomly selected person is homozygous or heterozygous for a disease allele. The Hardy–Weinberg distribution (*Box 10.1*) describes the relationship of genotype frequencies to gene frequencies. The Hardy–Weinberg distribution makes it possible to calculate the frequency of carriers of recessive conditions in a population, without having to sample a large number of people and genotype them in the laboratory. Along with the basic mendelian rules, it is the central tool for assessing genetic risks.

The bean–bag model that we use in *Box 10.1* to derive the Hardy–Weinberg distribution illustrates an important precondition of the distribution. The probability that the second bean will be $\underline{A}$ or $\underline{a}$ must be entirely independent of whether the first bean was $\underline{A}$ or $\underline{a}$. In genetic terms, the genotype distribution will

BOX 10.1

The Hardy–Weinberg distribution

Suppose there are two alleles, A and a in a population (there may or may not be others as well; it doesn't matter). Say the gene frequency of A is p and the gene frequency of a is q. p and q will sum to 1 if A and a are the only alleles in the population; if there are other alleles $p+q$ will be less than 1. The Hardy–Weinberg distribution predicts that the frequencies of the three possible genotypes are:

AA	Aa	aa
p^2	$2pq$	q^2

People sometimes state this as $p^2 + 2pq + q^2 = 1$. This is wrong. The Hardy–Weinberg distribution is not an equation. It describes the relation between gene frequencies and genotype frequencies. p^2, $2pq$ and q^2 only add up to 1 if those two alleles are the only alleles in the population, so that everybody must be either AA or Aa or aa. If there are three alleles in the population (say, A, a and a_1, with frequencies p, q and r) the frequencies of AA, Aa and aa are still p^2, $2pq$ and q^2, but there are also other genotypes in the population, The total distribution is:

AA	Aa	aa	Aa_1	aa_1	a_1a_1
p^2	$2pq$	q^2	$2pr$	$2qr$	r^2

The basis of the Hardy–Weinberg distribution can easily be seen by doing a little thought experiment. Imagine all the genes in a gene pool as a large collection of beans in a bag. A proportion p of the beans are of type A and a proportion q are of type a. Eyes shut, reach into the bag and pick a bean. The chance it is A is p, and the chance it is a is q. Pick a second bean. Again the chance it is A is p, the chance it is a is q (we assume there are enough beans in the bag that removing the first one did not significantly change p or q). The chance both beans were A is p^2; the chance both were a is q^2. The chance the first bean was A and the second a is pq; similarly the chance you picked first a then A is qp. Overall, the chance you picked one A and one a is $2pq$.

be Hardy–Weinberg only if there is **random mating**. Random mating does not mean free love; it just means that you don't ask your beloved's genotype before you pop the question. This is not as far-fetched as it sounds. There are many ways in which people tend to select mates based partly on genotype. There is **assortative mating** for height, intelligence, deafness and many other phenotypes that are at least partly genetic. The effect of assortative mating is to increase the proportion of homozygotes for each allele in the population, and decrease the proportion of heterozygotes, compared to the predictions of Hardy–Weinberg.

Assortative mating is mainly important in clinical genetics in the context of inbreeding. Relatives share genes, and so if you marry a relative rather than an unrelated person you increase the chance that your partner will have alleles in common with you. If you carry an allele for a recessive condition there is an increased chance that your partner will also carry it, and thus an increased risk of having a child with the condition, compared to an outbred couple. This is discussed further in *Section 10.3* in relation to the **Choudhary family (Case 3)**.

Using Hardy–Weinberg to calculate carrier risks

Suppose the sister of a boy with cystic fibrosis is getting married. She knows the disease is genetic, and she wants to know the risk that she might have an affected child. She is healthy, but of course it is quite likely that she is a carrier of cystic fibrosis (see below for the exact probability). This has no implications for her own health, but her children would be at risk if her partner happens also to be a carrier. Calculating the risk that her partner is a carrier is the same as calculating the probability that a person, picked at random from the population, is a carrier. Hardy–Weinberg enables us to do this.

If we ignore the extensive allelic heterogeneity among cystic fibrosis mutations, and classify all alleles as A (functional) and a (non-functional), with frequencies p and q, the proportions of the genotypes are:

<u>AA</u>	<u>Aa</u>	<u>aa</u>
p^2	$2pq$	q^2

Cystic fibrosis affects one birth in 2000 in Americans of Northern European origin (it is less frequent among Hispanics, African–Americans and Asian Americans). Therefore q^2 is $1/2000$. Hence q is the square root of $1/2000$, which is nearly $1/45$. One allele in 45 at the *CFTR* locus is a; the remaining $44/45$ must be A (we had decided to classify *all* alleles as A or a, so in this case $p+q=1$). We can now calculate the carrier frequency: $2pq = 2 \times 44/45 \times 1/45 = 1/23$, approximately. Assuming random mating, there is a 1 in 23 chance the girl's partner is a carrier.

For an X-linked condition the calculation is even simpler. If hemophilia A affects one boy in 5000 in a certain population, what proportion of the women are carriers? Males can only be A or a, so the frequency of the disease allele is simply equal to the proportion of males who are affected:

	Females			Males	
<u>AA</u>	<u>Aa</u>	<u>aa</u>		<u>A</u>	<u>a</u>
p^2	$2pq$	q^2		p	q

The carrier frequency among women is $2 \times 4999/5000 \times 1/5000$ or 1 in 2500.

For a rare condition, the frequency of the normal allele can usually be approximated to 1, which makes the calculation easier. However, it is important to note that for rare autosomal recessive conditions, a significant proportion of cases are the offspring of consanguineous marriages. This is not a major factor with cystic fibrosis in the USA or UK, because cystic fibrosis is a relatively common disease. But the rarer a condition is, the higher is the proportion of cases where consanguinity is a factor. Ignoring this and simply assuming a Hardy–Weinberg distribution can lead to serious over-estimation of carrier frequencies for very rare diseases (see below).

Changing gene frequencies

Gene frequencies can change from generation to generation for a number of reasons:

- New mutations increase the number of disease alleles in the gene pool. There can also be back mutation, changing a disease allele into a normal allele. However, for loss of function mutations, the process is largely uni-directional. Any one of a large number of possible sequence changes can convert a functioning gene into a non-functioning one, but only a very specific back-mutation can restore the function of a non-functional allele.

The ratio of forward to back mutation rates is likely to be of the order of 1000 : 1. Other mutations may well occur to non-functional alleles, but the allele remains non-functional.

- Natural selection will remove disease alleles from the gene pool if the disease is such that affected people are less likely to reproduce. Artificial selection might have a similar effect (see *Section 10.4*).
- A large influx of migrants from a population with substantially different gene frequencies could change the gene pool.
- Every population is made up of a finite number of individuals. Those that actually reproduce every generation comprise only about one-third of the total census size. Reproducers are never exactly representative of the former generations for purely statistical reasons, and this introduces chance fluctuations of gene frequencies at every generation. These changes will accumulate over time, because at every generation children are formed by the gametes produced in the last generation. The smaller the size of the population, the greater the random fluctuations that will take place at every generation, and the more rapidly changes will be observed over generations.

Whatever the initial genotype frequencies in a population, one generation of random mating is enough to establish a Hardy–Weinberg distribution. If, when a population is surveyed, the distribution is seen to differ significantly from Hardy–Weinberg, this might mean one of several things:

- *The survey methodology is flawed*. This is seen most often when a new DNA polymorphism is being checked. A non-Hardy–Weinberg distribution of genotypes probably means that the genotyping method is producing errors and needs to be improved to make it reliable.
- *Selection has already occurred*. A genotype that causes substantial prenatal or infant mortality will be under-represented in a sample of adults.
- *There is significant assortative mating*. This might be simple inbreeding, or perhaps the population is not freely interbreeding, but consists of two or more groups that have different gene frequencies and that largely breed among themselves (population stratification).

Note that if you are using a chi-squared test to check whether genotype numbers fit Hardy–Weinberg, with two alleles there is only one degree of freedom, even though you have three observed and expected numbers. That is because once you have fixed q, everything else in the expected numbers follows.

Factors determining gene frequencies

People sometimes imagine that dominant characters should be common and recessive ones rare. Actually there is no connection between the gene frequency of an allele and whether it causes a dominant or recessive phenotype. Huntington disease is one example among many of a rare dominant; blood group O is a common recessive.

For a neutral character where selection plays no role, the gene frequencies reflect the frequencies in the founders of that population, modulated by genetic drift if, at any time, the breeding population was reduced to small numbers. Most common neutral DNA polymorphisms (SNPs or microsatellites, see *Chapter 9*) fit this category. Occasional mutations will introduce some random variation by changing one allele into another. As explained in *Chapter 7*, deamination of methylated cytosines has tended, over evolutionary time, to convert CpG sequences systematically into TpG, but this effect on gene frequencies is only noticeable on an extremely large timescale.

For diseases, the gene frequencies reflect additional factors. Recurrent mutations tend to increase the pool of loss of function alleles, while selection acts to remove disease alleles from the population. For dominant and X-linked diseases selection is very effective, because everybody (dominant), or all males (X-linked) who carry the disease allele have the disease and so are exposed to selection. For autosomal recessive conditions, selection acts much more slowly, because most of the disease alleles are in healthy heterozygotes, who are not subject to selection. For this reason, alleles for recessive diseases can persist for very many generations in a population, even if the disease is very severe. This leads to important **founder effects** in many populations. If a population, however numerous today, derives from a small number of founders, or passed through a bottleneck when only a few individuals contributed to the next generation, then any recessive allele that was present in one of the founders is likely to be present at high frequency in the modern population. Equally, if a normally common recessive condition happened to be absent from the small pool of founders, it will be rare or absent in the modern population (*Figure 10.2*).

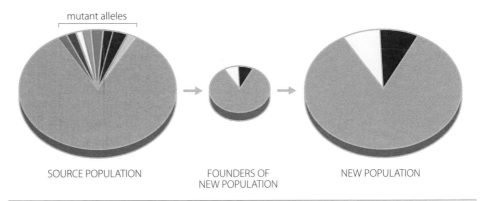

Figure 10.2 – **Founder effects.**

Founder effects are seen in many populations. For the reasons explained above, they affect the frequencies of recessive conditions but not usually of dominant or X-linked conditions. *Table 10.1* shows some examples, and *Disease box 10* describes in more detail some diseases characteristic of one such population, Ashkenazi Jews.

Heterozygote advantage

There is a second reason why a recessive condition may be common in a population. The classic case is sickle cell disease. This is common in many populations where

Table 10.1 – Diseases common in certain populations, probably because of a founder effect

Disease	OMIM	Mode of inheritance	Population	Comments
Diastrophic dysplasia	222600	AR	Finns	90% of Finnish cases have a splice donor mutation in intron 1
Aspartylglucosaminuria	208400	AR	Finns	Carrier frequency 1 : 30; 98% have p.Cys163Ser mutation
Neuronal ceroid lipofuscinosis	256730	AR	Finns	Single mutation, p.R122W, found in 97% of Finnish cases
Hermansky–Pudlak syndrome	203300	AR	Puerto Ricans	Carrier frequency 1 : 21; much rarer in most other populations
Bardet–Biedl syndrome	209900	AR	Bedouin	Two non-allelic forms, BBS2 and BBS3 both relatively frequent
Myotonic dystrophy	160900	AD	Quebec – Sanguenay	Prevalence 1 : 500, 30–60 × prevalence in most other populations
Butyrylcholinesterase deficiency	177400	AR	Alaskan Eskimos	Deficiency allele frequency 0.1. Three different alleles reported in this population
Usher syndrome type 1C	276904	AR	French-Acadians in Louisiana	43/44 cases homozygous for a c.216G>A mutation
Hereditary motor and sensory neuropathy, Lom type	601455	AR	Bulgarian gypsies	The OMIM entry gives an interesting commentary

Note that all diseases are autosomal recessive (AR) except for myotonic dystrophy.

falciparum malaria is or was recently endemic, but is absent from populations where malaria was not frequent. The driving force is that heterozygotes are relatively resistant to malaria. Thus in historical times normal homozygotes often died of malaria, and sickle cell homozygotes died of their disease, leaving the heterozygotes to contribute disproportionately to the next generation (*Figure 10.3*).

Even a very small degree of heterozygote advantage, continued over many generations, can greatly influence the gene frequencies. If, relative to Aa heterozygotes, a proportion s_1 of aa and a proportion s_2 of AA homozygotes fail to reproduce, at equilibrium the ratio of gene frequencies, q/p, is s_2/s_1. For cystic fibrosis s_1 is effectively 1 (we are talking about conditions during the past, not today) while we calculated above that q/p is $1/45$ for people of Northern European origin. It follows that s_2 must also be about $1/45$. In other words, in order to account for the high proportion of people of Northern European origin who are carriers of cystic fibrosis, carriers must have enjoyed a 2% reproductive advantage over

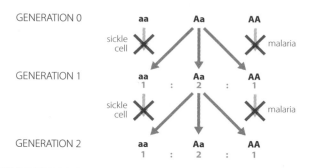

Figure 10.3 – Heterozygote advantage.
A hypothetical extreme example in which everybody with sickle cell disease (aa) fails to reproduce because of their disease, while all normal homozygotes (AA) fail to reproduce because of malaria. Only heterozygote × heterozygote matings contribute to the next generation. Regardless of how many generations the selection continues, at birth every generation always consists of 25% sickle cell homozygotes, 50% heterozygotes and 25% normal homozygotes. No real situation is this extreme.

normal homozygotes during past centuries. Such an advantage is too small to be easily detectable in survey data, and its nature is controversial.

Heterozygote advantage or founder effect?

If a disease is common in a certain population because of a founder effect, we would expect most affected people to have exactly the same ancestral mutation. On the other hand, if heterozygote advantage has been the mechanism, a whole range of mutations might be common. A good example is β-thalassemia in Jews from Kurdistan. The carrier frequency is as high as 20%, but 13 different β-globin mutations have been described in this small group. Clearly, heterozygote advantage (presumably resistance to malaria) has been the driving force here. On the other hand, among the Amish of Lancaster County, Pennsylvania, the rare recessive Ellis–van Creveld syndrome (OMIM 225500) is relatively common, with a gene frequency of 0.07. All affected people in nine families studied had the same sequence changes in each copy of the *EVC* gene on chromosome 4. All could trace their ancestry back to one couple, Samuel King and his wife, who immigrated in 1744. This is an example of a founder effect. In this particular case the founder is relatively recent, so the shared ancestry is demonstrable genealogically. In most cases it has to be inferred by identifying a shared haplotype of non-pathogenic polymorphisms on the chromosomal segment carrying the mutant gene. As it happens, the *EVC* mutation in the Amish families is always accompanied by a second, non-pathogenic sequence change in the *EVC* gene. The change is not found on non-mutant chromosomes. This provides additional confirmation that we are looking at copies of a single ancestral chromosome.

There are several examples of isolated populations where more than one mutation causing a certain recessive disease is relatively common. Heterozygote advantage is a likely explanation, but there may also be an observational bias. Mutations are normally identified by studying affected people, not by screening a whole population. If one disease allele is fairly common, there will be plenty of people heterozygous for that allele. Whenever such a person happens to carry another disease allele they will be affected, and so both their disease alleles will be identified. Thus a common recessive disease allele provides a mechanism for bringing the rarer alleles in a population to medical attention. But as some of the Jewish diseases in *Disease box 10* illustrate, sometimes the effects of heterozygote advantage, founder effects and genetic drift are hard to disentangle.

10.3. **Investigations of patients**

| CASE 21 | Ulmer family | 253 | **261** | 284 | 389 |

- Hannah, a 6-month-old baby girl
- Ashkenazi Jewish origin
- Tay–Sachs disease
- Test the sibs?

Tay–Sachs disease is a lysosomal storage disease (see *Section 8.2*) caused by lack of hexosaminidase A. Because of the enzyme deficiency, G_{M2} ganglioside accumulates in lysosomes in retinal ganglia and other neurons, leading to death, usually at age 2–4 years. The disease is known from all ethnic groups, but is about 100 times more common in Ashkenazi Jews compared to most other groups. About 1 in 30 North American Jews is a carrier, compared to perhaps 1 in 300 people in most other populations. This has led to carrier screening programs being set up specifically in Jewish communities in the USA and several other countries, as described in *Chapter 11*. As their families led entirely secular lives and were not part of any Jewish community, Rachel and Uzi had missed out on screening.

Having learned about Tay–Sachs disease, Rachel and Uzi were very concerned to know whether either of their healthy children was a carrier and pressed for them to be tested. The geneticist contended that it was unethical to test young children. Any test result would have no implications for the child's health or management. The time to offer a test was when the child was of an age to make an independent informed choice. They might prefer not to know, and it was wrong to close off that possibility for them when there was no compensating benefit in testing a child. The geneticist did point out that each child had a 2 in 3 risk of being a carrier (not 1 in 2 – see *Box 10.2*).

The risk a healthy sib is a carrier

If two carriers of an autosomal recessive disease have a child, the chance is 1 in 4 that it will be affected, 1 in 2 that it will be a carrier, and 1 in 4 that it will be homozygous normal. However, the chance that a healthy sib of an affected child is a carrier is not 1 in 2, but 2 in 3. As the figure shows, we know the child is not affected, so it must be one of the three in the shaded box.

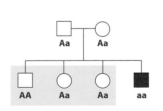

This is an interesting example of how hard it can be to spot an error when the error consists of giving the right answer to the wrong question.

- The right question is, what is the risk that a healthy sib is a carrier? Answer 2 in 3.
- The wrong question is, what is the risk that any child of a carrier couple will be a carrier? Answer 1 in 2 – but this is not the question the parents asked.

Rachel and Uzi thought they might have more children, and if so they would want prenatal diagnosis. To prepare for this possibility, mouthwash samples were taken from both of them and the *HEXA* gene checked. Three *HEXA* mutations together make up over 90% of all Tay–Sachs mutations in Ashkenazi Jews (*Table 10.2*). Rachel and Uzi each carried one of those mutations. Rachel had a mutation of the intron 12 splice site and Uzi had a 4 bp frameshifting insertion in exon 11. Hannah was a compound heterozygote for these two loss of function mutations.

Table 10.2 shows the results of a survey that looked just for the three major Ashkenazi mutations in Tay–Sachs carriers. In non-Jewish populations these mutations are not particularly common, and other work has demonstrated the expected wide assortment of individually rare mutant alleles. The situation in Ashkenazi Jews is interesting. As explained above, if the high frequency of Tay–Sachs disease were just a founder effect we would not expect more than one mutation to be common. This is discussed further in *Disease box 10* at the end of this chapter.

Table 10.2 – **Distribution of hexosaminidase A mutations**

Mutation	Percentage in Ashkenazi carriers (*n* = 156)	Percentage in non-Jewish carriers (*n* = 51)
4 bp insertion in exon 11	73	16
Intron 12 splice site mutation	15	0
p.Gly269Ser in exon 7	4	3
Unidentified	8	81

Data of Paw *et al.* (1990) cited in OMIM entry 272800.

| CASE 3 | Choudhary family | 3 | 9 | 66 | 242 | **262** | 389 |

- Girl (Nasreen) aged 8 months, parents Aadnan and Mumtaz
- Deaf
- Parents are first cousins
- Pedigree suggests autosomal recessive deafness

In this highly inbred family there had been a question whether Nasreen's deafness was autosomal recessive, and whether her two uncles, Waleed and Mohammed, were deaf from the same cause or some other cause. This question was eventually answered (*Section 9.3*) by exploiting the family structure to perform autozygosity mapping. This highlighted a candidate gene, *TMIE*, for mutation analysis. The causative mutation was identified, allowing testing and exact counseling for all the family members who wished it. This was particularly important for Waleed and his cousin Benazir, who were planning to marry.

The autozygosity mapping required a special test in the laboratory, and before she felt able to request it, the geneticist wished to calculate whether this extra investigation could make a substantial difference to her counseling. She decided to calculate what the likelihood was that a child of Waleed and Benazir would be deaf, assuming all the family deafness was autosomal recessive. She wanted to compare this with the low likelihood of recurrence if the cases in the family were coincidental. On the recessive hypothesis, Benazir's brother Aadnan (Nasreen's father – individual I, in *Figure 10.4*) was a carrier. Therefore, one of Benazir's and Aadnan's parents was a carrier – presumably their mother, since she was the link into the other side of the family. Thus Benazir's carrier risk would be 1 in 2, and the overall risk that a child of hers and Waleed's would be deaf was 1 in 4. This calculation showed that there was a large uncertainty in the risk – high if the family condition was genetic and recessive, much lower if not. It was therefore felt justifiable to expend some effort in the laboratory to try to resolve the uncertainty.

For more general genetic counseling of consanguineous couples, we need to calculate coefficients of relationship and of inbreeding.

- The **coefficient of relationship of two people** is the proportion of their alleles that they share by virtue of having one or more definable common ancestors.

Calculating the effects of inbreeding

What proportion of their genes do relatives share?

For close relatives the answer may be intuitively obvious:

- parent and child share half their genes (always)
- full sibs (same two parents) share half their genes (on average)
- half-sibs (one parent in common) share one-quarter of their genes (on average)
- uncles / aunts and nephews / nieces share one-quarter of their genes (on average)
- first cousins share one-eighth of their genes (on average)

If these figures are not intuitively obvious, or where the relationship is more complicated, Sewall Wright's path coefficient method is easy to follow and reliable:

(1) draw the pedigree showing only the common ancestor(s) and the links to them
(2) choose one path between the two relatives, through a common ancestor and count the number of links
(3) if that path has *n* links it contributes $(1/2)^n$ to the coefficient of relationship
(4) if there is more than one possible path, do the same for each path
(5) add together the contribution of each path

This is illustrated below for the simple cases of full sibs and first cousins, to show that it does indeed produce the right answer. A more complicated example is shown in *Figure 10.4*.

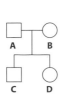

Full sibs:

Pathway	Contribution
C–A–D	$(1/2)^2 = 1/4$
C–B–D	$(1/2)^2 = 1/4$
Total:	$1/2$

First cousins:

Pathway	Contribution
E–C–A–D–F	$(1/2)^4 = 1/16$
E–C–B–D–F	$(1/2)^4 = 1/16$
	$1/8$

BOX 10.3

- The **coefficient of inbreeding of a person** is the proportion of loci at which the individual is expected to be homozygous because of the consanguinity of the parents. It is half the coefficient of relationship of the parents. Equally, it is the probability that at any given locus the individual receives two alleles that are identical by descent.

The easiest method for doing the calculation is Sewall Wright's path coefficient method (*Box 10.3*). *Figure 10.4* shows how Nasreen's coefficient of inbreeding could be calculated. Using the path coefficient method, the coefficient of relationship of Aadnan and his wife Mumtaz is calculated as $^{10}/_{64}$ – a bit closer than the $^{1}/_{8}$ of first cousins. The coefficient of inbreeding of Nasreen is therefore $^{5}/_{64}$. Note that even quite highly inbred pedigrees produce relatively moderate coefficients of inbreeding. Without resorting to incest, it is difficult to invent a pedigree where a child has a coefficient of inbreeding as high as $^{1}/_{4}$. Mouse geneticists use repeated brother–sister matings over many generations to produce highly homozygous lines. Only the pharaohs of ancient Egypt are recorded as trying the same thing in humans.

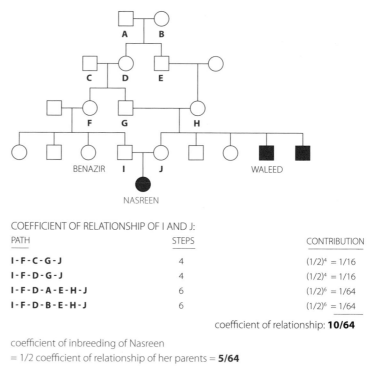

COEFFICIENT OF RELATIONSHIP OF I AND J:

PATH	STEPS	CONTRIBUTION
I-F-C-G-J	4	$(1/2)^4 = 1/16$
I-F-D-G-J	4	$(1/2)^4 = 1/16$
I-F-D-A-E-H-J	6	$(1/2)^6 = 1/64$
I-F-D-B-E-H-J	6	$(1/2)^6 = 1/64$

coefficient of relationship: **10/64**

coefficient of inbreeding of Nasreen
= 1/2 coefficient of relationship of her parents = **5/64**

Figure 10.4 – Calculation of the coefficient of inbreeding of Nasreen Choudhary (Case 3).
Because there is more than one inbreeding loop, it is not easy to do this calculation intuitively. The path coefficient method is used to calculate the coefficient of relationship of Nasreen's parents.

10.4. **Going deeper ...**

The frequencies of genetic diseases in a population depend on the opposing effects of mutation and selection, working on whatever frequencies were present in the initial founder population.

For dominant and X-linked diseases mutations normally have a short half-life.

- In the extreme case of a lethal dominant condition, every case must be a new mutation. The parents would not be parents if they were themselves affected. Note that genetic lethality means inability to pass on one's genes, and not necessarily physical lethality.
- A mutation will usually persist for only one or a few generations if it causes a dominant condition that reduces a person's chance of passing on his genes, even if it does not wholly prevent reproduction. An unusual appearance or a mild disability can be quite enough to reduce a person's chances of success in the marriage market. A classic survey of achondroplasia (OMIM 100800) provided a perfect illustration. In 1941 ET Mørch surveyed 94 075 consecutive births in Denmark and noted 10 achondroplastic babies. Only two of them had an achondroplastic parent, so he assumed that 80% were new dominant mutations. He also surveyed achondroplastic adults in Denmark and found that, although achondroplastic people are perfectly fertile, they had on average only 20% the number of children that was normal in the population. Mørch's data have been questioned because he may have unwittingly included cases of clinically similar recessive skeletal dysplasias in his newborn survey. Maybe his figures are best regarded as a thought experiment. The principle remains clear and valid. Neurofibromatosis I (*Disease box 1*) illustrates this: about 50% of cases are new mutations.
- For an X-linked recessive condition, selection is effective only against affected males. If a population has roughly equal numbers of XX females and XY males, one-third of all X chromosomes are in males (*Figure 10.5*). For a genetically lethal condition such as DMD, this means that one-third of all DMD mutant alleles are wiped out each generation. Since DMD is still with us, this loss must be roughly balanced by fresh mutations. If the rates of mutation and selection balance out, one-third of cases of DMD would be fresh mutations. This has major implications for risk estimation. We cannot assume that the mother of an isolated DMD boy is a carrier – the chance is 2 in 3. Only if she also has an affected brother or other maternal relative is she an obligate carrier (as with **Judith Davies** in **Case 4**).

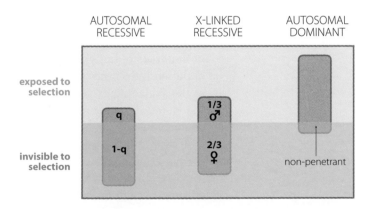

Figure 10.5 – Conditions with different modes of inheritance have different degrees of exposure to natural selection.
See text for calculations.

For recessive characters, selection works on mutant alleles only when they are in homozygous form. The ratio of genes in homozygotes to those in heterozygotes is $2q^2 : 2pq$ ($2q^2$ because there are two mutant alleles in each homozygote). Assuming p is very close to 1, the ratio simplifies to just q (*Figure 10.5*). In other words, for a typical recessive with $q = 0.01$, the mutant alleles are exposed to selection only 1% of the time. Over evolutionary time selection will be effective, but mutant alleles can easily persist over a few dozen generations.

The result of these different dynamics of selection is that serious dominant and X-linked conditions are likely to show a high proportion of new mutations and extensive allelic heterogeneity, while for most recessives, mutation can be discounted when considering families and individual mutant alleles may be quite common in a population. These considerations apply best to loss of function conditions, where in principle there can be extensive allelic heterogeneity. Dominant conditions may be the result of gain of function mutations, in which only one or a few specific mutations may be able to cause the condition.

Clinical geneticists are naturally most concerned with conditions that are both common and serious, and all such conditions must have somehow escaped being wiped out by natural selection. Possible mechanisms include the following.

- A very high mutation rate. DMD is an example. Probably the remarkable structure of the dystrophin gene (*Chapter 3*) contributes to this.
- Heterozygote advantage for a recessive condition. Thalassemia (Case 14, Nicolaides family) is a clear example. As mentioned above, cystic fibrosis (Case 2, Brown family) must also have some heterozygote advantage, otherwise it could not be so common. In fact, unless there is evidence of a high mutation rate, as in congenital adrenal hyperplasia (Case 19, Stott family), it is reasonable to suppose that most of the more common severe recessive conditions in any large population, probably have some slight degree of heterozygote advantage.
- Symptoms mostly appear after reproductive age. Huntington disease (Case 1, Ashton family) is a classic example, as are the familial breast and colon cancers described in *Chapter 12*.
- Selection during spermatogenesis. As mentioned above, most cases of achondroplasia are new mutations, yet the condition is relatively common. The mutation rate is fairly high to account for this. This is only mildly surprising until we remember that only one very specific change, p.Gly380Arg in the FGFR3 protein will produce achondroplasia (see *Box figure 6.1*). Most A→a mutation rates are the sum of the rates of mutation of hundreds of individual nucleotides, but for achondroplasia the whole mutation rate is the rate of this one specific change. The mutation rate at the nucleotide concerned is many orders of magnitude higher than the mutation rate at almost any other specific nucleotide in the entire genome. Inspection of the sequence does not suggest any reason for such an extraordinarily high mutability. The answer is believed to be that the mutation rate is not actually especially high, but cells in the male germ-line that carry the mutation are at a proliferative advantage, and so contribute disproportionately to the production of sperm.

What is the chance the offspring of a consanguineous marriage will have a recessive disease?

Consider Jack and Jill who are first cousins. Suppose the gene frequency of a disease gene is q. The chance that Jack is a carrier is $2pq$. For a rare disease p is virtually 1, so Jack's carrier risk is very nearly $2q$. Jill shares $1/8$ of her genes with Jack by virtue of their relationship. That is to say, for any allele in Jack, there is a 1 in 8 chance that Jill has the same allele, inherited from a common ancestor. Therefore if Jack is a carrier, the chance that Jill is a carrier is $1/8$. If they are both carriers, the chance of a child being affected is 1 in 4. Overall the risk is $2q \times 1/8 \times 1/4 = q/16$. *Table 10.3* shows that the rarer a condition is, the greater is the relative risk for first cousins compared to unrelated people.

Table 10.3 – **Inbreeding and the risk of a recessive disease**

Disease gene frequency	Risk of affected child – unrelated parents	Risk of affected child – first cousin marriage	Relative risk for first cousins
q	q^2	$q/16$	$1/16q$
0.01	1 in 10 000	1 in 1600	6.25
0.005	1 in 40 000	1 in 3200	12.5
0.001	1 in 1 000 000	1 in 16 000	62.5

The calculation is only valid for rare diseases because it assumes the frequency of the normal allele is effectively 1, and it assumes that the only way first cousins would both carry a disease gene is if they both inherit it from a common ancestor.

Another way of looking at this, is that the rarer a recessive condition is, the greater the proportion of cases that are the offspring of consanguineous marriages. As mentioned before, this means that Hardy–Weinberg calculations of carrier frequencies are likely to be misleading when applied to rare recessives.

Can we abolish genetic disease?

Clinical geneticists are very clear that their goal is not to wipe out genetic disease, and their output must not be measured by the number of abnormal pregnancies terminated. Their goal is to enable people with genetic diseases, or at risk of them, to lead as normal lives as possible, including having families. Nevertheless, health planners might find it attractive if a by-product of genetic services were a reduction in the frequency of genetic disorders.

The discussion of mutations and selection above shows that abolishing genetic disease is not a generally realistic aim. Most serious dominant conditions have a high proportion of new mutations, while for recessives, the great majority of mutant genes are in healthy heterozygotes. If a country's dictator decided to sterilize all people with serious genetic diseases, this would not prevent fresh cases appearing in the next generation. Even continued over many generations this program could not succeed in its aim. A few dominant late-onset conditions such as Huntington disease could be largely prevented, but the only way to prevent recessive diseases would be to sterilize all carriers. This would rebound badly on the dictator and his family. Although carrier frequencies for individual recessive conditions are typically of the order of 1 in 100, OMIM lists thousands of different conditions, and every one of us is a carrier for several lethal recessive conditions. A sterilization program could prevent genetic disease only by sterilizing the dictator, along with the rest of the human race.

A slightly different question is whether medicine is storing up long-term problems by effectively combating natural selection (see *Box 10.4*).

BOX 10.4

Should treated people repay their debt to society by not having children?

Consider a treatable genetic condition such as phenylketonuria (PKU; see **Case 22, Vlasi family** in *Chapter 11*). Untreated phenylketonurics are severely mentally retarded and are likely to spend their lives in an institution. When the treatment works, an affected person is enabled to live a normal life, including having children. Genetically the person is still homozygous for the mutation, and any child will inevitably inherit a mutant allele. The treatment is expensive – should there be a bargain? Should we say that we agree to fund the treatment, but in return the treated person should agree not to pass on his or her mutant genes?

Most clinicians would find such a proposition deeply distasteful – but they may have at the back of their mind an uneasy feeling that as responsible physicians, perhaps they ought to face the question. The question should indeed be faced – because when it is examined, it goes away. We showed above that for a recessive condition the proportion of all mutant alleles that are present in affected people is q, where q is the gene frequency. In the UK, PKU affects about one person in 10 000. Thus q is 0.01. In other words, agonizing about whether or not a treated phenylketonuric has the right to pass on his genes is agonizing about 1% of the problem while ignoring the other 99%. Since we know we can have no influence on the 99%, it is pointless to worry about the 1%. Of course, each time a treated phenylketonuric passes on a mutant allele rather than failing to reproduce, that must marginally increase the frequency of mutant alleles in the next generation. Continued over 100 generations, a treatment program might double the gene frequency. Most people would feel that humanity has rather more serious problems to face over the next 2500 years than a doubling of the frequency of PKU mutant alleles.

DISEASE BOX 10

Jewish diseases and Finnish diseases

Ashkenazi Jews and Finns are the two best-studied examples of populations with strong founder effects. Both have high levels of education and well developed medical services that provide good data on the range and frequency of genetic diseases. *Table 10.1* listed some Finnish diseases, and *Box table 10.1* in this section shows some Ashkenazi Jewish diseases. Motulsky (1995) provides a good concise review of Jewish diseases.

Both populations have expanded greatly from a fairly small number of founders.

Box table 10.1 – Some diseases that are unusually prevalent among Ashkenazi Jews

Disease	OMIM number	Mode of inheritance	Carrier frequency	Comments
Tay–Sachs disease	272800	AR	$1/30$	Three fairly common Ashkenazi mutations – see **Case 21 (Ulmer family)** and *Chapter 11*
Familial dysautonomia	223900	AR	$1/30$	Very few non-Jewish cases reported; 99.5% of Jewish cases have the same splicing mutation
Gaucher disease	230800	AR	$1/15$	Two common Ashkenazi mutations p.Asn380Ser (75%) and c.84insG (15%); p.Leu444Pro also frequent
Canavan disease	271900	AR	$1/40–1/60$	Two common Ashkenazi mutations, p.Glu285Ala and p.Tyr231STOP
Fanconi anemia complementation group C	227645	AR	$1/90$	Most Ashkenazi cases have a splice site mutation in intron 4
Niemann–Pick disease Type A	257200	AR	$1/80$	Three mutations account for 65% of Ashkenazi cases
Bloom syndrome	210900	AR	$1/200?$	Most Ashkenazi cases have the same mutation, deletion of ATCTGA and insertion of TACATTC at nucleotide 2281
Familial breast cancer	113705 (*BRCA1*); 600185 (*BRCA2*)	AD	Total 2.5%	Three common Ashkenazi mutations: c.185delAG (1% of population), c.5382insC (0.15%) in *BRCA1*; c.6174delT (1.5%) in *BRCA2*
Torsion dystonia 1	128100	AD	$1/1000–1/300$ affected	Genetics heterogeneous; many Ashkenazi and non-Jewish patients have the same 3 bp deletion

- Of the 13–14 million Jews in the world, about 80% are Ashkenazi, descendants of a population that migrated to the Rhineland in Germany in the ninth century, and later moved into Poland, Lithuania, Belarus and surrounding regions. Ashkenazim have been distinct from Sephardic Jews, who are primarily from Spain, Portugal and North Africa, for over 1000 years. Until a few hundred years ago, Sephardim constituted the majority of all Jews, and their communities in Spain and Portugal may have existed since Roman times. The Ashkenazi population probably comprised a few thousand individuals in the early modern period. Motulsky (1995) suggests that a small prosperous merchant class may have contributed disproportionately to succeeding generations, producing very strong founder effects.

- In Finland there were two phases of expansion, either of which could have produced strong founder effects: one in prehistoric times soon after the south of the country was first settled, and another in the seventeenth century when pioneer groups populated the largely empty north (De la Chapelle, 1993).

There has been controversy over whether the distribution of alleles in Ashkenazi diseases can be explained just in terms of population history. With a simple founder effect, one might expect one mutant allele, on one specific marker haplotype, to explain all the excess cases of a disease (excess over the levels found in other populations). That is what we see in familial dysautonomia, Fanconi anemia and Bloom syndrome. But in Tay–Sachs, Gaucher, Niemann–Pick and Canavan diseases, two or more alleles are relatively common. This has been taken as evidence of heterozygote advantage. It is noteworthy that three of the four diseases listed are lysosomal storage diseases (Tay–Sachs, Gaucher and Niemann–Pick disease), and in fact another lysosomal storage disease, mucolipidosis IV, is also relatively common in Ashkenazim. Is this just coincidence, or could there be something about being a carrier of a lysosomal storage disease that was advantageous at some time in the history of this population?

A natural observational bias could explain some of the data. For example, three different *BRCA1/2* mutations are fairly common in Ashkenazim and rare elsewhere (see *Chapter 12*). This seems remarkable – but it may be just an initial random fluctuation, amplified by the strong population expansion. Before demanding a special explanation, we should remember all the other genes where we don't find common Ashkenazi mutations. Maybe it is not so remarkable that one gene in a thousand should show a random fluctuation large enough to produce the present distribution.

10.5. **References**

De la Chapelle A (1993) Disease gene mapping in isolated human populations: the example of Finland. *J. Med. Genet.* **30**: 857–865.

Motulsky AG (1995) Jewish diseases and origins. *Nat. Genet.* **9**: 99–101.

Paw BH, Tieu PT, Kaback MM, Lim J and Neufeld EF (1990) Frequency of three Hex A mutant alleles among Jewish and non-Jewish carriers identified in a Tay-Sachs screening program. *Am. J. Hum. Genet.* **47**: 698–705.

10.6. **Self-assessment questions**

(1) 200 unrelated people were typed for a single nucleotide polymorphism that has two alleles, C and T. 87 people were CT, 93 TT and 20 CC. What are the gene frequencies of the C and T alleles? Is the population in Hardy-Weinberg equilibrium?

(2) Usher syndrome Type 1 is an autosomal recessive deaf–blindness syndrome that affects one person in 100 000 in a population. Although all cases are clinically indistinguishable, genetic analysis has shown that mutations in several different genes can cause Usher syndrome (locus heterogeneity). What is the carrier frequency, (a) if all cases are due to mutations at a single locus, and (b) if homozygosity at any one of 10 different loci contributes equally to the overall incidence?

(3) Inability to taste low concentrations of bitter substances such as phenylthiourea and perhaps some types of cabbage is (usually) an autosomal recessive trait. People can be classified as tasters and non-tasters. 64% of people in a population dislike spring greens and won't eat them because they taste unpleasantly bitter. What is the frequency of the taster allele?

(4) It is known that erythropoietic protoporphyria behaves as a dominant condition with reduced penetrance, but molecular analysis has shown that affected people are all compound heterozygotes, having a rare non-functioning allele and a common low-functioning allele ($q = 0.11$ in France). If the condition affects 1 person in 30 000 in France, what is the frequency of the non-functioning allele? What is the risk that an affected person, married to an unaffected person, will have an affected child?

(5) A woman's only son has Duchenne muscular dystrophy. She has no brothers or sisters, and there is no history of the disease in the rest of the family. What is the chance her daughter is a carrier?

(6) The healthy sister of a boy with cystic fibrosis marries an unrelated man whose family has no history of the disease. Both are of Danish stock. She is pregnant. What is the risk the child will have cystic fibrosis? If she had consulted you beforehand, would you have advised her not to have children?

(7) An autosomal recessive disease affects one person in 40 000. A woman's marriage breaks up under the stress of caring for her affected child. She finds solace with a sympathetic cousin; eventually they marry and now she is pregnant. What is the risk their child will be affected?

(8) Fred has an extremely rare autosomal recessive disease. What is the chance that both of his grandfathers are carriers?

(9) Waleed and Benazir (*Figure 10.4*) marry and have a deaf son, Aziz. Deaf people often prefer to marry a deaf partner, and Aziz marries Nasreen Choudhary. What is the chance their first child will be deaf? Calculate the coefficient of inbreeding of this child. Apart from deafness, is this child at high risk of other recessive conditions?

After working through this chapter you should be able to:

- Distinguish between screening and diagnosis
- Describe the parameters commonly used to define the performance of a screening program
- Describe the technical, social and ethical requirements that a screening program should fulfil
- Give examples of prenatal, neonatal and postnatal screening programs, and discuss their advantages and disadvantages to individuals and to society

11.1. **Case studies**

CASE 22	Vlasi family	**273**	280	389

- Valon, a 6-year-old boy
- Serious learning problems
- Small, microcephalic, blue eyes, fair skin and hair, eczema; hyperactive
- ? Phenylketonuria

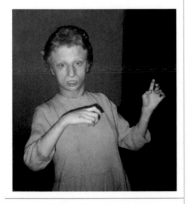

Figure 11.1 – A patient with untreated PKU.

Valon, aged 6 years, was the only child of Adem and Flora Vlasi. They had had a very unsettled life. Valon was born in Kosovo. The family lived in a remote rural area where only basic medical care was available. Soon after he was born the political situation became unstable and the family moved several times before entering Australia as refugees. Over the years, Adem had been worried about Valon's progress but Flora said the problems were likely to be due to all the moves he had experienced and the fact that he had not been to school. When they settled and Valon was enrolled in school, the teachers recognized at once that he had serious learning problems. They arranged for assessment by an educational psychologist and suggested that the family doctor refer him to a pediatrician. In the clinic the doctor was surprised to see that Valon had a condition he had only read about in textbooks. Valon was small and microcephalic and had blue eyes, very fair skin and hair, as well as eczema. He was hyperactive and when restrained he rocked his body. The pediatrician also thought that Valon had a musty smell about him in spite of him being well cared for by his parents. The doctor strongly suspected that Valon had phenylketonuria and arranged for measurement of phenylpyruvic acid in a urine sample and phenylalanine levels in a blood sample.

11.2. **Science toolkit**

Screening versus diagnostic tests

The word 'screening' is often used loosely as a synonym for testing, but the essentials of a true screening program are that it is applied to a whole population. In contrast to diagnostic tests, where a person has a problem and approaches the clinician for a test, screening is usually a top-down process, offered by some organization to a large cohort of people (probably defined by age, reproductive state, or ethnic origin). In any genetic screening program, ethical considerations are at least as important as technical questions. In this section we will consider some of the more straightforward technical matters, and return to some more general questions in the final section of this chapter.

Most screening tests do not result in a definite diagnosis, but serve to define a high risk group of people, who are then offered a definitive diagnostic test (*Figure 11.2*). Usually this involves setting an arbitrary cut-off point (*Figure 11.3*). This is always a compromise. Setting the cut-off too high means missing an unacceptably large proportion of the target group, while setting it too low means exposing too many people to further investigation, most of whom will turn out not to be affected. Even screening programs for mendelian disease such as phenylketonuria or cystic fibrosis are subject to these compromises. A DNA test might give an immediate diagnostic answer, but screening programs rarely rely on mutation analysis as the first line of investigation. *Box 11.1* shows some of the measures used to define the validity of a screening test.

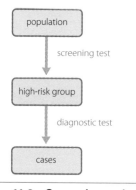

Figure 11.2 – Screening and diagnostic tests.

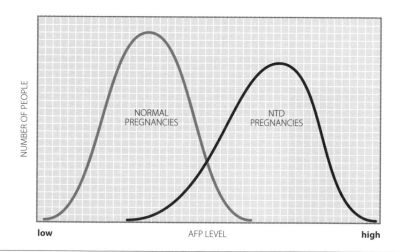

Figure 11.3 – A typical screening test.
The level of alpha-fetoprotein (AFP) in the serum of a pregnant women is an indicator of the risk that her fetus has a neural tube defect (spina bifida or anencephaly). A raised level of AFP in the mother's blood indicates a higher risk, but the distributions in normal and affected pregnancies overlap. An arbitrary cut-off is used to select about 5% of women for further investigation. This involves detailed ultrasound examination and/or amniocentesis (see *Chapter 14*). Most women with raised AFP eventually deliver normal babies.

BOX 11.1

Parameters of a screening test

Considering, for example, the AFP test shown in *Figure 11.3*, women can be positive or negative on the test, and can have a fetus with or without a neural tube defect (NTD). In the table, a, b, c and d are actual numbers of women in each category.

	Fetus has NTD	**Fetus does not have NTD**
Positive on test	a	c
Negative on test	b	d

Sensitivity of test = proportion of affected picked up = a / (a+b)

Specificity of test = proportion of all unaffected that are true negatives = d / (c+d)

False positive rate = proportion of all tests that give a false positive result = c / (a+b+c+d)

False negative rate = proportion of all tests that give a negative result = b / (a+b+c+d)

Positive predictive value – proportion of all positives that are affected = a / (a+c)

Odds ratio = odds of being a case after a positive test (a:c) compared to odds of being a case after a negative result (b:d) = (a/c) / (b/d) = ad / bc

Relative risk = risk after a positive test compared to general population risk or risk after a negative test = [a / (a+c)] / [(a+b) / (a+b+c+d)] or [a / (a+c)] / [b / (b+d)]

When might screening be done?

Genetic screening tests (*Figure 11.4*) fall into three groups.

- Prenatal screening – pregnant women in the UK, for example, are usually offered screening for Down syndrome, sickle cell disease and thalassemia. A general fetal anomaly screen uses a careful ultrasound examination of the fetus to look for structural anomalies. This should pick up most NTDs, in addition to other abnormalities, making a separate AFP test unnecessary. Screening for Down syndrome is discussed in relation to **Case 8 (Howard family)** in *Section 11.3*. Many individual mendelian and chromosomal conditions are also detectable prenatally, but these are not population screening tests; they are offered to individual couples who are known to be at high risk because of their family history.
- Newborn screening – as described in the next section, in many countries all newborn babies are screened for phenylketonuria. A variety of other tests may also be routinely offered (see *Section 11.4*). The list differs in different countries and often from institution to institution within a country. In the UK, national newborn screening programs are in place for phenylketonuria, cystic fibrosis, sickle cell disease, hypothyroidism, medium chain acyl-CoA dehydrogenase deficiency, hearing, and various problems detectable by clinical examination. In many other countries the list is much longer (see *Section 11.4*)

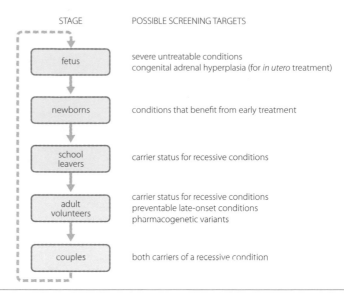

STAGE   POSSIBLE SCREENING TARGETS

fetus — severe untreatable conditions / congenital adrenal hyperplasia (for *in utero* treatment)

newborns — conditions that benefit from early treatment

school leavers — carrier status for recessive conditions

adult volunteers — carrier status for recessive conditions / preventable late-onset conditions / pharmacogenetic variants

couples — both carriers of a recessive condition

Figure 11.4 – **When might screening be done?**

- **Adult screening** – this is most likely to be for carrier status for recessive, diseases – for example Tay–Sachs carrier screening in Ashkenazi Jews (see *Section 11.3*, **Case 21, Ulmer family**). Particular groups of adults may be screened for other genetic risk factors, though this is usually conducted through family tracing rather than true population screening. For example, people with a strong family history of breast cancer are screened for *BRCA1/2* mutations (see *Chapter 12*), and people with high cholesterol levels may be screened for genetic hypercholesterolemia (see *Disease box 11*). As described in *Chapter 8*, screening for pharmacogenetic variants affecting drug metabolism is mandated for a few drugs, and may perhaps become more common over the coming years.

For some conditions there are a variety of different ways in which screening might be offered. Carrier screening for a recessive condition might be performed on newborn infants, on school leavers, on couples of childbearing age selected by general practitioners, on pregnant women and their partners, or on anybody who cares to visit a drop-in centre. Each approach has its advantages and drawbacks. Points to consider include:

- can the subjects give properly informed consent?
- how easy is it to access the group to be screened?
- how relevant will the information be at that time to the person screened?
- what are the practical and ethical implications of a positive result?
- what will the program cost, and do the benefits justify the cost?

These considerations are discussed a little further in *Section 11.3* in relation to Tay–Sachs carrier screening.

Who should be screened?

Screening can be offered to the whole population or to specific groups. Singling out particular groups for screening may become politically fraught, no matter how sound the epidemiological case for doing so. When Down syndrome testing was restricted to older women because of their higher risk (see *Table 2.1*), some younger women who subsequently had a baby with Down syndrome complained that they had been unfairly discriminated against. Plans to screen specific ethnic groups have often caused trouble. In the UK, all babies are screened for sickle cell disease, and carrier screening is offered to all women early in pregnancy, even though the risk for white native British people is extremely low; however, the methodology used depends on the risk level in the local population.

In other cases screening is based on family history. This is done partly for economic reasons. Scanning the entire *BRCA1* and *BRCA2* genes for mutations is very expensive and, in the British NHS, testing is prioritized based on family history. These tests, and cascade screening (see *Disease box 11*) represent a halfway house between family-based clinical genetics and population screening.

How should screening be done?

A DNA test is seldom the best screening test. The cheap and rapid DNA tests that would be suitable for large-scale screening always check for specific mutations (see *Chapter 5*). However, what we usually want to know is whether *any* mutation is present, not just certain specific ones. For loss of function conditions with extensive allelic heterogeneity, it is usually more efficient to use a functional test for large-scale screening. PKU screening is based on measuring the level of phenylalanine in a blood spot; Tay–Sachs screening normally measures the ability of the affected enzyme to break down an artificial substrate; and cystic fibrosis screening relies on measuring the level of immunoreactive trypsin, although cystic fibrosis carrier screening would necessarily use a DNA test.

11.3. **Investigations of patients**

| CASE 8 | Howard family | 26 | 38 | 69 | 102 | **277** | 389 |

- Helen – new-born daughter of Henry and Anne (33 years old)
- Down syndrome
- Risk of recurrence if they have more children?

Antenatal screening for Down syndrome (and other chromosomal anomalies) has been available for many years. Until the 1980s the screening test consisted of asking the mother's age. As *Table 2.1* shows, the risk of having a baby with Down syndrome rises sharply for older women. Over a certain cut-off (normally in the range 35–38 years, depending on resources available) women were offered a definitive diagnostic test. The diagnostic test is chromosome analysis of fetal cells obtained by amniocentesis or chorion villus biopsy. These procedures are invasive, unpleasant for the woman, and carry a 0.5–2% risk of causing a miscarriage. They are only appropriate for women at the highest risk.

Screening by maternal age alone has low sensitivity. Although the individual risk is higher for a woman over 38, there are so many more pregnancies among younger women that the majority of babies with Down syndrome are in fact born to younger women. Current screening protocols use a combination of ultrasound findings and maternal serum biochemical markers to improve the sensitivity. The ultrasound test measures the fluid under the skin of the neck of the fetus (nuchal translucency). Several substances in the mother's blood may be assayed. These include alpha-fetoprotein (AFP), beta-human chorionic gonadotrophin (hCG), unconjugated estriols (uE3), pregnancy-associated plasma protein A (PAPP-A), and inhibin A. For each, the distribution of levels in Down syndrome pregnancies (after adjustment for gestational age and maternal weight) is rather different from that in normal pregnancies. In the large US FASTER study (Malone *et al.*, 2005) median second trimester values for Down syndrome pregnancies, as multiples of the median for normal pregnancies, were 0.74 (AFP), 1.79 (hCG), 0.72 (uE3) and 1.98 (inhibin A). All the Down syndrome and normal distributions overlap strongly, so that none of the levels is diagnostic by itself, but in combination, and including the mother's age, they give a composite risk figure that is far more predictive than age alone. Women whose composite risk is greater than some predetermined cut-off, typically 1:250, are offered the diagnostic test.

No one protocol is best for all circumstances. Deciding what cut-off to use involves a trade-off between sensitivity and false positive rate. Any increase in sensitivity will be accompanied by a decrease in specificity. *Table 11.1* shows illustrative data from the FASTER study. First trimester screening allows women with positive results to have chorion villus biopsy and a less traumatic procedure for any termination of the pregnancy. But some women book too late for this, and in others the nuchal translucency cannot be assessed because of the lie of the fetus or the mother's high body mass. These women may be offered a serum 'triple' or 'quadruple' test at 15–20 weeks using hCG, uE3, AFP and, in the quadruple test, inhibin A. A two-stage fully integrated protocol has the best performance on paper, but requires women to turn up for both phases of the screen and drags out the process. The FASTER study recommended first trimester screening where practicable. Similar guidelines are recommended by the UK National Institute of Health and Clinical Excellence (NICE): all pregnant women in the UK should be offered a screening test with a detection rate above 75% and a false positive rate of less than 3%.

Women such as Helen's mother Anne, who had a previous child with Down syndrome, would normally be offered a diagnostic test regardless of their age or

Table 11.1 – **Peformance of different protocols for antenatal screening for Down syndrome**

Protocol	Test sensitivity (%)		
	75	85	95
NT, PAPP-A and hCG at 12 weeks	1.4	4.8	21
Quadruple test at 15–20 weeks	3.1	7.3	22
Fully integrated test	0.2	0.8	5.0

Figures show the percentage of false positive test results with different screening protocols and cut-off thresholds. The test sensitivity is determined by the threshold value of the composite risk that is chosen for declaring the screening result positive. NT is nuchal translucency assessed by ultrasound. Quadruple test: maternal serum AFP, hCG, uE3 and inhibin A. Fully integrated test: NT + PAPP-A at 12 weeks followed by quadruple test in second trimester.
Data taken from the FASTER study (Malone *et al.*, 2005).

objective risk level. Although the recurrence risk for a younger woman is low, their anxiety level is naturally very high after having had an affected baby, and it would be cruel to refuse them the test.

There is considerable debate about the most appropriate test to use once fetal cells have been obtained (*Box 11.2*). As described in *Chapter 4*, Anne Howard opted for interphase FISH testing, and received a reassuring normal result within 2 days – but she had to understand that this did not mean that her fetus was chromosomally normal, only that it had the correct number of copies of chromosomes 13, 18 and 21.

BOX 11.2

What is the best prenatal diagnostic test for Down syndrome?

After antenatal screening by one of the methods described above, women whose risk of a Down syndrome baby is above the cut-off are offered a diagnostic test. Fetal cells are obtained by amniocentesis or chorion villus biopsy, as described in *Chapter 14*. What is the best way of analyzing these cells?

- *Traditional karyotyping*, as described in *Chapter 2*, can detect every chromosome abnormality, but arguably this is not desirable. While autosomal trisomies are always pathological, detecting some other abnormalities would present the couple with very difficult decisions that they might prefer not to have to face. Some, such as Turner syndrome or XYY have well understood but relatively minor consequences, while the effects of others, such as *de novo* apparently balanced rearrangements or mosaicism for a small unidentified extra chromosome (a 'marker'), are unpredictable. Is it perhaps better not to know? *Box figure 11.1* shows some data found by full karyotyping.

- *Molecular tests* check specifically for the common trisomies of chromosomes 13, 18 and 21. The technique used may be interphase FISH or QF–PCR (see *Chapter 4*). Both these methods can be applied to uncultured cells, avoiding the long wait required while the fetal cells are grown up for conventional cytogenetics.

In one UK survey, full karyotyping took 12 days and cost £253 per test; quantitative PCR took 24 hours and cost £30 per test. But around 10% of the abnormalities missed by the rapid test have a poor prognosis. Some of these will be picked up on routine ultrasound examination, and some will abort spontaneously, but some will result in live-born abnormal babies. A common strategy is to get a quick result with QF–PCR and back this up with full karyotyping, but some laboratories use just QF–PCR.

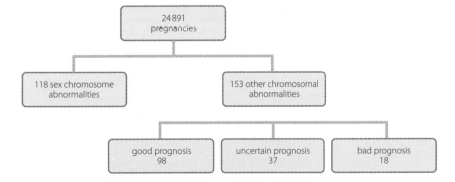

Box figure 11.1 – Chromosomal abnormalities found by full karyotyping of prenatal samples that would not have been detected by molecular trisomy testing.
Data on 24 891 women tested because of increased risk of Down syndrome, from Ogilvie *et al.* (2005).

- Valon, a 6-year-old boy
- Serious learning problems
- Small, microcephalic, blue eyes, fair skin and hair, eczema; hyperactive
- ? Phenylketonuria
- Testing for subsequent baby?

When the family came to Sydney, Flora was already 6 weeks pregnant. Having learned that Valon had a serious genetic disease, she and Adem were extremely worried about the risk of the new baby being affected. With all their other problems, they felt they could not cope with a second affected child, and they discussed terminating the pregnancy despite their general reservations about abortion. When their family doctor explained that even if the baby was affected (a 1 in 4 risk), it could be treated, they immediately asked for the treatment for Valon – but the doctor explained that the treatment was only effective if started very soon after birth (see *Chapter 14*). So they asked if the new baby could be tested as soon as it was born, and were assured that it would be.

Flora delivered a healthy girl, and mother and baby were discharged from hospital. A few days later the midwife visited them at home. As well as checking on the health and progress of mother and baby, she pricked the baby's heel and collected a blood spot on to a special card (a Guthrie card). This is standard practice for every baby born in many countries, regardless of family history. The card was sent to a central laboratory and here the level of phenylalanine in the blood was measured. Although it would have been easier to take the blood sample while the baby was still in the hospital, this was not done because, while it is *in utero*, a phenylketonuric baby's phenylalanine is cleared through the placenta by the mother (who is expected to be a phenotypically normal heterozygote) – see *Figure 11.5*. Only after the placental connection is broken does the phenylalanine level in a phenylketonuric baby start to rise. It takes a few days for an elevated level to become readily apparent. The optimal time is day 5, though in countries without integrated healthcare systems, the best course may be to take blood at 24–48 hours, while the mother and baby are still in hospital.

Laboratories may use various methods to check the phenylalanine level, including a bacterial growth assay, chromatography, fluorimetry, or tandem mass spectrometry. The latter has the advantage of allowing a number of other analytes to be measured at the same time (see *Table 11.4*). A DNA test is not used at this stage because there are many possible mutations in the *PAH* gene. A direct enzyme assay is not used because that would require a liver biopsy. Whatever the method, this is a screening test and not a diagnostic test. The cut-off for the screening test is usually set around 120

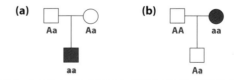

Figure 11.5 – While it is *in utero*, the level of phenylalanine in a fetus is determined by the mother's genotype and not its own.
(a) A phenylketonuric fetus develops normally *in utero* because the mother clears excess phenylalanine through the placenta. (b) Because the high level of phenylalanine in the maternal circulation crosses the placenta, the normal fetus of a phenylketonuric mother will be born severely brain-damaged and microcephalic unless the mother goes on a low phenylalanine diet throughout her pregnancy.

µM (normal range 58 ± 15 µM). Babies whose blood level is above the cut-off are called in for more specific testing. This involves more careful measurement of the blood phenylalanine level. In PKU this is typically above 1000 µM. A lower, but still elevated level is seen in babies with benign hyperphenylalaninemia. These babies develop normally without treatment. The screening test has a sensitivity of around 98–99% for PKU provided it is not performed too soon after birth. Babies proven to have PKU are put on a special diet, as described in *Chapter 14*. Careful adherence to the diet ensures that the child grows up with no or minimal cognitive impairment.

Phenylalanine hydroxylase requires an essential cofactor, tetrahydrobiopterin (BH_4). A small percentage of phenylketonuric babies have a genetic defect in the production or recycling of BH_4, rather than mutations in the *PAH* gene. These require a different treatment because BH_4 is required for several other amino acid hydroxylations. The laboratory work-up checks for these variant forms of PKU, and will often include DNA studies to define the mutations in the *PAH* gene.

| CASE 4 | Davies family | 4 | 10 | 67 | 104 | 155 | 186 | **281** | 389 |

- Boy (Martin) aged 24 months, parents Judith and Robert
- Clumsy and slow to walk
- Family history of muscular dystrophy
- Pedigree shows X-linked recessive inheritance
- Order diagnostic DNA test
- Frameshift mutation in the dystrophin gene
- Screening of all new-born boys?

Martin was not diagnosed until he was 2 years old, when his slow walking and clumsiness had become apparent. In some families, by the time the first affected boy is diagnosed there is already a second affected boy. This has led to the suggestion that all newborn boys should be screened for the disease. Technically this could be done reasonably cheaply by measuring the serum creatine kinase, which is strongly elevated in affected boys (see *Chapter 4*). Baby boys with a high creatine kinase could then be tested by a multiplex MLPA deletion screen (see *Figure 5.10*), which would pick up about two-thirds of cases. For the remainder a muscle biopsy might be required, to demonstrate the absence of dystrophin protein.

The proposal has been controversial. A small number of repeat cases would be avoided; on the other hand, making so grave a diagnosis so early, and when there is no useful treatment, robs the family of a couple of years of happy parenthood. There is also the question of how many unaffected boys whose creatine kinase was for some reason high would be subjected to muscle biopsy, and how serious the psychological trauma would be for parents whose baby initially tested positive, but was eventually shown to be unaffected. Neonatal DMD screening has so far been limited to some small local pilot programs, for example in Wales.

| CASE 2 | Brown family | 2 | 8 | 66 | 132 | 154 | **281** | 389 |

- Girl (Joanne) aged 6 months, parents David and Pauline
- ? Cystic fibrosis
- Order molecular test?
- Define mutations in CFTR gene
- Universal newborn screening?

Both Joanne's parents David and Pauline come from quite large families (*Figure 1.8*). Their relatives are clearly at high risk of being carriers of cystic fibrosis. Since we now know what mutations are present in David and Pauline (*Chapter 5*), it is fairly simple for any relative who might so wish, to be tested for these two specific mutations. This is an example of **cascade screening** (see *Disease box 11*). Because cystic fibrosis mutations are common in the general population, it is prudent also to test for a panel of the commonest mutations, just in case anybody happens to be a carrier coincidentally, having inherited a mutant gene from a different ancestor from the ones who were the source of David's or Pauline's mutations.

As the commonest severe recessive disease in many populations of European origin, cystic fibrosis has been considered for general population screening as well as cascade screening. This could include newborn screening to detect affected babies and/or screening adults to detect carriers. The argument for newborn screening is that early treatment improves the prognosis. In both the USA and the UK, this argument has been accepted and universal newborn screening is recommended. The method is based on measurement of immunoreactive trypsin (IRT), which is raised in cystic fibrosis. *Figure 11.6* shows the flow-chart for the British scheme.

For carrier screening it is necessary to use a DNA test, because carriers are entirely normal biochemically. The problem here is the very large number of mutations (over 1000) that have been described. As pointed out in *Section 5.4* it is easy to screen for a specific mutation but hard to test a gene for *any* possible mutation. The *CFTR* gene has 27 exons (see *Figure 3.8*) and there is currently no way of scanning the entire sequence of such a gene at a cost low enough to use in population screening. Because of founder effects and heterozygote advantage (*Chapter 10*) a few specific mutations make up the bulk of all cystic fibrosis mutations in any particular community. Any carrier screening protocol therefore involves a trade-off between cost and sensitivity. Testing for the few commonest mutations is cheap but misses some proportion of carriers. Testing for many mutations is expensive, and however many individual mutations are checked, the sensitivity will never be 100%. *Table 11.2* shows the distribution of *CFTR* mutations detected by one large UK laboratory.

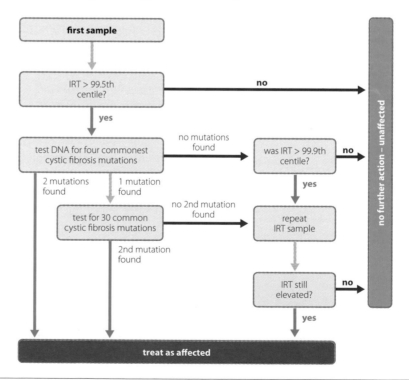

Figure 11.6 – Flowchart of a British scheme for screening newborn babies to allow early identification and treatment of those with cystic fibrosis.
IRT, immunoreactive trypsin.

Inevitably, some couples who have tested negative will actually both be carriers, with a 1 in 4 chance of having an affected baby. Almost all of these will be couples where one partner was recognized to be a carrier, but the other carried a rare mutation and was a false negative on the test. If the carrier frequency is 1 in 23 (*Chapter 10*) and the sensitivity of the screening test is 0.9, then about 1 person in 25 will be found to be a carrier. Given the smaller number of such people compared to the number initially screened, it is possible to test the partner for a larger panel of mutations to try to minimize the number of false negatives. Ultimately, one criterion for a screening program might be that the risk for a positive–negative couple should be no greater than the initial risk for any couple before screening. It could then be argued that the program has left nobody in a worse position than they were in before screening. For a carrier frequency of 1 in 23, this requires a 99.8% sensitivity for testing the partner of a known carrier (so that the risk of a false negative is 1 in 500). The figures in *Table 11.2* suggest that reaching 99.8% sensitivity would be a challenge.

Table 11.2 – Distribution of *CFTR* mutations in 1754 cystic fibrosis chromosomes analyzed in Manchester, UK

Mutation	Exon	Number found	Percentage of cystic fibrosis	Cumulative %
p.F508del	10	1420	81.0	
p.Gly551Asp	11	62	3.5	84.5
p.Gly542X	11	20	1.1	85.6
c.621+1G>T	Intron 4	17	1.0	86.6
c.1898+1G>A	Intron 12	16	0.9	87.5
p.Arg553X	11	13	0.7	88.3
p.Arg117His	4	13	0.7	89.0
p.Arg560Thr	11	11	0.6	89.6
c.3272−26A>G	Intron 17a	10	0.6	90.2
c.3659delC	19	9	0.5	90.7
p.Asn1303Lys	21	8	0.5	91.2
c.1717−1G>A	Intron 10	7	0.4	91.6
c.2711delT	14a	7	0.4	92.0
Other detected		114	6.5	98.5
Unknown		27	1.5	
Total		**1754**		**100.0**

A sensitivity of 90% could be achieved by testing for the commonest nine mutations; 95% sensitivity would require testing for 26 mutations.
Data courtesy of Dr Martin Schwartz, St Mary's Hospital, Manchester.

CASE 21   Ulmer family   253   261   **284**   389

- Hannah, a 6-month-old baby girl
- Ashkenazi Jewish origin
- Tay–Sachs disease
- Test the sibs?
- Screening for Tay–Sachs disease?

Among Ashkenazi Jews the carrier frequency for Tay–Sachs disease is 1 in 30. Because of this, carrier screening programs have been established in the USA and many other countries, starting in the early 1970s. *Table 11.3* shows some statistics. In countries where the Ashkenazi community have embraced carrier screening enthusiastically, the majority of affected babies are now born to non-Jewish couples.

Table 11.3 – **Tay–Sachs carrier screening among Ashkenazi Jews, 1971–1998**

Country	Number tested	Carriers	Carrier–carrier couples
United States	925 876	35 372	795
Israel	302 395	7277	380
Canada	65 813	3301	62
South Africa	15 138	1582	52
Europe	17 725	1127	37
Brazil	1027	72	20
Mexico	655	26	0
Argentina	84	5	0
Australia	3334	102	4
Total	**1 332 047**	**48 864**	**1350**

Data from Chapter 153 (Gravel *et al.*) of *Metabolic and Molecular Basis of Inherited Disease* edited by Scriver *et al.* (2001) and reproduced here with permission from The McGraw-Hill Companies.

Screening uses a biochemical test, measuring the ability of hexosaminidase A in serum to hydrolyze an artificial substrate MUG (an *N*-acetyl glucosamine derivative of 4-methyl umbelliferone). DNA testing is not used for population screening because not all carriers have one of the common Ashkenazi mutations (see *Table 10.2*). A more definitive diagnostic test is required after a positive screening result. About 2% of Jewish and 35% of non-Jewish people identified as carriers by the screening test in fact carry a so-called pseudodeficiency allele. Such alleles encode a variant form of the enzyme that is inactive against the artificial substrate used in the screening test, but retains enough activity against G_{M2} ganglioside to be non-pathogenic. Screening for Tay–Sachs disease is usually combined with screening for a variable selection of the other 'Jewish diseases' listed in *Disease box 10*.

There are various ways in which a carrier screening program could be implemented, and various actions that might follow a positive test result. Which one is adopted is very much a matter for the community concerned. Whatever protocol is adopted, screening should be voluntary and requires fully informed consent.

- **Testing babies or children** is unethical and inefficient. The child cannot give proper consent and the result has no implications until many years later, by which time it may well have been forgotten.
- **Testing school leavers** raises issues of just how far consent is truly voluntary, and requires careful handling to avoid stigmatization of carriers. Some Orthodox communities try to solve the stigmatization problem by giving the results to a match-maker and not to the individual tested (see below).
- **Testing young single adult volunteers** minimizes problems of consent but will miss some fraction of the target group.
- **Testing couples** identifies the small number of at-risk couples without worrying the much larger number of carriers whose spouse is a non-carrier (compare the last two columns of *Table 11.3*). But it removes the possibility of choosing not to marry a carrier. In some Orthodox communities where marriages are semi-arranged, the match-maker has the results of testing young single people for a range of recessive conditions, and will indicate if a proposed marriage would be risky.

11.4. **Going deeper ...**

What conditions should we screen for?

Technically, the possibilities for genetic screening seem almost unlimited – certainly they are already vast, and are increasing every year. In practice, however, what is on offer is very much more limited. Apart from the inevitable time-lag in bringing new developments into service, there are four main technical reasons why genetic screening is not more widespread (social and ethical factors are considered later).

- If you work through *Self-assessment questions 1–3*, you will see that the positive predictive value of a test may be very low, even if the test performs well in the laboratory. It is technically difficult, as well as economically questionable, to screen for rare conditions.
- A DNA variant may be indisputably associated with increased risk of a disease, but may be responsible for only a small fraction of the overall risk. Many DNA single nucleotide polymorphisms are associated with an increased risk of developing a common complex disease, but for almost all of them the odds ratio is so low as to make any prediction useless, even when the combined data from all known susceptibility factors are used. The **Population Attributable Risk** (*Box 11.3*) is an important consideration

---

The Population Attributable Risk

This is the proportion of the total disease risk in the population that is attributable to the factor in question. It is sometimes called the Population Attributable Fraction. If the PAR is low, it calls into question the value of screening for the factor.

If the overall risk in the population is r, but a proportion p of the population have a variant that gives them an additional risk of R, on top of the general risk, then the PAR for that variant is pR/r.

BOX 11.3

in any screening program. If a variant explains only 5% of the total risk, what is the point of screening for it? If that 5% is concentrated in a few individuals who have a very high risk, it might be valuable for those individuals to know – but this is approaching the situation for mendelian diseases, where testing is mainly family-based. If the variant is common, so that the extra risk is spread across a large proportion of the population, there seems little value to anybody in knowing.

• It is important to consider not just the *relative risk* but also the *absolute risk*. Even a high relative risk may not be too worrisome if it translates into a low absolute risk. An example is Factor V Leiden (OMIM 227400). This is a well-authenticated risk factor for venous thromboembolism, for example, among long-haul airline passengers and oral contraceptive users. The *relative* risk among oral contraceptive users is high (around 15) but the *absolute* risk still quite low, because oral contraceptive users are generally young and the risk of embolism is very age-dependent.

• In general, there is no point in screening unless a positive result leads to some useful action. This might mean lifestyle changes, prophylactic drugs to reduce the risk, or maybe increased surveillance, for example, to pick up a cancer at an early stage when it is still treatable. Sometimes genetic testing is done simply to provide people with information for planning their future as, for example, in predictive testing for Huntington disease, but normally a screening test should lead to some practical outcome.

The Office of Genomics and Disease Prevention at the Centers for Disease Control and Prevention in the USA has provided a framework that can be used for assessing any genetic (or other) test, not just a screening test. This ACCE framework suggests a test should be assessed against four sets of criteria.

• **Analytical validity**: how accurately does the test measure what it is supposed to measure? For a DNA test this might translate into asking what proportion of all mutations in a gene are picked up by the test protocol.

• **Clinical validity**: how accurately does the test detect or predict the presence or absence of disease? For example, most people with hereditary hemochromatosis (OMIM 235200) have mutations in both copies of their *HFE* gene, usually p.Cys282Tyr and/or p.His63Asp. But testing for these mutations has low clinical validity because the great majority of homozygotes or compound heterozygotes for the mutations do not have clinical hemochromatosis.

• **Clinical utility**: how useful are the test results in providing clinical benefits? Everybody with Type 1 Waardenburg syndrome (OMIM 193500) has a mutation in the *PAX3* gene. The test has high analytical and clinical validity – but detecting the mutations does not provide much obvious clinical benefit to most patients, beyond satisfying their curiosity.

• **Ethical, legal and social implications**

Population-based screening programs, where individuals opt out rather than opt in, need to be funded by the state or insurance companies. Funders will evaluate any proposed scheme critically against technical, financial and ethical criteria.

The criteria used are usually based on a set formulated by Wilson and Jungner in a 1968 report for the World Health Organization (see *References*). *Box 11.4* shows a selection of the criteria used by the UK National Screening Committee. In the directly marketed sector the arguments may look very different. Companies will offer a genetic test if they see a likely profitable market for it, regardless of

BOX 11.4

Criteria used by the UK National Screening Committee

For a complete list of the 22 criteria see www.screening.nhs.uk/criteria.

The condition:

(1) The condition should be an important health problem.

(2) The epidemiology and natural history of the condition ... should be adequately understood...

(3) All the cost-effective primary prevention interventions should have been implemented as far as practicable.

(4) If carriers of a mutation are identified as a result of screening, the natural history of people with this status should be understood, including the psychological implications.

The test:

(5) There should be a simple, safe, precise and validated screening test.

(7) The test should be acceptable to the population.

(9) If the test is for mutations, the criteria used to select the subset of mutations to be covered by screening, if all possible mutations are not being tested, should be clearly set out.

The treatment:

(10) There should be an effective treatment or intervention for patients identified through early detection, with evidence of early treatment leading to better outcomes than late treatment.

The screening programme:

(13) There should be evidence from high quality randomised controlled trials that the screening programme is effective in reducing mortality or morbidity. Where screening is aimed solely at providing information to allow the person being screened to make an 'informed choice' (e.g. Down syndrome, cystic fibrosis carrier screening) there must be evidence from high quality trials that the test accurately measures risk. The information that is provided about the test and its outcome must be of value and readily understood by the individual being screened.

(14) There should be evidence that the complete screening programme (test, diagnostic procedures, treatment / intervention) is clinically, socially and ethically acceptable to health professionals and the public.

(15) The benefit from the screening programme should outweigh the physical and psychological harm (caused by the test, diagnostic procedures and treatments).

(16) The opportunity cost of the screening programme (including testing, diagnosis and treatment, administration, training and quality assurance) should be economically balanced in relation to expenditure on medical care as a whole (i.e. value for money).

(17) All other options for managing the condition should have been considered (e.g. improving treatment, providing other services), to ensure that no more cost-effective intervention could be introduced...

(20) Evidence-based information, explaining the consequences of testing, investigation and treatment, should be made available to potential participants to assist them in making an informed choice.

(22) If screening is for a mutation, the programme should be acceptable to people identified as carriers and to other family members.

whether or not it might result in useful actions or long-term benefits. This has resulted in various companies offering 'lifestyle' genetic screening – testing for variants associated with increased risk of some common disease, coupled with advice on how to mitigate any increased risk (see *Box 11.5*). Profitability may, however, depend on being able to pass part of the cost on to somebody else. Somebody in the UK who gets a disturbing test result from an internet-based company, will probably expect their family doctor and NHS genetics service to deal with their worries.

Newborn screening is the least ethically contentious area of population screening, because the targets are treatable conditions and the aim is to ensure early treatment to avoid irreversible damage. In every advanced country newborn babies are screened for a variety of conditions where early diagnosis has the potential to improve outcome. Screening (except for hearing) uses a blood spot taken from a heel prick. Babies testing positive are then referred for a definitive diagnostic test. Blood sampling has to wait until some time after delivery, because until the placental connection is broken, the baby's blood chemistry will be heavily influenced by the mother (see *Figure 11.5*). In the USA, the sample is normally taken 24–48 hours after birth. In the UK every new mother is visited at home by a midwife after 5 days to check on the health of the mother and baby, and the heel prick is done at that visit.

In 2005 the American College of Medical Genetics recommended screening for the 29 conditions listed in *Table 11.4*. A further 25 conditions are listed as secondary targets – these would often be detected in the course of the primary screen and should be reported, but are not actively sought because they do not have documented treatments, or the natural history is insufficiently well understood. Later, severe combined immunodeficiency disease was added to the list of core conditions, and T-cell deficiencies to the list of secondary targets. Each state or region devises and operates its own screening program, with varying coverage of the recommended 30 conditions. Up-to-date summaries are available from the National Newborn Screening and Genetics Resource Center (see www.marchofdimes.com/peristats). Currently (July 2010) nearly all babies born in the USA live in states that require screening for 21 or more disorders.

In the UK the policy is more conservative and cautious. Nationwide screening programs are in place for only five conditions: phenylketonuria, cystic fibrosis, medium chain acyl-CoA dehydrogenase deficiency, hypothyroidism and hemoglobinopathies. Screening for other conditions depends on local initiatives. This shorter list is dictated partly by cost, but also by the very stringent requirements used by the UK National Screening Committee for approving a screening program (*Box 11.4*). For most of the rarer biochemical disorders, the diagnosis is not made, and treatment not started, until the baby comes to attention because it is sick. Perhaps the universal free National Health Service reduces the risk of a sick baby slipping through the net and not being diagnosed.

Attitudes towards prenatal screening, or screening children or adults for carrier status or risk of developing a late-onset condition, are more engrained in local cultures. Criteria 7, 14, 15, 20 and 22 of the UK NSC set cover ethical and social issues. Screening is an expression of the desires and values of the society in

BOX **11.5**

'Lifestyle' genetic testing

Searching the internet, you can easily find companies offering to genotype you for certain common DNA variants in order to help you decide your most healthy lifestyle. The offer may focus on some particular aspect, producing a 'cardiac risk profile' or 'obesity risk profile', for example. More recently, many companies have been offering whole genome scans, genotyping you for 500 000 or so SNPs and reporting all those that have been associated with disease susceptibility. All these offers are based on reports of associations between common DNA polymorphisms and risk of specific diseases. The reports are likely to be by reputable scientists in peer-reviewed journals. Impressive though the list of references may look, there are several questions you need to ask.

(a) Has the association been validated? Only a minority of reported associations are validated in independent datasets.

(b) Has it been validated in your ethnic group? Many identified risk factors are specific to certain ethnic groups.

(c) What is the risk ratio? That is, does the variant increase your risk by a factor of 20, 5, 2 or 1.1? Almost certainly the answer will be much nearer 1.1 than 20. Note that odds ratios are not relative risks – work through *Self-assessment question 4* to be clear on this. Almost certainly the answer will be much nearer 1.1 than 20. Do you care about a 10% increase in your risk? It is important to distinguish between the statistical significance of an effect and its size. A large survey can identify a highly significant association (that is, there is no doubt that it is real) with a quite trivial risk ratio. Note incidentally that it is well known that initial risk ratios almost always come down in subsequent studies, even when the risk is confirmed.

(d) What is the population attributable risk?

(e) Will the predictions take your family history and your own clinical data into account? Despite the technical success of genome-wide association studies, for almost every disease all reported DNA variants collectively account for only a very small proportion of the overall heritability. Family history remains a much better predictor than SNP genotypes.

As the cost of DNA sequencing continues to tumble, companies will increasingly offer whole exome or whole genome sequencing, rather than SNP genotyping; the paper by Ashley *et al.* (2010) gives a foretaste. This approach may perhaps have the potential to reveal rather more significant risks than those revealed by SNP genotyping (see *Chapter 13*). It will take a few years before we know whether that will in fact happen. Meanwhile, it would be prudent to read the paper by Janssens and van Duijn (2008) before parting with your money.

Assuming a test is satisfactory by all these criteria, the question remains, so what? From a public health point of view, there is a risk that 'lifestyle' genetic testing may simply dilute universally valid messages about the need to eat sensibly, get some exercise and stop smoking. Companies looking at market opportunities may be less bothered by such thoughts – but no company could risk saying to people who come out as low risk on their test that they can therefore cheerfully indulge in an unhealthy lifestyle. The lawyers would have a field day. A person's reported risk may be below the population average, but it is not zero. Some people given a low risk for a particular disease will nevertheless succumb to that disease. Therefore, quite regardless of the test result, the advice from the company must be the same routine healthy living advice, just delivered a bit more emphatically for high-risk people. It might therefore be argued that such testing has no ethical implications. The same advice may be available to everybody free of charge, but some people will only take notice of it if they have paid $250 and received a scientific-looking piece of paper. The public health question is, what is the balance between those who would be motivated to act appropriately by receiving advice of a high risk and those who would act inappropriately on receiving advice of a lower risk?

Table 11.4 – The 29 conditions for which the American College of Medical Genetics (2005) recommends that every newborn baby should be screened

Condition	OMIM number	Treatment
Medium chain acyl-CoA dehydrogenase deficiency	201450	Nutritional supplements; avoid fasting
Congenital hypothyroidism	**	Oral thyroid hormone
Phenylketonuria	261600	Low-phenylalanine diet
Biotinidase deficiency	253260	Daily oral biotin
Sickle cell anemia	603903	Vigilant medical care, avoid infections
Congenital adrenal hyperplasia	201910	Genital surgery; hormone replacement
Isovaleric acidemia	243500	Low protein diet, nutritional supplements
Very long chain acyl-CoA dehydrogenase deficiency	201475	High carbohydrate, low fat diet; supplements; avoid fasting
Maple syrup urine disease	248600	Low protein diet
Galactosemia	230400	Avoid milk and dairy products
HbS/β thalassemia	141900	As for sickle cell anemia
HbS/C disease	141900	As for sickle cell anemia
Long chain 3-hydroxyacyl-CoA dehydrogenase deficiency	609016	High carbohydrate, low fat diet; supplements; avoid fasting
Glutaric acidemia Type I	231670	Low protein diet with oral carnitine
Hydroxymethylglutaric aciduria	246450	High carbohydrate, low fat, low protein diet; avoid fasting
Trifunctional protein deficiency	609015	Low fat diet, supplements, avoid fasting
Multiple carboxylase deficiency	253270	Oral biotin
Methylmalonic acidemia (mutase deficiency)	251000	Vitamin B_{12} and other supplements; low protein diet
Homocystinuria	236200	Diet, supplements including vitamins B_6 and B_{12}
3-methyl crotonyl-CoA carboxylase 1 deficiency	210200	Low protein diet
Hearing loss	**	Communication strategy; hearing aids, maybe cochlear implant
Methylmalonic acidemia (cblA or cblB deficiency)	251100	Vitamin B_{12}, low-protein diet
Propionic acidemia	606054	Low-protein diet, supplememts
Carnitine – acylcarnitine translocase deficiency	212138	Carnitine
β-keto thiolase deficiency	203750	Vigilant medical care, low-protein diet
Citrullinemia	215700	Low-protein diet, supplements
Argininosuccinic aciduria	207900	Low-protein diet, supplements
Tyrosinemia Type I	276700	NTBC (see *Section 14.4*)
Cystic fibrosis	219700	Vigilant medical care

They are listed in order of priority, based on frequency, severity, effectiveness of treatment and practicality of screening. Some rare conditions rank high because they can be added in to a multiplex tandem mass spectrometry, or high performance liquid chromatography screen, for very little extra cost. ** Congenital hypothyroidism and hearing loss have many causes, not all genetic.

which it takes place. Antenatal screening will have little place in a society where abortion is unacceptable under any circumstances, even though the two are not necessarily linked. Some societies are more accepting of abnormal people, or more fatalistic about abnormalities, while in others the desire for a normal child is very strong. Views on individual responsibility, and on the relative values of individual freedom and public health will affect the acceptability of specific programs. Attitudes to children are important – how far do parents own their children, and have the right to know about their genetic make-up, or how far must children's autonomy be respected, and no tests performed until the child is old enough to give properly informed consent? It is a general principle that screening should be voluntary and needs informed consent. People must in general be free to opt out of screening if they wish. This does not simply mean that they can decline testing; it also means that if, say, after declining prenatal testing they have an affected child, they should not be in any way blamed or penalized. But do parents who object to PKU screening have the right to risk condemning their child to life in an institution?

In Britain, the Greek Cypriot community have taken up screening for β-thalassemia with enthusiasm, whereas the Pakistani community, also at high risk, have by and large not wanted it. In Israel there is said to be a strong popular demand for every possible screening test, whereas in the UK the approach is much more cautious. For example, a chain of British high-street stores stopped offering a set of 'lifestyle' tests after public disquiet about the implications – even though many would argue that such tests are no more harmful than a horoscope, and at worst, only a waste of money. According to the stores, the reason for discontinuing the offer was lack of public interest which, if true, reflects better on the good sense of the British public.

Concerning the economics of screening, it is interesting to see how Criterion 16 in the UK NSC list is rather cautiously worded. Assessing the financial benefits of a screening program usually involves balancing the immediate costs of screening against claimed savings in the longer term. This is a difficult area, though of course a vital one in many areas of policy. It is handled using *discounted cash flow*. To compare a present cost with a saving in 10 years' time, the present cost is treated as an investment, whose value in 10 years is calculated using compound interest. The choice of interest rate to use (the discount rate) can have a major effect on the outcome, but different types of institution may have different views about the relevance of potential savings in the distant future. Moreover, these calculations have their limitations as guides to action. Applied to normal childbearing, the discounted cash flow method suggests that reproduction is financially disastrous for society: it is very unlikely that an individual's contribution to society in taxes as a working adult can ever repay the discounted cost of his delivery, upbringing and education.

If the cost calculations look reasonable, the decision on whether to implement a screening program revolves round public demand and social acceptability. Since public opinion is never unanimous about such issues, decisions are in the end political.

Familial hypercholesterolemia

We are all familiar with a high cholesterol level as a sign of unhealthy eating – but about 1 person in 500 has an extremely high cholesterol level as a result of a genetic condition and regardless of diet. Familial hypercholesterolemia (FH; OMIM 143890) is an autosomal dominant condition. In most populations it is the commonest of all clinically significant mendelian conditions. Heterozygotes typically have serum cholesterol and LDL-cholesterol levels of 250–450 and 200–400 mg/dl (normal range 150–250 and 75–175 mg/dl, respectively). They develop tendon xanthomata (subcutaneous cholesterol deposits) and suffer coronary artery disease in mid-life, with many premature deaths from myocardial infarction. Rare homozygous affected people have these features to a more extreme degree.

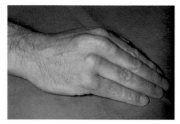 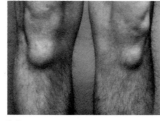 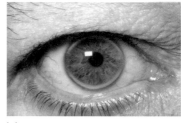

(a) (b) (c)

Cholesterol deposition in patients heterozygous for familial hypercholesterolemia. (a, b) Tendon xanthomata, and (c) corneal arcus. Photos courtesy of Dr Paul Durrington, Manchester Royal Infirmary.

Michael Brown and Joseph Goldstein won the 1985 Nobel Prize for Medicine for their work on FH that has led to a detailed understanding of cholesterol homeostasis (see *References* for further information). They demonstrated that FH was usually caused by mutations in the low density lipoprotein receptor (*LDLR*) gene. This cell surface receptor imports cholesterol-containing LDL into liver cells, where it represses endogenous cholesterol synthesis as part of a homeostatic mechanism. The mutant receptor is either absent or fails to bind LDL, depending on the particular mutation, leading to uncontrolled endogenous production of cholesterol. Sometimes FH can be caused by mutations in either of two other genes:

- some people produce LDL that is not recognized by the LDL receptor because a mutant *APOB* gene encodes an abnormal form of the lipoprotein
- occasional patients have gain of function mis-sense mutations in *PCSK9*, a gene encoding a protein-processing enzyme that is part of the homeostatic mechanism.

The normal action of internalized LDL is to repress 3-hydroxy-3-methylglutaryl coenzyme A (HMG CoA) reductase, which catalyzes the rate-limiting step in cholesterol synthesis. In FH patients, statin drugs are used to inhibit the enzyme. This is a very effective clinical management, which can normalize cholesterol levels and health risks. Because the condition is common, has serious health implications and can be effectively treated, there is a good case for screening the whole population for FH. However, the resource implications are considerable. Screening based on cholesterol levels and tendon xanthomata has poor sensitivity, especially in younger people. DNA-based screening is expensive because the *LDLR* gene on chromosome 19p13.2 has 18 exons and several hundred different mutations have been described.

Since this dominant condition affects large extended pedigrees, a very cost-effective method of ascertaining large numbers of affected people is to test relatives of known affected cases, a procedure known as **cascade screening** or cascade testing. The principle was mentioned earlier in connection with testing relatives of **Joanne Brown (Case 2)** for cystic fibrosis mutations. The best developed cascade screening program for FH, in the Netherlands, has run since 1994. Relatives are contacted directly by a genetic field-worker. Family tracing is exceptionally thorough, leading to an average of 25.7 relatives per proband being tested. Of those who turned out to be affected, only 39% were already on statins. Details of this and other programs are reviewed by Hadfield and Humphries (2005).

Studies of the Dutch program have demonstrated very clear clinical benefits: 93% of affected people ascertained through the program subsequently took statins, thus greatly reducing their risk of premature death. Various ethical issues can be raised. The direct contacting of relatives is considered ethically problematic in some countries and instead probands are left to suggest to their relatives that they might benefit from talking to a geneticist. This avoids some problems, but greatly decreases the number of relatives tested per proband. There are questions about identifying affected children – does the benefit of early treatment outweigh the risk of stigmatization or impaired self-image? It is also necessary to think about insurance implications for people contacted out of the blue. Logically, underwriting should be based on the phenotype – the actual cholesterol level in the treated patient – and not on the genotype. Since statin treatment is effective, this should largely dispose of the insurance issues. Careful studies of the Dutch program have shown none of the predicted ill effects, though it is possible that this partly reflects the admirable qualities of Dutch society, and might not be so easily replicated elsewhere.

11.5. References

Ashley EA, Butte AJ, Wheeler MT, *et al.* (2010) Clinical assessment incorporating a personal genome. *Lancet*, **375**: 1525–1535.

Hadfield SG and Humphries SE (2005) Implementation of cascade testing for the detection of familial hypercholesterolaemia. *Curr. Opin. Lipidol.* **16**: 428–433.

Janssens ACJW and van Duijn CM (2008) Genome-based prediction of common diseases: advances and prospects. *Hum. Molec. Genet.* **17**: R166–R173.

Malone FD, Canick JA, Ball RH, *et al.* (2005) First-trimester or second-trimester screening, or both, for Down's syndrome. *New Engl. J. Med.* **353**: 2001–2011.

Ogilvie CM, Lashwood A, Chitty L, Waters J, Scriven PN and Flinter F (2005) The future of prenatal diagnosis: rapid testing or full karyotype? An audit of chromosome abnormalities and pregnancy outcomes for women referred for Down syndrome testing. *Br. J. Obstet. Gynac.* **112**: 1369–1375.

Wilson JMG and Jungner G (1968) *Principles and Practice of Screening for Disease*. World Health Organization, Geneva.

Useful websites

For information on newborn screening in the USA see: www.marchofdimes.com/professionals/14332_1200.asp.

For information on screening programs in the UK see: www.screening.nhs.uk/policydb.php.

The Brown-Goldstein lab website at UT Southwestern Medical Center tells a fascinating story of their Nobel Prize-winning work on cholesterol regulation: www4.utsouthwestern.edu/moleculargenetics/pages/brown/past.html

11.6. **Self-assessment questions**

(1) A hypothetical disease is caused by mutations in the *IGNO* gene. One person in 100 carries a mutation. You have a genetic testing protocol that detects 80% of all mutations. You receive 10 000 blood samples from newborn babies – but 1% of the samples were taken into contaminated tubes that give a false positive result on your test. What is the positive predictive value of your test?

(2) A scientist has been studying people who suffer severe adverse effects of a certain drug. In the general population 1 person in 10 000 suffers these effects. He has identified a DNA polymorphism that is strongly associated with the risk. In blind testing in the laboratory, $^{99}/_{100}$ people who had shown the adverse drug reaction tested positive for the variant, while only $^{1}/_{100}$ people who had taken the drug without ill-effects tested positive. He proposes to screen the entire 1 million population of his city for the variant. Calculate the positive predictive value of his test.

(3) Repeat the calculation of the previous question, assuming the adverse reaction occurred in 1 person in 10 rather than 1 in 10 000. What does this tell us about the potential of screening in general?

(4) Two DNA variants are each associated with a 50% increase in the chance of having a certain disease. For each variant, draw up a 2×2 table as in *Box 11.1*, with numbers from testing 1000 cases and 1000 controls, and calculate the odds ratio, assuming variant A is present in 50% of the normal population and variant B is present in only 5%.

(5) Assuming an incidence of neural tube defect of 1:100 pregnancies tested, use the curves in *Figure 11.2* to estimate the sensitivity and positive predictive value of the MSAFP test, using cut-offs of:

(a) everybody above the normal mean value

(b) everybody above the minimum abnormal value

(c) everybody above the maximum normal value

(6) In cystic fibrosis carrier screening, some couples will have one partner test positive and the other negative. Calculate the sensitivity required of a screening test so as to ensure that such couples are at no greater risk of really both being carriers than they were before any screening was done. Assume the carrier frequency in this population is 1 in 40.

(7) You are a health administrator charged with establishing a population screening program for carriers of cystic fibrosis (who make up 1 person in 25 in your population).

(a) Decide at what stage in their life and under what circumstances people should be tested; write a brief justification of your choice.

(b) You have proposals from two companies for performing the high-throughput genotyping. One offers to test a limited panel of mutations, covering 70% of all mutations; the other tests a larger panel covering 90% of all mutations. Naturally the costs are different, but before you can make decisions you need to know the likely results. For each option, calculate the expected outcomes from screening 1 million people, in terms of cystic fibrosis births avoided and cystic fibrosis births to couples who were not both carriers on the screening test.

12 | Is cancer genetic?

After working through this chapter you should be able to:

- Describe carcinogenesis as an evolutionary process within an individual
- Define oncogenes and tumor suppressor genes, giving examples
- Describe the types of genomic instability found in cancer cells and the roles of cell cycle checkpoints in avoiding these
- List the essential capabilities of malignant tumors and describe the types of somatic genetic change that lead to their development, including activation of oncogenes or inactivation of tumor suppressor genes by somatic mutation, epigenetic changes, deletions leading to loss of heterozygosity, and chromosomal rearrangements leading to fusion genes
- Describe at least three inherited cancer syndromes and discuss their relationship to common sporadic cancers
- Describe the roles of genetics in diagnosis, treatment and prevention of cancer

12.1. Case studies

CASE 23	Wilson family	**295**	313	389

- ? Familial breast cancer

Wendy Wilson saw a television program about breast cancer running in families that raised her concerns about her own family history. She had mentioned her worries some years before to her family doctor but had been reassured. Her mother Wanda had developed the disease at the age of 42 years and sadly died when she was 44 years old. Her mother's sister Amy who lived in New Zealand also developed breast cancer in her 40s but after surgery and chemotherapy was well 7 years later. The previous Christmas Wendy had received a card from an elderly great aunt in which she mentioned that one of her grandsons was undergoing treatment for breast cancer as well, and expressed her shock that a man could be affected. Wendy got in touch with her brother William and sister Veronica and they decided they should look into things in more detail. Veronica was the family genealogist and before long had contacted several relatives they had lost touch with. They found one of Wanda's cousins had died at a young age of breast cancer. The television program had mentioned that tests for familial breast cancer were available through genetic clinics so Wendy made an appointment with her family doctor to ask for a referral. At the surgery Wendy gave as many details as possible to the doctor and he consulted the online guidelines provided by the genetics center. Wendy's family fulfilled the criteria for a high risk and so a referral was made. Before the appointment the genetic counselor from the center contacted Wendy to draw up a family tree. She also asked Wendy for details of her mother and where she was treated so that her medical records could be obtained to confirm the details of her illness.

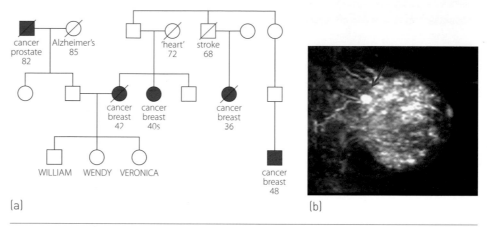

(a)
(b)

Figure 12.1 – (a) Pedigree of the Wilson family, showing types of cancer and age at diagnosis. (b) Carcinoma of the breast detected in a 40-year-old woman by magnetic resonance imaging. This lady had a *BRCA1* mutation. Photo. courtesy of Dr Gareth Evans, St Mary's Hospital, Manchester.

| CASE 24 | Xenakis family | **296** | 317 | 389 |

- Family history of bowel problems
- ? FAP

Christos was one of three children born in Cyprus in the 1960s to Xavier and Demi Xenakis. Xavier started having bowel symptoms at the age of 41 but didn't go and see his doctor until he became really unwell. At the hospital, bowel cancer with liver metastases was diagnosed and only palliative treatment was possible. He died later that year, and soon afterwards Christos moved to Seattle to open his own restaurant with his wife and young son and daughter. Demi came to live with them. Life was very busy but the restaurant did well. At an insurance medical examination some years later, Christos mentioned that he had recently noticed some rectal bleeding which he thought might be due to hemorrhoids. Because of the family history the doctor recommended that Christos had a sigmoidoscopy and to everyone's concern this revealed multiple polyps.

The surgeon explained that this indicated Christos had Familial Adenomatous Polyposis (FAP) and that the only sensible treatment was to remove the colon, since it was inevitable that cancer would develop in one or more of the polyps. While Christos was still in hospital, the surgeon recommended he be referred to the genetic clinic when he was recovered to find out about risks for his children, and also about screening tests that they could have in due course. After a few months the family attended the genetic clinic. The counselor explained dominant inheritance, and they worked out that each child was at 50% risk of having inherited the mutated gene. They learned that genetic testing would be possible if a mutation was found in Christos and that, in children who were at risk or who were found to be mutation carriers, regular sigmoidoscopies were offered from 10 years of age.

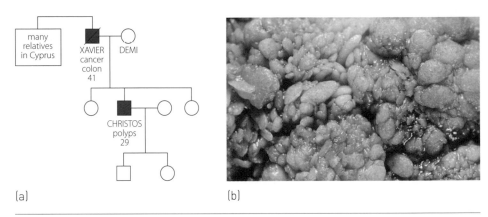

(a)   (b)

Figure 12.2 – Familial adenomatous polyposis coli.
(a) Pedigree of the Xenakis family. (b) Part of a surgically resected colon with polyps. Photo. courtesy of Medical Illustration Department, Manchester Royal Infirmary.

12.2. **Science toolkit**

Natural selection and the evolution of cancer

Imagine an isolated wood in which a population of voles lives. One vole acquires a heritable mutation that makes it able to reproduce faster than the other voles. When you visit the wood 100 vole generations later you would expect to find that most of the voles were descendants of that one faster breeding mutant. Exactly the same simple Darwinian argument applies to the cells of your body. Cell division is under genetic control. If one cell acquires a mutation that makes it divide faster than others then, all things being equal, its descendants will take over your body. Thus cancer is not a specific disease with one cause, and one cure waiting to be discovered. All things being equal, it is simply the natural end-point of evolution within the body of any multicellular organism. Greaves (2007) provides a detailed and thoughtful, if somewhat speculative, exploration of this issue.

Fortunately, all things are not equal. Multicellular organisms could not survive if they did not have mechanisms to control and repress the evolution of their somatic cells, at least until their reproductive life is over. Over the billion years through which they have been evolving, multicellular organisms have developed sophisticated and many-layered defenses against rogue cells. Cell growth is tightly controlled. Most somatic cells do not have the capability of dividing indefinitely. Any cell that behaves inappropriately and whose antisocial behavior cannot be remedied is made to kill itself (**apoptosis**). In an important paper, Hanahan and Weinberg (2000) listed six functional capabilities that a malignant tumor needs to acquire in order to develop and survive (*Box 12.1*). Acquiring each capability means overcoming a separate regulatory mechanism or line of defense in the organism. Consistent with this, classic studies of the age-specific incidence of the common epithelial cancers suggested that four to seven independent events were needed to generate a malignant tumor.

BOX 12.1

The six essential capabilities of a malignant tumor

According to Hanahan and Weinberg (2000), a malignant tumor needs to acquire the following six capabilities during its development:

- ability of cells to divide independently of external growth signals
- ability of cells to ignore external anti-growth signals
- ability of cells to avoid apoptosis
- ability of cells to divide indefinitely without senescence
- ability to stimulate sustained angiogenesis
- ability to invade tissue and establish distant secondary tumors

Tumors contain a diversity of cells and these capabilities probably belong to only a small population of cancer stem cells. Acquiring each capability is likely to require a specific genetic or epigenetic change in order to circumvent a regulatory mechanism. Possible exceptions are the ability to divide indefinitely, if the founding cell is already a stem cell, and the ability to metastasize – it is controversial how often this is a specifically acquired capability and how often it is just a frequent result of acquiring the other five capabilities.

Overcoming the defenses

Given typical mutation rates, the chance of any cell in a person's body sequentially acquiring six specific mutations would appear to be negligibly low. Assuming a mutation rate of 10^{-6} per gene per cell, the chance of a cell picking up six successive specific mutations is 10^{-36}. There are only of the order of 10^{14} cells in a human body, so it would appear that the defenses against cancer are impregnable. Since we know that one person in three will nevertheless develop cancer, there has to be some way round the defenses.

The trick is that the mutations early in the process must somehow greatly increase the probability of later mutations. They can do this in either of two ways.

- They can give the cell a growth advantage. If the mutant cell can generate 1000 mutant daughter cells, the chance that one mutant cell will acquire the next mutation has increased 1000-fold. Pathologists have long known that tumors develop through stages that are marked by increasing growth potential, and that rapidly dividing tissues are the ones most likely to develop tumors. It is believed that the founding cells of many tumors have stem cell-like properties, so that they already have unusual growth potential.
- They can increase the general mutation rate by destabilizing the genome. All cancer cells show one of two types of genomic instability:
  (i) **chromosomal instability** – most tumor cells have bizarre karyotypes with grossly abnormal numbers of chromosomes and many structural rearrangements (*Box 12.2*);
  (ii) **microsatellite instability** – a few tumors are chromosomally normal, but DNA testing shows that normal checks on the accuracy of DNA replication have been lost (see below).

As a result of these changes, the early stages of tumorigenesis are likely to produce a growing population of cells with a great variety of random mutations, making fertile ground for subsequent developments. One of the great challenges in understanding tumorigenesis is to distinguish **driver mutations,** that are causally implicated in the process, from the many incidental but irrelevant **passenger mutations.** The genes that harbor driver mutations are classified as **oncogenes** or **tumor suppressor genes.** The classification is primarily dependent on the type of mutation required – gain of function or loss of function – but this in turn depends on the normal function of the gene. Broadly speaking, oncogenes are genes whose normal role is to stimulate cell division, while the normal role of tumor suppressor (TS) genes is to restrain cell division.

Chromosomal instability in cancer cells

Cancer cells usually have grossly abnormal karyotypes with many gains, losses and rearrangements. Solid tumor cells normally give very poor chromosome preparations that are difficult or impossible to analyze using conventional cytogenetic techniques. M-FISH or SKY are multicolor versions of chromosome painting (see *Section 4.4*) that make each original chromosome appear in a different color. These methods allow detailed analysis of the cytogenetic changes in individual cancer cells. As an example, here is the karyotype recorded for the human HT29 colon carcinoma cell line by Dr T Reid:

67–71,XX,del(X)(p11.2)[19], del(3)(p21)[11], der(3)ins(3;12)(p12;?)[16], der(3)del(3)(p25) ins(3;12)(p12;?)[5], der(3)t(X;3)(?;qter)[11], i(3)(q10)[21], del(4)(q31.3) [21], +der(5)t(5;6)(q11;?)[10], del(6)(q12)[9], t(6;14)(q21;q13)[15], der(6)t(6;14)(q21;q13)[5], +del(7)(p15)[17], −8[20], der(8)i(8)(qter->q10::q10->q24::hsr::q24->qter)[21], +11[20], −13[9], der(13)i(13)(q10)del(q14)[11], der(13)t(5;13)(p13;p11.1)[12], i(13)(q10)[18], −14[21], −14[4],+15[20], der(17)t(17;19)(p11;p11)[21], i(18)(p10)[19], −19[13], i(19)(q10)dup(19)(q13.1q13.4)[19], +i(20)(q10)[21], −21[21], der(?22)t(17;?22;17)[20]

21 cells were analyzed. The chromosome number varied between 67 and 71. The numbers in square brackets are the number of cells having each specified abnormality. This and many other cases can be viewed as 'Skygram' karyotype diagrams on the National Cancer Institute website at http://www.ncbi. nlm.nih.gov/sky/

BOX 12.2

Living for ever: the importance of telomeres

Cancer cells are immortal: they have acquired capability number 4 in *Box 12.1*. HeLa cells, a standard laboratory cell culture workhorse, have been growing vigorously in culture since their unfortunate donor, Henrietta Lacks, died of cervical cancer in 1951 (see Skloot, 2010). Ordinary human cells won't do this. They grow in culture for a few dozen divisions, but then they stop growing, a condition called senescence. Cells with certain cancer-related mutations (in *TP53* and *RB1*, see below) avoid senescence. After some further divisions they reach a stage called crisis. Crisis is marked by death of the great majority of the cells. The few survivors have acquired extensive chromosomal rearrangements and the immortality of cancer cells.

These events are related to a problem with replicating chromosome ends. Recall that the two strands of the double helix are anti-parallel, and that DNA strands can only grow in the 5′→3′ direction (*Box 3.2*). One strand of the double helix has a free 5′ end. When this strand is used as a template for synthesis of a complementary strand, the polymerase moves towards the end of the strand and there is no problem extending the new strand up to the end of the template (*Figure 12.3a*). The other, with a free 3′ end, has problems. When this strand is used as a template, the polymerase moves in the direction from the end towards the interior of the template, against the direction of movement of the replication fork. The new strand is made discontinuously in 100–200 nt segments (**Okazaki fragments**). Each fragment starts with a short (10 nt) RNA primer. The last primer does not necessarily start on the very last nucleotide of the chromosome, and even if it did, the 10 nt corresponding to the primer would be lost as the primer is removed when the Okazaki fragments are ligated together. Thus a linear DNA double helix inevitably loses some sequence at the end each time it is replicated.

Bacteria solve this problem by having circular chromosomes; eukaryotic cells use **telomeres**. Human chromosomes end with about 10 kb of repetitive sequence, $(TTAGGG)_n$. With each round of cell division the telomere shortens by 50–100 nt. Within limits, this doesn't matter because the telomeric repeats contain no genetic information. Repeated division will lead to complete loss of telomeres. One function of the telomeres is to protect chromosome ends against DNA repair mechanisms that recognize broken DNA ends and try to join them together (*Figure 12.3b*). This is what happens to cells in the post-senescence crisis.

Every cell of our body is descended by a chain of cell divisions from the original fertilized egg, which in turn is descended through a chain of cell divisions from the zygotes that created our parents, and so through an unbroken chain of cell

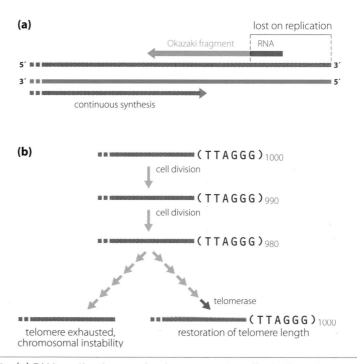

Figure 12.3 – (a) DNA replication mechanisms cannot replicate the extreme 3′ end of a molecule. (b) Telomeres of human chromosomes contain tandemly repeated TTAGGG units. Some repeats are lost each time a cell replicates its DNA. Continued loss in cultured cells leads to chromosomal instability. In the germ-line and in cancer cells, telomerase can restore telomeres to full length.

divisions through the generations and back through time right to the very dawn of life. So how do we still have telomeres? The answer is that certain cells possess an enzyme, **telomerase**, that can restore telomeres to full length. Telomerase adds TTAGGG units using its own inbuilt RNA template, and is therefore not dependent on an external template. Telomerase restores telomere length in the germ-line of each generation. Normal somatic cells lack telomerase (the gene is there but not expressed) – but most cancer cells possess it. Reactivation of telomerase is an important step in acquiring the capability to divide indefinitely. Equally, of course, telomerase looks like an excellent target for an anticancer drug – though the results of trials have been disappointing.

Oncogenes

The oncogene story begins with investigations of cancer viruses in the 1970s. Viruses never cause cancer in the way they cause flu – cancer is never infectious and no virus causes cancer in every infected person. Nevertheless, a few cancers in humans and animals are causally associated with the presence of certain viruses – for example, cervical cancer is associated with human papilloma virus. In the laboratory, **acute transforming retroviruses** could be recovered from certain animal tumors. These viruses were non-infectious but were able efficiently to transform cells in culture into cells that, when transplanted into recipient animals, formed tumors. Retroviruses have a very simple RNA genome consisting of just three transcription units (*Figure 12.4*). When the genomes of acute transforming retroviruses were analyzed they were seen to contain an extra gene, the oncogene. Several dozen oncogenes were identified through studies of such viruses, and named after the animal tumors from which the viruses were isolated (see *Table 12.1*). Other oncogenes were discovered by identifying DNA fragments from tumor cells that could transform mouse cells in tissue culture, causing them to grow in a manner similar to tumor cells.

These discoveries led to a brief flurry of speculation that all cancer might be the result of infection by oncogene-carrying viruses, and so might be preventable by vaccination. This beguiling idea lost its luster when it was discovered that normal

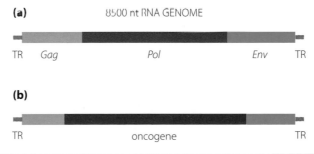

Figure 12.4 – (a) A retrovirus. The RNA genome comprises three transcription units, *gag*, *pol* and *env*. There are short terminal repeats (TR). (b) An acute transforming retrovirus. In a random processing error, part of the viral genome has been replaced by a cellular proto-oncogene. Over-expression or random mutations may render the cellular gene oncogenic when the virus enters a host cell. The viral genes are partially deleted and the virus is unable to replicate.

Table 12.1 – **Viral oncogenes and their cellular counterparts**

Gene	Animal source	Cellular proto-oncogene	
		Location	**Function**
ABL	Abelson murine leukemia	9q34	Signal transduction (tyrosine kinase)
ERBB2	Avian erythroblastic leukemia	17q21	Signal transduction (receptor tyrosine kinase)
FES	Feline sarcoma virus	15q26	Signal transduction (tyrosine kinase)
FMS	Friend murine leukemia	5q33	M-CSF receptor tyrosine kinase
HRAS	Harvey rat sarcoma	11p15.5	Signal transduction (small GTPase)
KRAS	Kirsten mouse sarcoma	12p12	Signal transduction (small GTPase)
MYB	Avian myeloblastosis	6q22	Transcription control (nuclear protein)
MYC	Avian myelomacytosis	8q24	Transcription control (nuclear protein)
SIS	Simian sarcoma virus	22q12	Platelet-derived growth factor B chain
SRC	Rous chicken sarcoma	20q12	Signal transduction (tyrosine kinase)

cells contained homologs of viral oncogenes. Some complex viruses do indeed contain virus-specific oncogenes, but the acute transforming retroviruses are in fact transduction vectors: they pick up genes at random from an infected cell and deliver them into the next cell they infect. The transduced gene replaces part of the normal viral genome, so the viruses are replication-defective.

Clearly there must be some difference between the oncogene in the virus, which transforms cells, and the normal cellular version, which does not. Viral oncogenes are activated versions of the cellular genes (**proto-oncogenes**). The proto-oncogene terminology is often ignored in current research literature and the genes are usually simply called oncogenes – but the distinction between activated and non-activated forms is crucial.

Function and activation of oncogenes

A great breakthrough in molecular understanding of carcinogenesis was achieved when the normal functions of cellular oncogenes were identified, starting in the early 1980s. As *Table 12.1* shows, the normal, non-activated versions of these genes have roles in the control of cell proliferation. Given their normal function, it is entirely understandable that pathogenically activated versions of these genes should be oncogenic. Activation involves a gain of function. This can be achieved in a variety of ways.

- *Point mutations* – as always, a gain of function requires a specific mutation. For example, bladder cancers may have the mutation p.Gly12Val in the *HRAS* (proto)oncogene. The three human *RAS* genes (*KRAS*, *HRAS*, *NRAS*) encode small GTPases which activate the RAS →RAF → MEK →MAPK intracellular signaling cascade (see *Disease box 8*). Gain of function mutations produce a hyperactive version of the GTPase that triggers excessive expression of the target genes.

- *Amplification* – some tumors contain many tandemly repeated copies of oncogenes, sometimes in the form of small extra chromosomes, sometimes as duplications within a chromosome. The *MYC* oncogene, for example, is frequently amplified in tumors.

- *Chromosomal rearrangements* can bring together exons of two distant genes to make a novel chimeric gene. As mentioned above, cancer cells usually have many chromosomal abnormalities. Much painstaking research has been dedicated to identifying changes that are specific to particular tumor types, and distinguishing them from the large numbers of random changes. Most of the changes have been identified in leukemia, which is easier to study than solid tumors. *Table 12.2* gives examples and *Box 12.3* illustrates one well-known case. These rearrangements are exceptionally interesting because cloning the breakpoints reveals the chimeric genes and has been a route to discovery of many oncogenes. Some genes are involved in many different rearrangements – the *MLL* gene at 11q23 has been noted with over 30 different fusion partners in leukemia patients. Tests for specific rearranged genes are an important part of molecular diagnosis of cancer. Often, as in the case of the **Tierney family (Case 20)**, defining the chimeric oncogene provides a guide to prognosis and treatment. Research into the function of the chimeric gene also provides an important entry into understanding the biology of the tumor.

- *A chromosomal rearrangement can up-regulate expression of an oncogene* by moving it into a transcriptionally highly active region of chromatin. The classic case is Burkitt's lymphoma, a childhood tumor particularly affecting the jaw and found mainly in Africa. Incidence is associated with infection by malaria and Epstein–Barr virus. Tumor cells have a characteristic somatically acquired balanced reciprocal translocation, t(8;14)(q24;q32), *Figure 12.5*. The effect of the translocation is to move the *MYC* oncogene from chromosome 8 to the neighborhood of the *IGH* immunoglobulin heavy chain gene on chromosome 14. Unlike most tumor-specific rearrangements, the move does not create a chimeric gene, but it places the MYC gene under the influence of a powerful B-lymphocyte-specific enhancer (see *Section 6.2* for a description of enhancers). Thus B lymphocytes, but not other cells with the translocation, greatly over-express *MYC*. The result is a lymphoma. Sometimes an alternative translocation moves *MYC* to the immunoglobulin light chain gene regions on chromosomes 2 or 22.

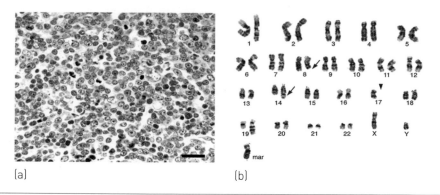

(a) (b)

Figure 12.5 – Burkitt's lymphoma.
(a) Histology, and (b) a karyotype showing the characteristic 8;14 translocation. Additional chromosome abnormalities are also present, as is usually the case in neoplasia. Reproduced from *Molecular Cancer*, **2**: 30; © 2003 Duensing *et al.*; licensee BioMed Central Ltd.

Table 12.2 – Tumor-specific balanced chromosomal rearrangements that create chimeric genes

Rearrangement	Genes	Disease
t(1;22)(p13;q13)	*RBM15/MKL1*	Acute megakaryoblastic leukemia (FAB–M7)
t(2;13)(q35;q14)	*PAX3/FKHR*	Alveolar rhabdomyosarcoma
t(3;8)(p21;q12)	*PLAG1/CTNNB1*	Pleomorphic salivary gland adenoma
inv(3)(q21q26)	*RPN1/EVI1*	AML without maturation (FAB–M1)
t(4;11)(q21;q23)	*MLL/AFF*	ALL/lymphoblastic lymphoma
t(6;11)(q27;q23)	*MLL/MLLT4*	AMML (FAB–M4)
t(9;11)(p22;q23)	*MLL/AF9*	ALL/lymphoblastic lymphoma
t(11;19)(q23;p13)	*MLL/MLLT1*	ALL/lymphoblastic lymphoma
t(7;11)(p15;p15)	*NUP98/HOXA11, HOXA13, HOXA9*	AML with maturation (FAB–M2)
t(9;22)(q34;q11)	*BCR/ABL1*	Chronic myeloid leukemia
t(11;14)(q13;q32)	*IGH/CCND1*	Chronic lymphocytic leukemia, Mantle cell lymphoma
t(15;17)(q22;q12)	*PML/RARA*	Acute promyelocytic leukemia (FAB–M3)
t(12;16)(q13;p11)	*FUS/DDIT3*	Liposarcoma
inv(16)(p13q22)	*CBFB/MYH11*	AMML (FAB–M4)
t(X;18)(p11;q11)	*SS18/SSX1, SSX2, SSX4*	Synovial sarcoma
t(14;18)(q32;q21)	*IGH/BCL2*	Follicular lymphoma
t(12;21)(p13;q22)	*ETV6 (TEL)/RUNX1 (AML1)*	ALL/lymphoblastic lymphoma
t(8;21)(q22;q22)	*RUNX1/ETO*	AML with maturation (FAB–M2)

See http://cgap.nci.nih.gov/Chromosomes/RecurrentAberrations for a large database of rearrangements established by Dr Felix Mitelman. Rearrangements have been particularly defined in leukemias and lymphomas because in these conditions the cells are usually a single clone and are more amenable to cytogenetic analysis than those in solid tumors. ALL, acute lymphoblastic leukemia; AML, acute myeloid leukemia; AMML, acute myelomonocytic leukemia.

BOX 12.3

The Philadelphia chromosome and the chimeric *BCR–ABL* gene

Lymphocytes from 90% of patients with chronic myeloid leukemia (CML) contain an abnormal small chromosome, the Philadelphia (Ph[1]) chromosome (*Box figure 12.1*). It is a sufficiently constant feature of the disease to make the diagnosis of CML questionable in its absence. The Ph[1] chromosome was shown to be one product of a balanced reciprocal 9;22 translocation, t(9;22)(q34.1;q11.2). The translocation junction creates a novel chimeric gene on the Ph[1] chromosome by joining the 5′ part of the *BCR* gene from chromosome 22 on to the 3′ part of the *ABL* gene from chromosome 9. The resulting *BCR–ABL* gene always contains exon 1 of *BCR* and usually the next 10 or so exons, joined to exons 2–11 of *ABL* (*Box figure 12.2*).

ABL is a known oncogene, having been first identified in an acute transforming retrovirus isolated from the Abelson rat sarcoma (*Table 12.1*). Its product is a tyrosine kinase that is part of a signaling system controlling cell growth. Activity of the kinase is tightly controlled, probably in part by the domain encoded by exon 1. The chimeric gene is transcribed and translated; its product is a tyrosine kinase that is constitutively active. Such a gain of function in an important growth control could clearly tip a cell towards uncontrolled growth.

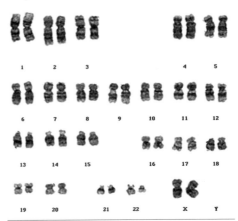

Box figure 12.1 – Karyotype of metaphase with t(9,22).
The abnormal chromosomes 9 and 22 (Philadelphia chromosome) are on the righthand side of each pair. Photo. courtesy of Dr Christine Harrison, University of Southampton.

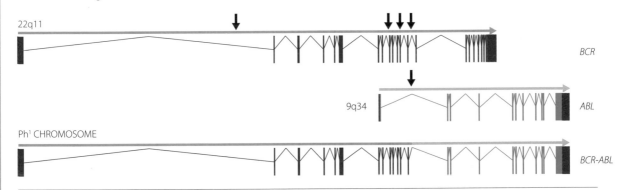

Box figure 12.2 – Joining the *BCR* and *ABL* genes to make the chimeric *BCR–ABL* gene.
The breakpoint in *BCR* can be in any of several different introns.

As mentioned in *Chapter 8*, because this abnormal tyrosine kinase is so characteristic of CML, a drug that specifically targets it has proved extremely effective at inducing remission in CML patients.

Tumor suppressor genes

The rare forms of cancer that are heritable have been hugely important in furthering our understanding of carcinogenesis. Back in 1971 Alfred Knudson formed a hypothesis about the relationship between the inherited and sporadic versions of a cancer. He hypothesized that the early rate-determining steps of carcinogenesis required the founder cell of a tumor to suffer two 'hits' – these might be simple mutations or some other genetic change. In sporadic cancers both hits were chance events, each with a low probability. In the familial version one hit was inherited. Every cell of a susceptible person carried one hit, so it only required one cell in the target tissue to suffer one further hit for the tumor to develop. The familial susceptibility was inherited from one parent as a dominant trait but the cellular phenotype that allows a cell to found a tumor is recessive, requiring two hits (this is a useful reminder that dominance and recessiveness are properties of phenotypes and not of genes or mutations, see *Figure 1.13*).

Knudson formulated his hypothesis in relation to retinoblastoma (RB), a rare childhood tumor of the retina. RB can be unilateral or bilateral, and an additional persuasive observation was that while the familial form is often bilateral, sporadic RB is always unilateral. A similar observation can be made about breast cancer. In familial RB there are sometimes multiple independent tumors in one eye. Clearly retinoblasts in people with familial RB have a strong tendency to become tumorigenic – though considering the size of the target cell population, the probability of such a transformation is compatible with typical mutation rates (*Figure 12.6*).

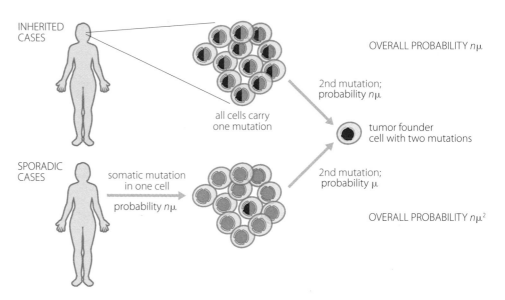

Figure 12.6 – The relation between sporadic and inherited forms of the same tumor. The target tissue contains *n* cells and the chance of one cell suffering a loss of function mutation in the tumor suppressor gene is μ.

Proving the two-hit hypothesis

A seminal paper in 1983 by Cavenee *et al.* showed how Knudson's hypothesis for RB could be confirmed, and set the agenda for the next 20 years of research into familial cancers. There was a suspicion that the 'hits' in RB might be on chromosome 13, because of a family in which familial RB co-segregated with an abnormality of that chromosome. Cavenee and colleagues collected cells and DNA from tumors in patients with sporadic RB. Using a combination of cytogenetic analysis and Southern blotting with probes from chromosome 13, they looked for differences between the tumors and the normal cells of the same patients. The cytogenetic analysis showed that some tumors had missing or extra copies of chromosome 13. The Southern blots showed that in some cases, where the normal (blood) DNA of a patient was heterozygous for a polymorphism, the tumor was homozygous. Correlating the cytogenetic observations and the occurrence of **loss of heterozygosity** in individual tumors, the researchers were able to put together a convincing description of chromosomal mechanisms for producing one of Knudson's 'hits' (*Figure 12.7*).

Later work added to the picture by showing that in inherited cases, the second hit always worked so as to eliminate the normal sequence. Tumor cells retained just the sequence that the patient had inherited from the affected side of his family. Some years later, when the *RB1* gene had been cloned and PCR made it possible to scan it for mutations, a variety of loss of function mutations were identified in the inherited RB-susceptibility allele. Acquired somatic mutations could also be demonstrated in the wild-type gene in tumors that had no relevant chromosome abnormality.

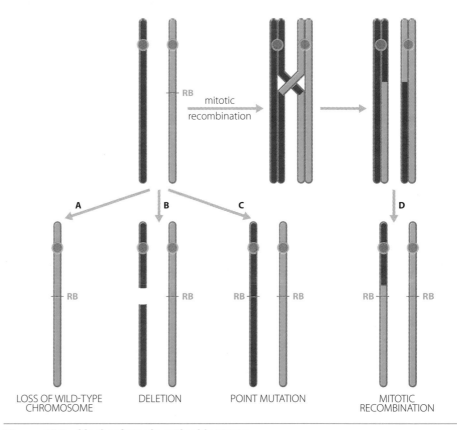

Figure 12.7 – Mechanisms in retinoblastoma.
The initial mutation (labelled RB) may be inherited or somatic. Mechanisms A, B and D result in loss of heterozygosity (in B, only for markers close to the *RB* locus; in D only for markers distal to the crossover). In Cavenee's original study, some tumors duplicated the remaining copy of chromosome 13 after loss of the wild-type chromosome by mechanism A.

The RB work confirmed the existence of TS genes and showed that the two-hit hypothesis explained the basis of familial cancer syndromes. It suggested two ways of identifying TS genes:

- identifying chromosomal regions of loss of heterozygosity in sporadic tumors by comparing tumor and constitutional (blood) DNA from the same patient
- mapping and positional cloning of the genes mutated in familial cancers

Loss of heterozygosity analysis turned out to be problematic. Fully developed tumors have innumerable chromosomal changes, mostly passenger mutations rather than drivers of tumorigenesis. Additionally, because the assays use pooled DNA from the heterogeneous cells of a tumor, usually with some stromal contamination, there is seldom a total loss of heterozygosity. Instead, allelic imbalances are seen, which may be difficult to interpret. Only with the introduction of genome-wide microarray-based methods (array-CGH and SNP chips, see *Section 4.2*) has this type of analysis realized its full potential. SNP chips have the advantage over array-CGH in that they can detect loss of heterozygosity even if there is no copy number change (for example, if a chromosome has been lost and its homolog duplicated). These techniques allow studies on a large enough scale to identify novel recurrent changes. For example, Beroukhim *et al.* (2010) used SNP chips to study copy number variants in 3131 tumors of 26 cancer types. In any one sample an average of 17% of the genome was amplified and 16% deleted, with an average of 24 gains and 18 losses per sample. Across a range of tumors 76 specific regions were amplified and only 25 of these contained known oncogenes. Of the 82 commonly deleted regions, only 9 contained known TS genes. While analysis of loss of heterozygosity thus had to await the development of new techniques to realize its potential, the family linkage approach quickly allowed the identification of the inherited susceptibility in many familial cancer syndromes. Once the gene responsible has been identified, sporadic tumors can be checked for mutations in the same gene. In this way a significant number of TS genes have been identified (*Table 12.3*).

The normal functions of tumor suppressor genes

TS genes act to restrain cell growth and are involved in a variety of checkpoints and controls; the two main areas are cell cycle checkpoints and control of apoptosis.

In a set of continuously growing cells the cell cycle can be divided into four stages (*Figure 12.8*). Progression through the cycle is controlled by a series of checks. These include:

- *the G1–S checkpoint* – cells should not be able to start replicating their DNA until all DNA damage has been repaired; cells with unrepairable damage are triggered to commit suicide by apoptosis
- *the S-phase checkpoints* operate while DNA replication is underway; different replication origins become active at different times during S-phase, and the checkpoints prevent initiation at new origins while there is DNA damage
- *the G2/M checkpoint* prevents cells from initiating mitosis when there is unrepaired DNA damage. A separate check in G2 (the decatenation checkpoint) prevents cells entering mitosis until the chromosomes are fully disentangled from one another.

Table 12.3 – **Familial cancer syndromes with inherited mutations in tumor suppressor genes**

Syndrome	OMIM number	Gene	Location
Retinoblastoma	180200	*RB1*	13q14
Familial adenomatous polyposis	175100	*APC*	5q21
Hereditary non-polyposis colon cancer (Lynch syndrome)	120435 120436	*MSH2* *MLH1*	2p22 3p21
Familial breast cancer	113705 600185	*BRCA1* *BRCA2*	17q21 13q12
Li–Fraumeni syndrome	151623	*TP53*	17p13
Gorlin syndrome	109400	*PTC*	9q22
Ataxia-telangiectasia	208900	*ATM*	11q23
Neurofibromatosis 1	162200	*NF1*	17q11
Neurofibromatosis 2	101000	*NF2*	22q12
Von Hippel–Lindau disease	193300	*VHL*	3p25
Multiple endocrine neoplasia 1	131100	*MEN1*	11q13
Multiple endocrine neoplasia 2	171400	*RET*	10q11
Familial melanoma	155601	*CDKN2A*	9p21

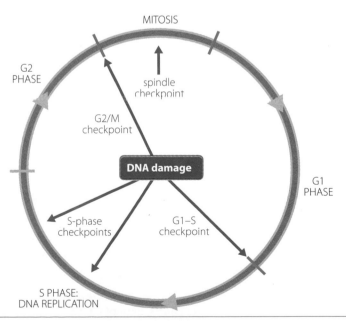

Figure 12.8 – **The cell cycle and its checkpoints.**

- *the spindle checkpoint* prevents the separation of chromatids in anaphase until every chromosomal centromere is attached to spindle fibers

The first three checkpoints represent different downstream responses to the machinery that detects DNA damage, especially double-strand breaks. This machinery involves several TS genes. Checkpoint mechanisms are strongly conserved through evolution. Much of our understanding of human cell cycle controls comes from studies of model organisms, especially yeast. The 2001 Nobel Prize for Medicine was awarded to Leland Hartwell, Tim Hunt and Paul Nurse for their work unraveling these controls (you can read their accounts of how they did it at <u>http://nobelprize.org/medicine/laureates/2001/</u>). Progress through the cycle is particularly controlled by cyclins, a family of proteins whose level in the cell fluctuates according to the phase of the cycle. Cyclins operate by activating a series of protein kinases, the cyclin-dependent kinases (CDKs). Specific CDK inhibitors counteract the cyclins.

The G1–S checkpoint in particular involves an impressive cast of TS genes (*Box 12.4*).

- *The RB protein (pRB)* binds and inhibits E2F, a transcription factor that activates expression of many genes required for moving through G1 phase into S phase. Phosphorylation of pRB by CDKs inactivates it and releases active E2F.
- *p53*, the product of the *TP53* gene, is normally bound by MDM2 which targets it for destruction. p53 stimulates transcription of *MDM2*, thereby regulating its own activity to a very low level. Various signals inactivate *MDM2*, or make p53 immune to its action allowing the p53 level to rise. Depending on the circumstances, this can either cause cell cycle arrest through the action of p21 or target the cell for apoptosis. p53 is inactivated by somatic mutations in a high proportion of all cancer cells; inherited mutations cause the Li–Fraumeni familial cancer syndrome.
- *p16 and p14^{ARF}* are both products of the same gene, *CDKN2A* (*Figure 12.9*). The use of alternative promoters and first exons causes the coding

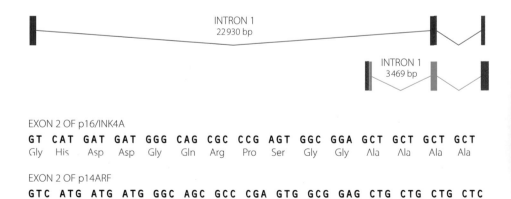

EXON 2 OF p16/INK4A

GT	CAT	GAT	GAT	GGG	CAG	CGC	CCG	AGT	GGC	GGA	GCT	GCT	GCT	GCT
Gly	His	Asp	Asp	Gly	Gln	Arg	Pro	Ser	Gly	Gly	Ala	Ala	Ala	Ala

EXON 2 OF p14ARF

GTC	ATG	ATG	ATG	GGC	AGC	GCC	CGA	GTG	GCG	GAG	CTG	CTG	CTG	CTC
Val	Met	Met	Met	Gly	Ser	Ala	Arg	Val	Ala	Glu	Leu	Leu	Leu	Leu

Figure 12.9 – The *CDKN2A* gene encodes two completely different proteins, p16 and p14^{ARF}, both of which function in cell cycle control.
CDKN2A is very often deleted in tumor cells. ARF, alternative reading frame.

BOX 12.4

The G1–S checkpoint

Progression through the cell cycle is primarily governed by the availability of specific cyclin proteins. These activate CDKs. The kinases act as effectors by phosphorylating a range of downstream targets; they are regulated by the availability of their cognate cyclins and by various inhibitors. Progression through G1 phase and into S phase is governed by cyclins D and E with their kinases. A complex network of upstream controls modulates their activity. *Box figure 12.3* shows only part of the network.

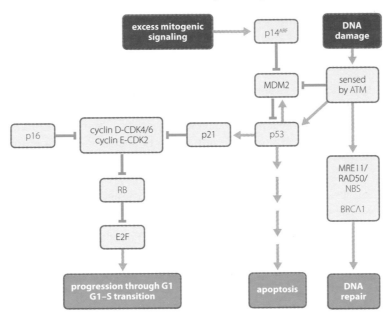

Box figure 12.3 – Some of the controls and interactions governing G1–S progress.
TS genes identified through familial cancers are shown in red. ▬▮ shows an inhibitory action, ▬▶ shows a stimulatory action.

sequence in exon 2 to be read in different reading frames for the two products, which end up sharing no amino acid homology. Remarkably, both function in cell cycle control. p16 is a CDK inhibitor. Inherited p16 mutations are found in some familial melanomas; these affect only the p16 product of the gene. Inherited mutations affecting only p14^{ARF} are very uncommon but the p14 promoter is often epigenetically silenced in tumors. Deletion of the whole *CDKN2A* gene is a very efficient way of disrupting cell cycle controls, and is a common occurrence in tumor cells.

- *ATM protein* is the primary sensor of DNA double-strand breaks. Activated ATM phosphorylates several proteins including MDM2 (inactivating it), and p53, CHK2, BRCA1 and the MRE11/RAD50/NBS DNA repair complex (all of which are activated by phosphorylation).

It is noteworthy that several TS genes encode extremely large proteins. Examples include the proteins encoded by *APC* (2843 amino acid residues), *ATM* (3056 residues), *BRCA1* (1863 residues), *BRCA2* (3418 residues) and *NF1* (2839 residues). There are counter-examples: the two products of the *CDKN2A* gene are a mere 156 and 173 residues long while some of the largest known proteins are muscle structural proteins like dystrophin (3685 residues), and titin (19 946 residues), that have no role in cancer. Nevertheless, the list in *Table 12.3* suggests that loss of function of genes encoding very large non-structural proteins is a frequent initiating event in tumorigenesis. Such proteins do in fact often have a structural role at the molecular, though not the microscopic, level. They interact with many other proteins and serve as scaffolds for assembling the large multi-protein machines that carry out many cellular tasks. Loss of function at such nodal points in the networks of interactions within cells may be a powerful way of disrupting normal cellular functions.

A desperate solution: apoptosis

Apoptosis is a specific active process that is triggered by various abnormal cellular states as well as being an important part of normal development (for separating the fingers of the hand in a developing embryo, for example). The mechanism involves activation of a cascade of proteolytic enzymes called caspases. Caspases can be activated through perturbations of mitochondria, with release of cytochrome c, or through the actions of FAS protein in conjunction with so-called death receptors. Such potent suicide machines naturally need to be kept under tight control, and the regulatory circuitry for apoptosis is extremely involved.

Among the conditions that can trigger apoptosis are irreparable DNA damage and excessive growth signaling. The p53 protein is a central link in these processes. It is activated by phosphorylation of specific residues and/or inactivation of its inhibitor MDM2. As shown in *Box 12.4*, p53 stimulates expression of the p21 protein which acts to promote cell cycle arrest. p53 also stimulates transcription of several proteins that are involved in both the mitochondrial and the FAS-mediated pathways of apoptosis. Because of its key role in all these processes, p53 has acquired the label 'guardian of the genome'. *TP53* is one of the most frequently mutated genes in all cancers.

12.3. Investigations of patients

| CASE 20 | Tierney family | 204 | 215 | **312** | 389 |

- 4-year-old boy, Jason
- Pale with extensive bruising and tachycardia
- ? Acute lymphocytic leukemia
- Bone marrow test and check diagnosis
- TPMT enzyme analysis prior to 6-mercaptopurine treatment

Childhood acute lymphoblastic leukemia (cALL) is a neoplasm of B cell precursors or stem cells. About 25% of cases have a balanced reciprocal 12;21 translocation, with breakpoints at 12p13 and 21q22.3. At the translocation junction, the 5′ portion of the *TEL* (*ETV-6*) gene and almost the entire coding sequence of the *AML1* (*RUNX1* or *CBFA2*) gene, are brought together to create a fusion gene. Loss of function experiments in mice show that both *TEL* and *AML1* are critical genes for hematopoiesis. Each gene encodes a transcription factor. *AML1* encodes the alpha subunit of core binding factor, a master regulator of the formation of hematopoietic stem cells. The fusion inhibits normal AML1-mediated transcriptional activity, resulting in alteration of the capacity of hematopoietic stem cells to self-renew and to differentiate. Both genes are found as fusion partners with a variety of other genes encoding kinases or transcription factors in both lymphoid and myeloid leukemias. The *TEL–AML1* fusion appears to be unique to B cell progenitor ALL.

The positions of the *TEL/AML1* breakpoints in the pale-staining subtelomeric chromosome regions make the translocation hard to spot by conventional karyotyping. Diagnosis is based on FISH. Interphase cells from Jason were hybridized to differently colored FISH probes for the *TEL* and *AML1* genes. One of the colored spots marking the *TEL* genes always lay adjacent to one of the *AML1* spots, confirming the presence of the *TEL–AML1* fusion gene (*Figure 12.10*). This was good news because individuals with *TEL* rearrangements usually show an excellent response to chemotherapy. As described in *Chapter 8*, the induction and consolidation treatments were successful, but there were initial problems with his long-term maintenance treatment because Jason had thiopurine methyltransferase deficiency which made him hypersensitive to one of the drugs used, 6-mercaptopurine. With a suitably low dose of the drug he remained healthy and disease-free.

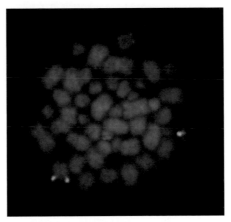

Figure 12.10 – Metaphase with *TEL–AML1* fusion.
The green signal is on the normal chromosome 12, one red signal is in the normal chromosome 21 and one is on the derived chromosome 12. The yellow *TEL–AML1* fusion signal is on the derived chromosome 21. Photo. courtesy of Dr Christine Harrison, University of Southampton.

| CASE 23 | | Wilson family | 295 | **313** | 389 |

- ? Familial breast cancer
- DNA analysis for mutation

Since one woman in eight in the USA or UK is likely to develop breast cancer at some time in her life, it is not surprising that many families have more than one case. Five to ten percent of affected women have a mother or sister with breast cancer, and about twice as many have either an affected first- or second-degree relative. Many of these represent chance coincidences, but statistical analysis suggests that in 5–10% of families the condition is truly familial. In 1990, linkage analysis in a large collection of multicase families pinpointed a possible susceptibility locus for early-onset breast cancer on chromosome 17. After 4 years of intensive work the *BRCA1* gene was identified by positional cloning. A further round of analysis in *BRCA1*-negative families led to identification of the *BRCA2* gene on chromosome 13.

BRCA1 and *BRCA2* are both large genes (*Figure 12.11*). *BRCA1* has 24 exons encoding a 1863 amino acid protein, and *BRCA2* has 28 exons encoding a 3418 amino acid protein. As mentioned above, such large proteins are likely to have multiple functions and many interacting partners. Our understanding of the roles of these proteins in the cell is still incomplete. One main role is

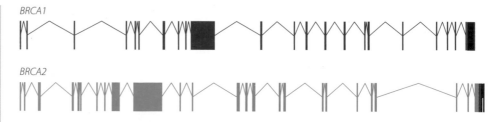

Figure 12.11 – Exon structure of *BRCA1* and *BRCA2* genes.
The two genes and proteins share no homology, and the expression array study shown in *Figure 12.18* suggests that they are involved in different pathways within cells. Both genes have one very large central exon (3426 and 4932 bp, respectively).

in detecting DNA damage and signaling its presence to cell cycle checkpoints. There is also evidence for roles of these proteins in transcription control. *BRCA1* and *BRCA2* behave as TS genes, in that familial cases often involve inherited loss of function mutations, and tumors in familial cases show loss or inactivation of the remaining wild-type allele. Curiously, however, sporadic breast tumors very seldom have *BRCA1/2* mutations, although 10–15% of sporadic tumors silence *BRCA1* epigenetically. It may be that although cells with two *BRCA1/2* mutations have a significant tumorigenic potential, those with a single mutation have no enhanced potential over normal cells. In that case, there may be alternative routes that have a higher probability of leading to a sporadic tumor.

The Breast Cancer Information Core of the National Human Genome Research Institute (http://research.nhgri.nih.gov/bic/) lists over 1600 *BRCA1* and 1800 *BRCA2* sequence changes. An unknown number of these are coincidentally discovered non-pathogenic variants. Most definitely pathogenic changes are small frameshifting deletions or insertions, splice site mutations, or deletions of one or more whole exons. They can be identified through sequencing or any of the standard methods for scanning a gene (*Chapter 5*). The whole exon deletions are best detected by MLPA (*Figure 5.9*). Like most premature termination mutations, these are expected to trigger nonsense-mediated decay of the mRNA, so that the mutations act as null alleles, producing no (or maybe very little) truncated protein.

Ashkenazi Jews are a special case. Three specific frameshifting mutations (c.185delAG and c.5382insC in *BRCA1*, and c.6174delT in *BRCA2*) are common in this population, presumably because of founder effects (*Chapter 10*). A survey of 5318 healthy Ashkenazi women found 120 (2.2%) were carriers of one or other of the three mutations. This frequency contrasts with the 0.2% frequency of all *BRCA1/2* mutations in non-Ashkenazi white women in the USA or UK. The high frequency of these specific mutations makes genetic testing among Ashkenazim important and relatively straightforward. Of course, excluding those three mutations does not remove the risk that some other *BRCA1/2* mutation, or a mutation in another gene, may be putting the person at high risk. Other populations, for example French–Canadians, Icelanders and Pakistanis, also have their own particular founder mutations.

The lifetime risk for a mutation carrier has been variously estimated at between 30% and 85%. This illustrates an interesting feature of susceptibility testing. The initial estimates were made in the large multi-case families in which the mutations were first found. But these families were selected for having many affected cases, and so the initial estimates of risk are from a biased set of families. Population-based surveys show a lower risk. Nevertheless, the risk is still substantial compared to the risk for people who do not carry the mutations, and possibly particularly so in women with a strong family history. Thus there is considerable demand for mutation screening. Because these are large genes, and loss of function mutations may be found anywhere within the gene, screening for mutations is laborious and expensive (although less so with the new massively parallel sequencing technologies described in *Chapter 5*). Clinicians need to prioritize families for screening, and this is done largely on the basis of the family history.

Markers of *BRCA1/2* mutations include:

- cases with unusually early onset
- bilateral cases (compare with the RB example)
- cases with male breast cancer (particularly a feature with *BRCA2* mutations)
- families with both breast and ovarian cancer (particularly a feature with *BRCA1* mutations)

None of these features is completely specific to *BRCA1/2* breast cancer, but risk indices have been developed based on these factors. *Table 12.4* shows one such index (Evans *et al.*, 2004). The indices allow physicians to assess the probability that any given case is likely to have a *BRCA1/2* mutation.

In the Wilson family, applying the scoring system of *Table 12.4* to the pedigree (*Figure 12.1a*) suggested there is an 18% chance of a *BRCA2* mutation, and a 15% chance of a *BRCA1* mutation if the *BRCA2* screen is negative. Note that no score is given for the prostate cancer in Wendy's paternal grandfather, because if the family problem is caused by an inherited *BRCA1/2* mutation, the pedigree shows that the problem is on Wendy's mother's side of the family. The presence of male breast cancer, and absence of ovarian cancer, strengthened the suspicion that this was a *BRCA2* family. The score was high enough to prioritize the family for DNA analysis.

A section of Wanda's excised tumor was recovered from the pathology lab archive and DNA was extracted. Testing eventually revealed a single nucleotide deletion in exon 18 of *BRCA2* in the tumor. The deletion of nucleotide 8525 in codon 2766 created a frameshift, leading to codon 2776 being read as a stop codon. No second mutation was identified in the tumor, although no check was made for loss of heterozygosity because there was no sample of Wanda's normal (blood) DNA for comparison. The presence of this mutation in the tumor strongly suggested that this was indeed a *BRCA2* family, because sporadic tumors rarely have *BRCA2* mutations.

Before family members could be offered mutation testing it was necessary to discover whether the mutation found in the tumor was a first or second hit – if

Table 12.4 – A scoring system to assess the likelihood of finding a *BRCA1* or *BRCA2* mutation in a family

Cancer, age at diagnosis (yr)	Points for *BRCA1*	Points for *BRCA2*
Female breast cancer, <30	6	5
Female breast cancer, 30–39	4	4
Female breast cancer, 40–49	3	3
Female breast cancer, 50–59	2	2
Female breast cancer, >59	1	1
Male breast cancer, <60	5 if *BRCA2* excluded	8
Male breast cancer, >59	5 if *BRCA2* excluded	5
Ovarian cancer, <60	8	5 if *BRCA1* excluded
Ovarian cancer, >59	5	5 if *BRCA1* excluded
Pancreatic cancer	0	1
Prostate cancer, <60	0	2
Prostate cancer, >59	0	1

Scores are summed for all cases in the family that are compatible with a dominantly inherited susceptibility. The total score is intended to represent the % chance of finding a mutation. Data from Evans *et al.* (2004) and reproduced here with permission from the BMJ Publishing Group.

it was the second hit, then the family mutation remained unidentified. Amy in New Zealand was contacted, and in discussion with Wendy agreed to provide a blood sample for testing. DNA was extracted by arrangement with Amy's local genetic service. Unlike blood, DNA is stable and can readily be sent around the world by normal mail. It was easy for Wendy's genetic center to test Amy's sample specifically for the c.8525delC mutation, and the result was positive. Now that the family mutation had been identified, Wendy, William and Veronica gave DNA samples for testing. The samples were tested just for the identified family mutation. This showed that Veronica and William carried the mutation but Wendy did not.

Wendy was naturally relieved at the news, but it was important in counseling her, to make sure she understood that she was still at the population risk of developing sporadic breast cancer, and would be wise to take part in the standard mammography screening program when she reached the eligible age. This was also an opportunity to point out to her that breast cancer risk is strongly influenced by lifestyle, and that women (including *BRCA1/2* mutation carriers) can reduce their risk by around 40% by weight loss and moderate exercise. Veronica carried the mutation and was therefore at high risk. Options for her included doing nothing, lifestyle changes, entering an enhanced surveillance program with annual mammography, taking Tamoxifen in the hope that this would reduce her risk, or the more radical step of prophylactic mastectomy. William was not at high risk himself of breast cancer because it is rare in males (his relative risk was very high, but the absolute risk was still low). On the other hand, although the relative risk of prostate cancer in *BRCA2* mutation carriers is only moderate, the absolute risk is high, and he was advised to have regular screening. Any daughter he had would also need counseling about her substantial risk of breast cancer.

| CASE 24 | Xenakis family | 296 | **317** | 389 |

- Family history of bowel problems
- ? FAP

The *APC* gene (OMIM 175100) on chromosome 5q21–22 was identified as the cause of FAP by positional cloning, guided by reports of an affected patient with a interstitial deletion of 5q. *APC* acts as a classic TS gene. Familial cases inherit one *APC* mutation and somatically inactivate the normal allele in their tumor. In addition, in contrast to the situation with *BRCA1/2* in breast cancer, mutation or loss of both alleles of *APC* is a common event early in the development of common sporadic colorectal cancers (see below).

The APC protein is another large (2843 amino acids) multifunctional protein. It appears to be involved in several different processes in the cell, including cell adhesion and interactions with the cytoskeleton. The function most clearly related to cancer is its role in the control of β-catenin levels. APC protein forms a complex with axin and glycogen synthase kinase 3β (GSK3β) that degrades β-catenin. The APC protein has three β-catenin-binding modules and seven 20-amino acid modules that down-regulate β-catenin levels (*Figure 12.12*). Cell signaling through the Wnt pathway inhibits formation of the complex, freeing the β-catenin to enter the nucleus. In the cell nucleus, β-catenin acts as a

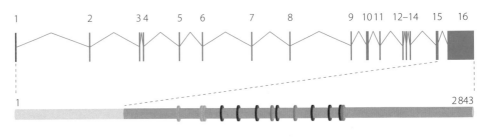

● β-catenin regulatory sequence
○ β-catenin-binding module
● axin-binding module

Figure 12.12 – The APC protein and its role in regulating β-catenin levels.
The protein has 2843 amino acid residues. Three 15-amino acid modules bind β-catenin and seven 20-amino acid modules down-regulate the level. The first 15 exons of the gene encode only 653 of the 2843 amino acids; all the rest are encoded by the large 3′ exon 16. Unusually, *APC* genes with a premature stop signal in any codon downstream of codon 640 produce a truncated protein, because nonsense-mediated RNA decay does not occur for stop codons in the last exon of a gene or about 50 nt upstream of the last splice site. Only truncations in the green shaded part of the protein would be eliminated by nonsense-mediated decay. Thus most mutations produce truncated APC proteins that can still bind β-catenin and have some limited ability to down-regulate it.

transcriptional co-activator, associating with the transcription factor TCF4 and promoting transcription of various target genes including cyclin D1 and the *MYC* oncogene. *APC* mutations allow the level of β-catenin to rise independently of the Wnt signal. Colorectal tumors that lack *APC* mutations may have gain of function mutations in β-catenin or loss of function mutations in axin that presumably have a similar end result.

APC functions as a classic TS gene, with either an inherited first hit and somatic second hit, or, in sporadic cases, two somatic hits. However, there is a very interesting relationship between the germ-line and somatic mutations. Both the position and type of the second hit depend on the position of the germ-line mutation. Nothing similar is seen in other familial cancer syndromes. Inherited mutations are almost exclusively nonsense (30%) or frameshifting (68%). Normally such mutations would invoke nonsense-mediated mRNA decay (*Section 6.2*), and there would be no protein product. *APC* is an exception because of the unusual exon–intron structure of the gene. As shown in *Figure 12.12*, exons 1–15 encode only the first 653 of the 2843 amino acids, all the remainder being encoded by the large exon 16. mRNA molecules with premature stop codons in the last exon of a gene, or within 50 nt of the last splice site, are generally exempt from decay (*Figure 6.3*). Therefore only stop codons before codon 640 of the *APC* gene would be expected to trigger nonsense-mediated decay. Most mutations in FAP are downstream of that point, and it seems likely that at least some of the truncated protein is produced. The properties of the truncated protein affect the selective advantage of a second hit. The relation between first and second hits can be summarized as follows (Albuquerque *et al.*, 2002):

• if the germ-line mutation produces a protein lacking all seven β-catenin regulatory sequences, the somatic second hit produces a protein having one, or occasionally two, such modules
• if the germ-line mutation produces a protein with one module, the somatic mutation usually removes them all, by truncation or allele loss
• in a patient whose germ-line mutation left two modules, the second hit in most of his tumors was a point mutation that removed all modules

Thus tumor cells always retain either one or two of the regulatory modules. The clear implication is that there is selection for a 'just right' level of β-catenin regulatory function. Perhaps complete loss would produce β-catenin levels that were sufficiently abnormal to trigger apoptosis in these relatively normal cells.

Christos Xenakis gave a blood sample, from which DNA was extracted for *APC* mutation testing. This showed that he was heterozygous for a nonsense mutation at codon 1309 of the *APC* gene (p.Glu1309X). This is a frequent germ-line mutation in FAP. It is highly penetrant, so that mutation carriers have a near-100% risk of developing colon cancer if untreated. Identifying it allowed at-risk family members to be tested. Christos's mother Demi contacted several relatives of her late husband in Cyprus to let them know about the newly discovered high risk in the family, and gave them a contact number of the Seattle geneticist for use by their local genetics service if any of them opted for testing. Meanwhile there were Christos's two young children to consider. Each was at 50% risk, and they would need annual sigmoidoscopy examinations from age 10 to check for development of polyps. All this could be avoided if a DNA test showed that the child had not inherited the mutation. The question arose whether to test them now or leave it until later. Testing now would mean that an at-risk child could grow up with the knowledge that he would need annual bowel screening and not have this suddenly sprung on him; postponing testing would mean that the child, by age 10, would be more able to understand and consent to the procedure.

This family illustrates some of the ethical arguments about DNA testing in children. Normally it is felt improper to test children for genetic susceptibility – for example in Case 21, Hannah Ulmer's parents were dissuaded from having their other children tested for Tay–Sachs carrier status. In the present case there are benefits for a child in being tested by age 10. For children at 50% risk of FAP, annual sigmoidoscopy surveillance needs to start around this time. It is clearly beneficial to a child to avoid this unpleasant procedure if he can be shown not to carry the family mutation. Only parental consent would be formally required for testing, but good practice would include discussing the issue with the child and obtaining consent as far as possible.

12.4. **Going deeper ...**

Hereditary non-polyposis colon cancer (Lynch syndrome)

FAP, the condition in the Xenakis family (Case 24), is not the only form of inherited susceptibility to colorectal cancer. Some families show a clear history of dominantly inherited early-onset colon cancer but do not have polyps. The susceptibility maps to chromosome 2p22 in some families and to 3p21.3 in others. A study of loss of heterozygosity in the tumors gave the first clue to the molecular events. Genotyping with microsatellite markers showed a quite unexpected effect: instead of loss of heterozygosity at specific chromosomal locations, the investigators found the tumors often showed additional novel alleles of the marker. Moreover, the effect was not specific to one particular chromosomal location, but was seen with microsatellites from all over the genome.

Microsatellites are short stretches of repetitive DNA sequence, often $(CA)_n$ (see *Chapter 9*). When DNA polymerase replicates such sequences it quite often makes mistakes, putting in an extra repeat unit or leaving one out. Such replication slippage occurs during PCR amplification, and is the cause of the extra bands ('stutter bands') seen when microsatellites are scored on gels (see *Figure 7.16b*). The same thing can happen when a living cell replicates its DNA, but *in vivo* proof-reading mechanisms detect mismatches between the template and the newly synthesized strand, and correct the errors. The microsatellite instability seen in hereditary non-polyposis colon cancer (HNPCC) is a result of failure of this **mis-match repair** (MMR) machinery.

The MMR machinery is quite highly conserved from *E. coli* through to man, and one route by which the human MMR genes were cloned was by searching for the human homologs of so-called mutator genes in yeast. Six genes are involved in the process in man (*Table 12.5*). Of these, mutations in *MSH2* and *MLH1* are the

Table 12.5 – Genes involved in mismatch repair

Gene	OMIM number	Location	Percentage of HNPCC
MSH2	609309	2p21	60%
MLH1	609310	3p22.5	30%
MSH6	600678	2p16.3	5% (atypical)
MLH3	604395	14q24.3	Rare or absent
PMS1	600258	2q32.2	Rare or absent
PMS2	600259	7p22.1	Rare or absent

Mutations in *MSH6* (*GTBP*) have been mainly described in women with endometrial cancer rather than colon cancer.

usual causes of HNPCC. They act as TS genes: one loss of function mutation can be inherited, and the remaining functional allele is inactivated in the tumor by somatic mutation or epigenetically (see below). Sporadic cases have both gene copies silenced somatically, by mutation or promoter methylation.

Why should a defect in a general mechanism like MMR specifically cause colon cancer? Partly the answer is that it can in fact cause other cancers. Microsatellite instability is sometimes seen in other tumors, especially gastric and endometrial tumors. Partly the answer can be found by looking for the likely consequences of a failure of MMR. Transforming Growth Factor B (TGFβ) is a strong inhibitor of cell proliferation in the colorectum. It acts through a cell-surface receptor of which the TGFBR2 (TGFβ receptor 2) protein is part. The *TGFBR2* gene contains a run of 10 consecutive A nucleotides in exon 3 of the coding sequence (*Figure 12.13*). MMR-deficient cells are liable to insert or skip one or more As. This creates a frameshift and renders the new copy non-functional. One survey found somatic *TGFBR2* mutations in the tumors of 100/111 cases of colon cancer with microsatellite instability. Several other relevant targets have been noted, that is, genes with relevant functions that contain microsatellite-like sequences.

```
743  TGC ATT ATG AAG GAA AAA AAA AAG CCT GGT GAG ACT TTC
120  Cys Ile Met Lys Glu Lys Lys Lys Pro Gly Glu Thr Phe
```

Figure 12.13 – Part of the sequence of exon 3 of the *TGFRB2* gene.
A run of 10 consecutive As makes replication of the gene vulnerable to defects in mismatch repair.

A rather similar effect has been suggested in the *APC* gene. A mis-sense variant, p.Ile1307Lys, is carried by about 6% of Ashkenazi Jews, and a much smaller proportion of other people. The variant appears to be a low-penetrance susceptibility allele for colon cancer, roughly doubling the normal risk. The DNA sequence change creates an unbroken run of As (*Figure 12.14*), suggesting a vulnerability to MMR defects. However, unlike with *TGFBR2*, there is no evidence that this run is preferentially mutated in HNPCC, so the susceptibility effect may operate at the protein level.

```
GCA  GAA  ATA  AAA  GAA  AAG      →      GCA  GAA  AAA  AAA  GAA  AAG
Ala  Glu  Ile  Lys  Glu  Lys             Ala  Glu  Lys  Lys  Glu  Lys
```

Figure 12.14 – The p.Ile1307Lys colon cancer susceptibility allele of the *APC* gene.
Note the run of 8 As created by the mutation.

The multistage development of cancer

Pathologists have long known that malignant tumors develop through stages marked by increasing growth and de-differentiation. FAP offers exceptional opportunities for studying the process. When the colon is surgically removed from an FAP patient, it often contains lesions showing every stage of tumor development. Vogelstein and colleagues (summarized in Kinzler and Vogelstein, 1996) analyzed such series, together with sporadic colon tumors, for mutations in candidate genes and loss of heterozygosity. They found some alterations that were often present in the early stages, and others that only appeared in later stages. Putting their observations together, they proposed the developmental scheme shown in *Figure 12.15*.

The earliest stages are the most critical, because these mutations must cause instability or a growth advantage in a relatively normal cell that still has most of its defenses intact. Probably there are only a small number of ways of achieving this, but a larger number of ways of developing once the initial stages are negotiated. Cells with HNPCC mutations may have a wider range of possible evolutionary paths towards cancer, but many of the same players are involved. Tumors lacking *APC* mutations often have mutations in other components of the same pathway, for example, β-catenin or axin. Tumors lacking *RAS* mutations commonly have mutations in the *BRAF* gene, which has similar functions. As mentioned above, TGFβ signaling is an important negative regulator of cell growth in the colon. Within the cell, the TGFβ receptor signals by phosphorylating serine or threonine residues in SMAD proteins. This pathway is commonly subverted in colorectal cancer, by *TGFBR2* mutations in cancers with MMR defects, or in non-HNPCC cancers by loss of chromosome 18 where the *SMAD4* gene is located.

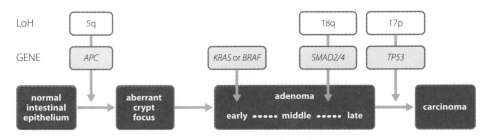

Figure 12.15 – A possible common pathway for the development of colon cancer.
The scheme (see Kinzler and Vogelstein, 1996) summarizes the way that some genes are often inactivated in early lesions, while others are inactivated only in late-stage lesions. There has been some controversy about the general applicability of this scheme, and there is no suggestion that every colon cancer has developed exactly in this way.

Broadening this approach, Vogelstein considered the balance between cell birth and cell death. Since adult tissues and organs remain a constant size, there must be some mechanism to regulate this balance. Vogelstein suggested that in each tissue there is one critical gene that governs the balance. He called such genes 'gatekeepers'. Mutations in tissue-specific gatekeepers would be initiating events in tissue-specific cancers. Once the tumor has initiated, progression will depend on the ability of the cell to maintain its defenses against disordered growth. He named the genes responsible for this as 'caretakers'. Thus tumors initiate with mutations in gatekeepers and progress with mutations in caretakers. This picture clearly fits colorectal cancer; how far it is generally applicable is debatable. At the very least, it is a nice tool for thinking about carcinogenesis.

Epigenetics in cancer

As we noted in *Chapter 7*, it is not clear how extensive is the role of epigenetic mechanisms in inherited disease. However, there is no dispute about their importance in cancer. Studies of DNA methylation in tumor cells show a somewhat paradoxical picture. On the one hand, the general level of methylation is reduced in many tumor cells compared to their normal counterparts. On the other, many CpG islands are hypermethylated. About half of all genes have a CpG island associated with their promoter (see *Chapter 7*). In normal cells these islands are not methylated, regardless of whether the related gene is active or silent. Promoter methylation (of isolated CpG dinucleotides) controls expression of genes that lack CpG islands, but not of those with islands. In cancer cells, however, genes that have CpG island promoters are often silenced by methylation. There is some evidence that tumors can be divided into those where many islands are methylated and those where this does not occur, implying the existence of some general mechanism favoring aberrant island methylation. It is claimed that tumors with extensive methylation of islands are clinically and etiologically distinct from those lacking this feature.

TS genes are silenced by promoter methylation at least as frequently as by mutation. The relative importance of these two routes varies from gene to gene. Several genes are known that are always silenced epigenetically and never by mutation, while for others the reverse is true, and for yet others both processes are common. For example *MLH1* is often silenced epigenetically, but *MSH2* never is. Jones and Baylin (2003) provide a review of this topic, with many examples and some speculation about mechanisms. One such speculation is that the hypomethylation of centromeres might predispose cancer cells to chromosomal instability. This is based in part on the observation that in ICF syndrome (OMIM 242860), deficiency of the *DNMT3B* DNA methyltransferase results in aberrant packing of centromeric heterochromatin (see *Disease box 2*).

Are familial breast and colon cancer really multifactorial conditions?

In the case of the Wilson family (Case 23), the result of mutation screening explained the strong family history. However, many multicase breast cancer families do not have mutations in either of the *BRCA1/2* genes. Mutations in *BRCA1* or *BRCA2* explain only around 25% of the overall familial tendency of breast cancer. Sustained searches have failed to reveal any *BRCA3* gene that could account for any significant proportion of the remaining cases. It seems likely that the remaining familial tendency is polygenic, made up of the combined effects of several low-penetrance loci. Several such loci have been identified, either by targeted analysis of known interactors with the BRCA1 or BRCA2 proteins, or by large-scale association studies of the type described in *Section 13.4* (*Table 12.6*).

All these variants together explain only a small extra part of the familial tendency of breast cancer. The functional gene variants are rare, while the SNPs are common but confer very modest extra risks. It is questionable whether genotyping women for any or all of these variants would have any clinical utility. They would make little difference to a woman's individual risk, but they might be used to fine-tune the age at which women are offered routine mammographic screening.

A somewhat similar but less striking situation is seen in colon cancer. The lifetime risk in the USA is 5–6%. About 20% of all colorectal cancer patients have two or more first or second degree relatives with colon cancer; 5–10% of cases show more or less mendelian inheritance. FAP and HNPCC account for about 4% of all colon cancers; the rest of the familial tendency is probably the effect of several low-penetrance susceptibility alleles.

Getting the complete picture: whole genome studies

Cancer research has moved decisively from studies of single oncogenes or TS genes to identifying the totality of somatic changes in tumor genomes. The use

Table 12.6 – Genetic variants associated with risk of breast cancer

Gene	Variant	Chromosomal location	Odds ratio
ATM	Loss of function	11q22.3	2.37
BRIP1	Loss of function	17q22	2.0
PALB2	Loss of function	16p12	2.3
CHEK2	c.1100delC	22q12.1	2.34
FGFR2	SNP rs2981582	10q26	1.26
MAP3K1	SNP rs889312	5q11.2	1.13
TNRC9	SNP rs51005538	16q12	1.11
LSP1	SNP rs1865582	11p15.5	1.07

Odds ratios are the odds of finding the specified variant in a woman with breast cancer compared to a healthy control (see *Box 11.1*). For *ATM, BRIP1* and *PALB2* the odds ratio refers to the overall frequency of loss of function mutations in cases compared to controls. For *FGFR2, MAP3K1, TNRC9* and *LSP1* the variants are SNPs identified in the study of Easton *et al.* (2007), which probably do not themselves increase risk, but mark chromosomal segments that contain an unidentified risk factor. See *Section 13.4* for further discussion of such data.

of SNP chips to study genome-wide copy number changes was mentioned earlier. Many laboratories are also now using next-generation sequencing to define whole genome sequences of tumors. If the normal genome of the host is also sequenced, a complete list of somatic mutations can be produced. In contrast to earlier work, the new studies give an unbiased picture of changes across the whole genome.

The first few published tumor sequences give a daunting impression of complexity. The mass of data obtained can be represented by a so-called Circos plot, as in *Figure 12.16*. *Table 12.7* gives a few example numbers. There are not only huge numbers of somatic changes – typically several tens of thousands per sample – but there is enormous diversity. Each tumor has its own individual set of variants,

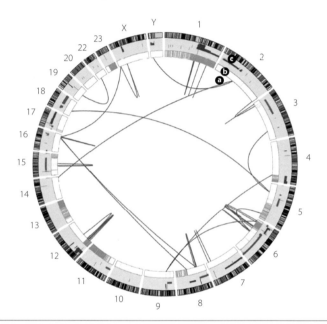

Figure 12.16 – Somatic changes in a primary non-small cell lung tumor from a cigarette smoker.
The outer circle of this 'Circos plot' shows the chromosomes, with their banding patterns, and the centromeres marked in red. (a) The innermost lines show structural rearrangements, red for interchromosomal and blue for intrachromosomal changes. (b) Regions of loss of heterozygosity and allelic imbalance are marked in green. (c) Copy number changes (red = gains, blue = losses). In addition to the changes shown here, 50675 point mutations were identified. Data of Lee *et al.* (2010) reproduced with permission from Nature Publishing Group.

Table 12.7 – Somatic changes identified by sequencing whole tumor genomes

Tumor	Type of sample	Total point mutations	Point mutations in gene regions	Genomic rearrangements	Copy number changes
Lung cancer	Cell line	22910	134	58	334
Melanoma	Cell line	33345	292	51	41
Breast cancer	Primary tumor	27173	200	34	155

Data from Ledford (2010).

with only modest overlap between tumors. Primary tumors, as distinct from cell lines, consist of a heterogeneous collection of cells; a full analysis will require single cell genome sequences. Clearly, very large panels of tumors will need to be sequenced to extract the biologically relevant changes from the sea of passenger mutations. It will also be necessary to incorporate studies of epigenetic changes, as these are known to be important in tumorigenesis.

Hopefully some of the heterogeneity can be resolved by looking at pathways rather than individual genes. The six capabilities listed by Hanahan and Weinberg (*Box 12.1*) can be acquired in innumerable different ways, but each one probably depends on subverting one or a few of the signaling pathways through which the behavior of a cell is controlled. *Figure 12.17* shows an example from a study of glioblastoma multiforme, a malignant brain tumor. In different tumors a variety of different mutations are seen, but all have the same effect of deregulating signaling from cell surface receptors through the RAS–MAPK pathway. Other mutations in the tumors similarly disrupt other vital systems. However, cell control seldom works through simple linear pathways, and a very sophisticated systems-level understanding of the network of interactions may be required before we can understand exactly how any given tumor cell has acquired those six capabilities.

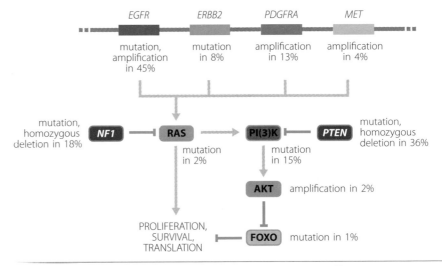

Figure 12.17 – Altered signaling in glioblastoma multiforme cells.
In different tumors different mutations all have the same effect of deregulating the responses of cells to signals at the cell surface receptors EGFR, ERBB2, PDGFRA and MET. Reproduced from Cancer Gene Atlas Research Network (2008) with permission from Nature Publishing Group.

An alternative to genome sequencing is to study the overall pattern of gene expression in a tumor compared to the corresponding normal cells. This is a step closer to the biology, and studies have demonstrated gene expression patterns ('signatures') that are characteristic of different tumor subtypes. Expression can be studied in either of two ways.

- *Using expression microarrays*. Bulk mRNA or cDNA from the tumor is dye-labeled and hybridized to a microarray, probably in a competitive assay to compare it with the repertoire of mRNA in the relevant normal tissue. The microarray carries oligonucleotides corresponding to unique regions of cDNA from every gene in the genome, and hopefully all the major splice variants. The University of Utah Genetic Science Learning Center (see *References*) has a useful animated website explaining from ground level the principles of expression array analysis in cancer.

- *Using next-generation sequencing of total cDNA from the tumor.* The sequence identifies expressed genes, and the relative level of expression is determined by counting the number of times a given cDNA features in the millions of short reads produced by the massively parallel sequencing (the read depth).

The raw data consist of a huge table, showing the hybridization intensity or read depth for every gene in every tumor studied. Patterns are extracted by hierarchical clustering. Tumors showing similar patterns of gene expression are shown in adjacent columns of the table, and genes showing similar patterns of expression are shown in adjacent rows. The result is often displayed as a 'heat map', in which cells are colored to indicate increased or decreased levels of gene expression, relative to the normal tissue. *Figure 12.18* shows an example that demonstrates the power of this approach to classify tumors into biologically related groups.

The goal of all the work described in this chapter is to find effective cures for cancer. To do this, it is necessary to understand what has gone wrong in any particular tumor and to identify the specific vulnerabilities of those tumor cells. In *Section 8.4* we saw how drugs are being developed to target tumors carrying specific mutations. The sequencing studies are showing just what a challenge it will be to make personalized treatment available for every cancer patient. Just as ordinary evolution has produced the immense diversity of species that inhabit our planet, so the random evolution of cell clones has produced an immense diversity of tumor cells. Perhaps expression data might provide physicians with a manageable halfway house between the simple classifications derived from tumor histology and the mind-numbing complexity revealed by sequencing. Some expression-based assays have already reached clinical practice. For breast cancer patients, looking for amplification of the *HER2* (*ERBB2*) receptor defines the responsiveness to Herceptin (see *Section 8.4*). The Mammaprint® assay uses expression levels of 70 genes to generate a signature that aims to predict which early-stage breast cancer patients are at risk of distant recurrences after surgery. How far either expression studies or DNA sequencing can usefully guide management of cancer in general remains to be seen.

Figure 12.18 – Expression profiling of ovarian tumors.
This heat map shows the expression pattern of 110 genes, selected from 7651 on the microarray, in 61 individual ovarian tumors. Each column is the data from one tumor, each row is the data for one gene. Expression levels are color-coded (green = significantly reduced expression, red = significantly raised expression). Results are clustered by hierarchical analysis to reveal common patterns. Eighteen of the tumors carried a *BRCA1* mutation, 16 had a *BRCA2* mutation and 27 had neither ('sporadic'). The expression profiles distinguish the *BRCA1* and *BRCA2* patterns, and show that different sporadic tumors fit one or other of these two patterns. Evidently *BRCA1* and *BRCA2* mutations cause ovarian cancer by different routes, and sporadic tumors follow one or other of these pathways. Reproduced from Jazaeri *et al.* (2002) with permission from Oxford University Press.

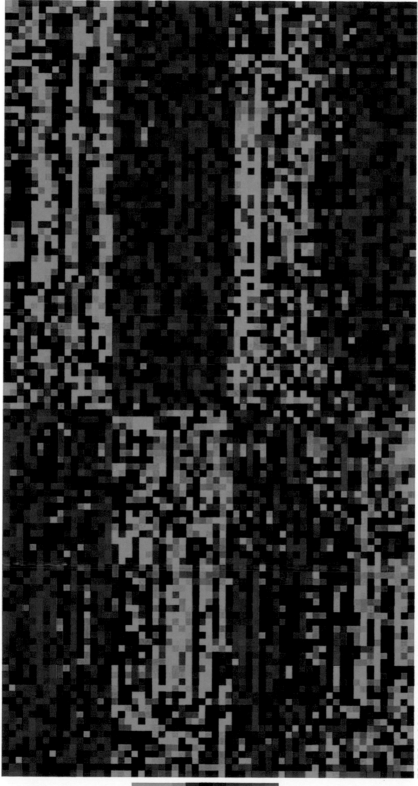

BRCA2 BRCA1 sporadic

PAK2 231951
NCSTN 199645
HGF 1219612
BAD 1286754
F23149_1 428507
DKFZP564C186 366353
UBL1 758495
GCAT 307094
RBBP4 773599
CALU 144881
RUNX1 263251
PTK2B 180298
FDFT1 25725
IL18R1 755054
P14L 809437
RALY 825583
KIAA0218 49404
MPI 50359
IL17R 842122
KIAA0008 357373
IL1B 491763
RAB3A 163579
HARS 43021
TUFM 34945
PEF 137353
GNB2 292213
SECRET 29054
SLC9A1 30272
NAGA 28985
MNAT1 38471
EST 124034
COVA1 588822
LOX 341680
MAPRE1 428223
FLJ22059 292223
ILK 292313
PISD 343609
PPIA 241900
EIF4A1 46171
KIAA0144 245015
TCEB2 52162
GART 502761
TAGLN2 45544
UBE1 898262
FLJ12442 32231
PPY2 210073
MAP2K3 45641
GTPBP1 826217
NM23-H1 176482
SF3B4 432564
AKT1 810331
PPP2R5A 41356
APMCF1 198904
ZNF173 755176
GS2NA 767994
AFP 74537
SLC25A11 878413
PPP1CB 485729
RBBP2 841655
SCYB5 198699
S100A4 472180
KIAA03 65 811029
SFRS11 204755
KDR 469345
SCYA4 205633
SCYA4 205633
RGS1 361323
RGS1 686248
RGS16 470132
RGS16 470132
SFRP4 841282
ENPP1 786041
PDGFRB 773439
BMP6 768168
MMP13 786029
CSRP2 75254
WNT2 149373
WNT2 149373
APEX 740907
POLR2A 740130
GOLGA1 34102
CSNK1E 854138
LOC51605 810343
ZNF211 346947
FOXO1A 628055
ZFP161 285742
ATP7A 687820
FLJ21940 810795
TNRC12 770000
TAL1 717727
NCOA1 609445
BRE 739993
RAB2L 741891
SAST 739625
ITGAE 665279
ARHGEF6 687990
TCF4 854581
TMEPAI 809824
CD36 243816
PTEN 322160
PDE6A 361840
CD83 564503
FLJ10701 430068
LOC51760 52226
SMG1 785605
WNT2 302286
IL7 701422
CRB1 248485
GABRP 563598
PLXNA2 303035
RNAC 125148
CUGBP1 25588
PON1 128143
RYBP 649654
CD36 243816
FLJ21661 80095

Z −2.5 −1.5 −0.5 0 0.5 1.5 2.5

von Hippel–Lindau disease

Patients with von Hippel–Lindau disease (OMIM 193300) are at risk of developing a variety of tumors (*Box table 12.1*). The most frequent causes of death are renal cell carcinoma or hemangioblastomas in the central nervous system. The disease is autosomal dominant, with an incidence of 1 in 35 000–45 000. 95% of gene carriers have developed one or more of the characteristic tumors by age 65. Because the different manifestations of the disease may be treated by different clinicians, the connection between them is not always made promptly, leading to delays in establishing the diagnosis. One role of clinical geneticists can be to act as a central point of reference for the family, and to co-ordinate the different surveillance programs that need to be put in place for family members.

Box table 12.1 – Patients with von Hippel–Lindau disease may develop a variety of tumors and require careful surveillance

Tumor	Frequency	Mean age at presentation	Screening	Age to start screening
Hemangioblastoma of CNS	60–80%	33 years	Annual craniospinal MRI	11 years
Hemangioblastomas of retina	60%	25 years	Annual ophthalmoscopy	Infancy
Endolymphatic sac tumors	11%	22 years	CT or MRI	When symptoms occur
Renal carcinoma	24–45%	39 years	Annual CT scan of abdomen	18 years
Pheochromocytoma	10–20%	30 years	Annual plasma or 24 hr urinary catecholamine	2 years

Data from Lonser *et al.* (2003).

The *VHL* locus was mapped to 3p25–26, and the gene was identified by positional cloning. It behaves as a classic TS gene. Patients inherit one loss of function mutation, and in their tumors the second copy is inactivated by mutation, deletion or methylation. 70–80% of sporadic renal clear cell carcinomas show inactivation of both copies of the gene. The gene is small (3 exons encoding a 213 amino acid protein) and mutation detection is relatively straightforward.

The expression of the disease varies between families (*Box table 12.2*). In some families affected people never seem to develop pheochromocytomas, while in other families these are frequent. This has led to the disease being divided into Types 1 and 2. Type 2 has been further subdivided into 2A, 2B and 2C. All forms are caused by mutations in the *VHL* gene. Loose genotype–phenotype correlations have been established: deletions and truncating mutations usually cause Type 1, while Type 2 families usually have mis-sense mutations. Particular mis-sense mutations are associated with the different sub-types of Type 2. Renal cell carcinoma is more frequent in Type 1 than in Type 2 families.

Box table 12.2 – Clinical subtypes of von Hippel–Lindau disease tend to breed true within families

Type	Pheo.	RCC	Hem.
1	–	+	+
2A	+	–	+
2B	+	+	+
2C	+	–	–

Pheo, pheochromocytoma; RCC, renal cell carcinoma; Hem, hemangioblastoma.

Investigation of the pathogenic mechanism has focused on the relation of the VHL protein to the HIF-1α (hypoxia-inducible factor 1α) protein. The VHL protein is part of an E3 ubiquitin ligase complex (VCB-Cul2) that controls the level of HIF-1α by degrading it when oxygen levels are normal (*Box figure 12.4*). HIF-1α is flagged for degradation by hydroxylation of specific proline residues in an oxygen-dependent reaction. VHL protein acts as the recognition component of the ubiquitin ligase: it directly binds hydroxylated HIF-1α. Pathogenic mis-sense mutations in VHL cluster in the HIF-1α-binding region of the protein. Under conditions of hypoxia HIF-1α is stabilized. It then acts as a multifunctional transcriptional activator. Among its many targets are VEGF (vascular endothelial growth factor), a powerful promoter of angiogenesis. It is noteworthy that the tumors in von Hippel–Lindau disease are all particularly highly vascularized. Other targets of HIF-1α include the growth factor TGFα and enzymes promoting glycolysis and glucose transport.

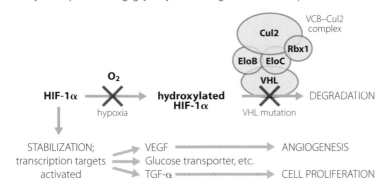

Box figure 12.4 – Hypoxia-inducible factor 1α causes major adjustments to cell metabolism in response to hypoxia.
Cul2, cullin-2; EloB, elongin B; EloC, elongin C; Rbx1, cullin regulatory protein. In VHL cells, HIF is constitutively active.

VHL protein appears to have other functions independent of HIF-1α (Barry and Krek, 2004). Although this protein is much smaller than the giant scaffold proteins encoded by some other tumor suppressor genes (see above), a surprising number of possible binding partners have been identified. VHL protein binds cyclin D1, leading to possible effects on the cell cycle. Effects on the extracellular matrix, via binding to fibronectin, and on the cytoskeleton via association with microtubules, may be significant in invasiveness and metastasis. In addition, VHL protein has recently been shown to bind directly to p53 and stabilize it against MDM2-mediated degradation.

12.5. References

Albuquerque C, Breukel C, van der Luijt R, *et al.* (2002) The 'just right' signaling model: *APC* somatic mutations are selected based on a specific level of activation of the β-catenin signaling cascade. *Hum. Molec. Genet.* **11:** 1549–1560.

Barry RE and Krek W (2004) The von Hippel–Lindau tumor suppressor: a multifaceted inhibitor of tumorigenesis. *Trends Mol. Med.* **10:** 466–472.

Beroukhim R, Murmel CH, Porter D, *et al.* (2010) The landscape of somatic copy-number alterations across human cancers. *Nature,* **463:** 899–905.

Cancer Genome Atlas Research Network (2008) Comprehensive genomic characterisation defines human glioblastoma genes and core pathways. *Nature,* **455:** 1061–1068.

Cavenee WK, Dryja TP, Phillips RA, *et al.* (1983) Expression of recessive alleles by chromosomal mechanisms in retinoblastoma. *Nature,* **305:** 779–784.

Easton DF, Pooley KA, Dunning AM, *et al.* (2007) Genomewide association study identifies novel breast cancer susceptibility loci. *Nature,* **447:** 1087–1093.

Evans DGR, Eccles DM, Rahman N, *et al.* (2004) A new scoring system for identifying a *BRCA1/2* mutation outperforms existing models including BRCAPRO. *J. Med. Genet.* **41:** 474–480.

Greaves M (2007) Darwinian medicine: a case for cancer. *Nat. Rev. Cancer,* **7:** 214–221.

Hanahan D and Weinberg RA (2000) The hallmarks of cancer. *Cell,* **100:** 57–70. *Readers who are not strong on cell biology may need to skip the detail, but this is an excellent introduction to a modern view of cancer.*

Jazaeri AA, Yee CJ, Sotiriou C, *et al.* (2002) Gene expression profiles of *BRCA1*-linked, *BRCA2*-linked, and sporadic ovarian cancers. *J. Natl. Cancer Inst.* **94:** 990–1000.

Jones PA and Baylin SB (2003) The fundamental role of epigenetic events in cancer. *Nature Rev. Cancer,* **3:** 415–428.

Kinzler KW and Vogelstein B (1996) Lessons from hereditary colorectal cancer. *Cell,* **87:** 159–170.

Ledford HL (2010) The cancer genome challenge. *Nature,* **464:** 972–974. *A news article discussing the potential and the problems of sequencing tumor genomes.*

Lee W, Jiang Z, Liu Z, *et al.* (2010) The mutation spectrum revealed by paired genome sequences from a lung cancer patient. *Nature,* **465:** 473–477.

Lonser RR, Glenn GM, McClellan W, *et al.* (2003) Von Hippel–Lindau disease. *Lancet,* **361:** 2059–2067.

Skloot R (2010) *The Immortal Life of Henrietta Lacks.* Crown Publishing Group, New York.

Useful websites

Cancer Gene Census provides a database of genes for which mutations have been causally implicated in cancer:
www.sanger.ac.uk/genetics/CGP/Census

University of Utah Genetic Science Learning Center section on expression analysis in cancer: http://gslc.genetics.utah.edu/units/biotech/microarray/

12.6. **Self-assessment questions**

(1) In relation to tumorigenesis, for each of the following statements decide if it is:
  (a) true of both oncogenes and tumor suppressor genes
  (b) true of oncogenes but not tumor suppressor genes
  (c) true of tumor suppressor genes but not oncogenes
  (d) true of neither tumor suppressor genes nor oncogenes.

  (1) May show nonsense mutations in sporadic cancers
  (2) May encode proteins involved in cell cycle regulation
  (3) Frequently mutated in familial and sporadic cancers
  (4) Often involved in loss of heterozygosity in sporadic cancers
  (5) Frequently mutated in familial but not sporadic cancers
  (6) May indirectly act to inactivate telomerase
  (7) Often involved in chromosomal rearrangements in sporadic cancers
  (8) May show inherited mis-sense mutations in familial cancers
  (9) Frequently mutated in sporadic but not familial cancers
  (10) May show gene amplification in familial and sporadic cancers

(2) Blood and tumor DNA was extracted from two unrelated children with retinoblastoma and typed for a 2-allele DNA marker that maps close to the *RB1* gene. One child has a family history of retinoblastoma while the other has a sporadic unilateral tumor. The genotypes were:

	Child A	Child B
Blood	Heterozygous 2–1	Homozygous for allele 1
Tumor	Homozygous for allele 2	Homozygous for allele 1

Mark each of the following statements as true or false:
(a) the result indicates that Child B has the sporadic form of the disease
(b) the result indicates that Child A has the familial form of the disease
(c) the result indicates that the tumor in Child B could be either homozygous or hemizygous for the marker
(d) the result indicates that if Child A has the inherited form of the disease, he inherited it on the chromosome that carries allele 2 of the marker

(3) Neurofibromatosis 2 (OMIM 101000) is the result of inherited and/or somatic mutations in the *NF2* tumor suppressor gene. Inherited NF2

shows 90% penetrance. Assuming a mutation rate of 3×10^{-5} per gene per cell, what is the size of the target cell population? What is the expected incidence of sporadic NF2?

(4) The *Figure* shows two families in which there are several cases of cancer (B, breast; O, ovarian; P, prostate; numbers are the age at diagnosis). Which of the two women marked with a question mark would you prioritize for *BRCA1/2* mutation screening?

(a)   **(b)**

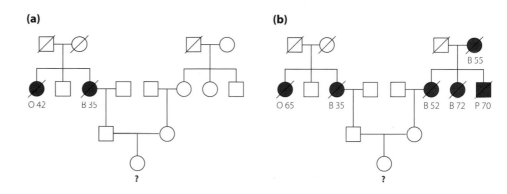

13 | Should we be testing for genetic susceptibility to common diseases?

After working through this chapter you should be able to:

- Describe the multifactorial nature of most human traits, both normal and abnormal, and the principles of multifactorial inheritance
- Explain quantitative trait loci
- Describe Falconer's threshold theory and use it to make qualitative predictions of risk
- Explain the uses and limitations of the concept of heritability
- Describe the principle of affected sib pair analysis
- Compare and contrast linkage and association as methods for identifying susceptibility factors
- Describe and explain the haplotype block structure of the human genome
- Describe the process and achievements of genome-wide association studies
- Discuss the 'missing heritability' problem and possible solutions
- Discuss the present and future prospects for testing healthy people to identify their genetic susceptibilities to common complex diseases

13.1. Case studies

CASE 25	Yamomoto family	**333**	346	389

- Family history of dementia
- ? Alzheimer disease
- Test for ApoE4?

Bill Yamomoto's mother had been getting increasingly forgetful. After a series of incidents including one when she left a pan on the cooker and set the kitchen on fire, it became clear that she was not coping with life on her own. She moved into sheltered accommodation in the same Californian town as Bill and his wife. She never adjusted to her new surroundings and soon required residential care.

Over the next 3 years her dementia progressed until she seldom recognized Bill and was unable to do anything for herself. It was almost a relief when she died at the age of 71 – as Bill said, 'my real mother died several years ago'.

When a friend of his wife said that Alzheimer disease was hereditary, Bill started to worry. He knew that his aunt Yumiko – his mother's sister who had always lived in the old family home in Hawaii – had been diagnosed with Alzheimer

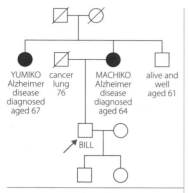

Figure 13.1 – **Pedigree of Yamomoto family.**

disease at the age of 67. His wife suggested he should to talk to his physician. The doctor told him that only the rare forms of the disease with onset before age 60 were inherited. Bill was still not entirely reassured.

Searching on the internet, he discovered that a genetic factor, ApoE4, was associated with susceptibility to the common late-onset form of the disease, and he came across companies offering to test for ApoE4. He wondered whether he should take the test, and decided to consult a geneticist. He wanted to know whether the test was reliable for somebody of Japanese ancestry like himself, and what he should do if the result was positive.

| CASE 26 | Zuabi family | **334** | 350 | 389 |

- Woman aged 52 years, Zafira
- Overweight; sedentary lifestyle; insatiable thirst
- Type 2 diabetes
- Test son

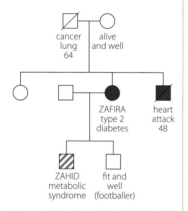

Figure 13.2 – **Pedigree of the Zuabi family.**

Zafira was 52 when she consulted her physician about a 3-month history of dizziness, headaches and blurry vision. She also mentioned that she had developed a terrible thirst, leading her to drink large amounts of water every day and produce correspondingly large amounts of urine. Her urine was found to contain sugar, and a fasting glucose test showed a level of 9 mmol/l. This confirmed the diagnosis of Type 2 diabetes (T2D). She was given a thiazolidenedione drug as the first line of treatment. Enquiry showed that she had an entirely sedentary lifestyle, and her body mass index (BMI) was 30; she was enrolled on a program of graded moderate exercise. Both exercise itself and weight loss help minimize morbidity in T2D.

The shock of diagnosis made Zafira think about her family. Her brother had died of a heart attack aged 48. He had been badly overweight and completely inactive, though she did not remember him drinking especially large amounts of water. When she learned that first-degree relatives of T2D patients were at high risk of developing the condition (her physician quoted a risk of 38% for a child of an affected parent), her thoughts turned to her elder son Zahid. He did not have overt disease, but he shared several risk factors. He went to work by car, took the lift to his office, spent all day sitting at his desk, enjoyed a good meal then spent the evening watching television. Not surprisingly he was overweight. He agreed to come for some tests. These showed that his BMI was 30 with a waist measurement of 99 cm. His fasting plasma glucose was 6.4 mmol/l, below the 7.0 threshold for T2D, but above normal. He was hypertensive (blood pressure 142/90 mmHg) and had dyslipidemia (triglycerides 1.9 mmol/l). His combination of obesity, impaired glucose tolerance, dyslipidemia and hypertension defined him as having the 'metabolic syndrome' (*Table 13.1*). This is a rather loosely defined but well-known precursor of T2D and a major risk factor for cardiovascular disease (reviewed by Eckel *et al.*, 2005). He was prescribed exercise and antihypertensive drugs.

Table 13.1 – **World Health Organization definition of the metabolic syndrome (1999)**

Feature	Measure
Diabetes	Fasting glucose > 7.0 mmol/l
Or impaired fasting glycemia	Fasting glucose 6.1–7.0 mmol/l
Or impaired glucose tolerance	
Or insulin resistance	Hyperinsulinemic
PLUS 2 or more of:	
Obesity	BMI > 30 or waist-to-hip ratio >0.9 (male) or 0.85 (female) (different figures may be appropriate for non-white people)
Dyslipidemia	Triglycerides ≥1.7 mmol/l
	HDL cholesterol (male) <0.9 or (female) <1.0 mmol/l
Hypertension	>140/90 mmHg
Microalbuminuria	Albumin excretion >20 µg/min

Other bodies have produced somewhat different but overlapping definitions. The list shows the complex of interacting characters that indicate susceptibility to T2D and cardiovascular disease. The prevalence of the syndrome rises with age among US adults, from 7% at age 20–29 to 44% at age 60–69. Prevalence is 50% in severely obese US youngsters, and is increasing at all ages and in most countries of the world.

13.2. **Science toolkit**

Two models of genetic determination

Traditionally, genetic characters have been divided into mendelian and **polygenic**. Polygenic conditions depend on the combined action of a very large number of genetic factors, each of which makes only a very small contribution to the final phenotype. Both categories, mendelian and polygenic, are conceptual models, useful tools for thinking about inheritance – but in reality, all conditions fall somewhere between the two. For any particular character, you need to decide what mix of the two conceptual models gives the best description, and then you need to add in environmental effects. *Figure 1.15* showed a linear spectrum of genetic phenotypes. Adding in environmental effects, the overall etiology of any disease might be represented by a point somewhere inside the triangle of *Figure 13.3*. 'Multifactorial' or 'complex' are useful non-committal terms for conditions that fall in the interior of the triangle.

Genes are always mendelian, but *characters* are never wholly dependent on the genotype at a single locus. Closer acquaintance with any mendelian disease reveals that these 'simple' conditions are actually not so simple. As described in *Chapters 6* and *8*, the quest for genotype–phenotype correlations seldom yields the desired neat result. The long road between a DNA sequence variant and an observable phenotype allows many additional players, environmental, genetic and simply chance ('stochastic'), to join the action. The concept of *penetrance* allows you to lump all these other factors together and not try to analyze them. Identified genes that influence the expression of a basically mendelian character are called **modifier genes**.

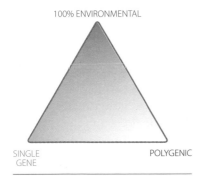

100% ENVIRONMENTAL

SINGLE GENE   POLYGENIC

Figure 13.3 – Etiology of diseases.
For any condition the overall balance of genetic and environmental determinants can be represented by a point somewhere within the triangle.

Dichotomous versus quantitative characters

You can divide all human characters into two sorts:

- dichotomous or discontinuous characters, like diseases and malformations, that you either have or do not have
- continuous or quantitative characters, that everybody has, but to differing degrees; examples would be height, weight or blood pressure.

Gene loci involved in determining continuous characters are called **quantitative trait loci (QTL)**. Some QTLs may be the result of the same simple loss of function or gain of function mutations that underlie most mendelian characters. However, in many cases QTL variants are likely to have more subtle effects on gene function. Variants in promoters or other control elements could result in small changes in the level of expression, as could copy number changes (*Section 2.4*). Sequence changes might slightly alter the stability of the mRNA or the balance of splice isoforms. The lactase gene variant responsible for persistence of intestinal lactase (see *Box 8.4*) might be a typical example. The same gene could cause a mendelian condition if it has a mutation of major effect, and act as a QTL with more subtle changes. Equally, a genetic change may have a major effect on one character and be a QTL for another.

Polygenic theory

Models of polygenic inheritance consider characters that depend on the combined action of a large number of genetic factors, each of which makes only a small contribution to the final phenotype. The main use of these models in human genetics is not to make predictions, but to provide a framework for thinking about complex genetic conditions. For any actual condition the framework needs to be populated by empiric epidemiological data. The two elements of the framework that are most relevant to clinical genetics are the concepts of **heritability** and of **thresholds**.

Heritability measures how much of the differences between people for a given trait are the result of the genetic differences between them, and how much are the result of differences in their environments. Mathematically, the heritability of a trait is the proportion of the total variance that is attributable to genetic factors. It is calculated (for continuous characters) from the correlation between relatives, and symbolized as h^2, reflecting its origin as a correlation coefficient. h^2 is a number between 0 (no genetic involvement) and 1 or 100% (no non-genetic factors).

In its simplest form, polygenic theory applies only to continuous, quantitative, characters. The geneticist DS Falconer used the concept of *thresholds* to show how polygenic theory could be extended to dichotomous characters (*Box 13.1*). For dichotomous traits, the heritability is estimated by comparing the incidence of a character in relatives of affected people with the incidence in the general population. In clinical genetics, thinking about thresholds helps make sense of the way risks for complex conditions, unlike risks for mendelian conditions, depend on family history.

BOX 13.1

Polygenic susceptibility to a disease

Although diseases are dichotomous characters (some people have the disease and others do not), threshold theory postulates that there is an underlying continuous susceptibility to the disease. Everybody has some susceptibility; most people have a middling susceptibility; a few have very high or very low susceptibility. The susceptibility is a typical polygenic character that depends on the combined small effects of many genes. Only people whose susceptibility exceeds a certain threshold develop the disease (see top part of *Box figure 13.1*).

If you have an affected relative, that person must have had a high genetic susceptibility. They have a 'bad hand' of high-susceptibility genes. You share genes with your relatives (see *Box 10.3*). You may be lucky and share only a few of your relative's high susceptibility genes, or you may be unlucky and share many. Overall, there will be a wide distribution of susceptibility among relatives of affected people, but the curve will be displaced towards the high-susceptibility end compared to the distribution in the general population (see bottom part of *Box figure 13.1*). Relatives of affected people are more likely than unrelated people to end up above the threshold. The closer the relationship, the more likely this is. Therefore complex diseases tend to run in families, but the tendency is much weaker than with mendelian diseases (*Table 13.2*).

Environmental effects can be incorporated into the model by supposing they move the threshold to a more or a less stringent value of the genetic susceptibility. Thresholds can be sex-specific. The classic example is pyloric stenosis. This is much more common in boys than girls (5M : 1F). The threshold must be lower in boys than girls, for some physiological reason. To be affected, a girl must have a particularly high susceptibility. On average, affected girls have higher susceptibility genes than affected boys. Therefore relatives of affected girls are at higher risk of pyloric stenosis than relatives of affected boys.

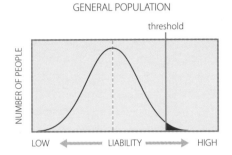

GENERAL POPULATION

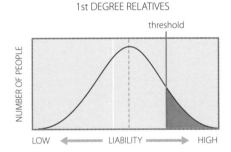

1st DEGREE RELATIVES

Box figure 13.1 – Distribution of susceptibility.
Distribution in the general population (top), with threshold. Distribution in relatives (bottom).

Although these models can be developed mathematically, they are mainly useful as qualitative tools for thinking about recurrence risks. They lead to the general rule:

> *In complex disease, the worse luck (many affected people; the less common sex affected) a family have had in the past, the greater is the risk of a recurrence.*

Note the complete contrast between complex and mendelian diseases in this respect. If by bad luck all your three children have cystic fibrosis, the risk your next child will be affected is still 1 in 4. But if you had two babies rather than one baby with a neural tube defect, the risk to the next baby changes from 1 in 25 to 1 in 12. Having a second affected child didn't change your risk, but it allowed us to recognize the high risk you always had.

The heritability is not a fixed property of a condition, like the mode of inheritance; it applies to a particular population at a particular time. The heritability of a trait can change with social changes. A century ago, the reason why some people suffered phenylketonuric mental retardation, while others did not, was wholly genetic. Nowadays those reasons are almost entirely environmental – lost samples, a family that couldn't be traced, or that were unable to make sure a homozygous child kept rigidly to the diet. A part-genetic condition that is associated with poverty and social deprivation will have a higher heritability in an egalitarian society than in one with great inequalities, because environmental differences are less in a more egalitarian society. The concept of heritability is often misunderstood, leading at times to its misuse in political arguments about whether or not to try to prevent a condition by social action. As long as its limitations are understood, heritability is a useful measure for researchers investigating a complex condition, because it gives a guide to the relevance of genetic factors under the circumstances prevailing at the time.

Investigating the genetics of complex diseases

Claims for genetic factors in complex disease need to be backed by evidence. This normally comes from three types of study.

- *Family studies* look at relatives of affected probands and ask how much more likely they are to be affected, compared to an unrelated person. The risk ratio is symbolized as λ, with a subscript denoting the relationship. For example, λ_s is the relative risk for a sib of a proband (*Table 13.2*). High values of λ suggest genetic factors – but it is important to remember

Table 13.2 – **Examples of recurrence risks for mendelian and multifactorial diseases**

Disease	λ_s	Lifetime risk (to age 80)
Cystic fibrosis	500	0.05%
Huntington disease	5000	0.01%
Celiac disease	60	3%
Multiple sclerosis	25	1%
Type 1 diabetes	15	6%
Type 2 diabetes	3–6	7–35%
Alzheimer disease (late onset)	4	35%
Breast cancer (females)	2	12%

λ_s is the relative risk for a sib of an affected proband, compared to an unrelated person. Compare the risks for the mendelian conditions (shaded rows) with the complex conditions. These are **empiric risks**, derived from surveys of families, not from theoretical calculations. They can vary between populations and also over time (the latter presumably because of environmental changes). When using such risks for counseling it is important to use risks derived from studies appropriate to the consultand's background. Data from Dr Alison Stewart, Cambridge.

that the same effect could be produced by shared family environment. Because we give our children their environment as well as their genes, it is not safe simply to rely on family studies, especially for behavioral traits.

- *Adoption studies* separate the effects of genes and family environment. For example, children of schizophrenic parents who were adopted at birth into unaffected families have a significantly increased risk of developing schizophrenia, compared to their adoptive sibs. This suggests that the familial tendency of schizophrenia is due, at least in part, to genetic factors rather than parental behavior.
- *Twin studies* look at affected people who have a twin. They compare monozygotic (MZ) and dizygotic (DZ) twins to see how often the co-twin is also affected. MZ twins share all their genes while DZ twins share on average half their genes; twins should share their environment to the same degree regardless of zygosity. Thus a higher concordance among MZ twins is evidence for genetic factors. MZ twins separated at birth and brought up in different environments form the perfect study, but their numbers are too small to provide anything more than fascinating anecdotes.

The end result of family, twin or adoption studies is an estimate (see *Figure 13.4*) of the heritability of the condition.

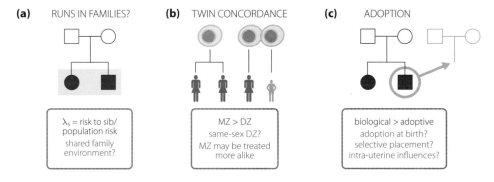

Figure 13.4 – Methods of demonstrating genetic effects in complex diseases, and reasons for caution in interpreting the results.

Linkage studies to identify susceptibility factors

Having decided that genetic factors do play a role in susceptibility to your chosen disease, the next step is to identify the factors. This is a great deal easier said than done. The first approach, in the 1990s, was through linkage analysis (*Chapter 9*). As with mendelian conditions, appropriate family members are typed for a large panel of genetic markers, and the data analyzed to find markers that co-segregate with the disease. However, the analysis is different. Standard lod score analysis requires the researcher to tell the computer the penetrance for each genotype, the gene frequencies, and the mutation rate. For mendelian diseases it is usually possible to make plausible guesses for these parameters, but there is no way this can be done for complex conditions. It is therefore necessary to use **non-parametric linkage analysis**.

Non-parametric analysis uses families with more than one affected person, and considers the extent to which the affected family members share genes. Genes, unlike characters, are always mendelian, and it is easy to calculate the expected sharing among any set of relatives. Affected relatives should show excessive sharing of any gene or marker that is involved in causing the disease, quite regardless of the mode of inheritance. The commonest approach uses affected sib pairs. Consider a pair of sibs with a mendelian recessive condition. *Figure 13.5* shows how they would share alleles at two marker loci, one closely linked to their disease locus and the other unlinked. *Table 13.3* generalizes this to other modes of inheritance, including complex disease. Even though a complex disease susceptibility factor is neither necessary nor sufficient for disease to develop, markers that are linked to a susceptibility locus should be shared by affected sibs more often than by chance. The result of analysis is a **non-parametric lod (NPL) score**, the significance of which is assessed according to the thresholds in *Box 13.2*.

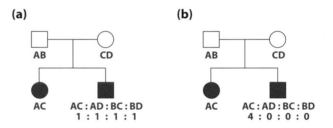

Figure 13.5 – Sharing of marker alleles by a pair of sibs who are both affected by a mendelian recessive disease.
(a) A marker that is on a different chromosome from the disease locus. (b) A marker that is closely linked to the disease locus. A, B, C, D represent different alleles at the marker locus.

Table 13.3 – Expected sharing of marker alleles by a pair of affected sibs

Marker	Sibs share no alleles	Sibs share 1 allele	Sibs share 2 alleles
Not linked to disease locus	¼	½	¼
Tightly linked to rare mendelian dominant	0	½	½
Tightly linked to rare mendelian recessive	0	0	1
Linked to common disease susceptibility locus	< ¼	> ½	> ¼

The figures for mendelian diseases assume that both sibs have the same alleles at the disease locus, which will normally be true as long as disease alleles are rare in the population. For a common disease susceptibility locus, one cannot predict the exact proportions, only the direction in which the proportions will deviate from the random expectation.

BOX 13.2

Thresholds of significance in genome-wide linkage studies

In *Section 9.2* we saw that the threshold for significance of a lod score is 3.0. The probability of getting so high a lod score if there is really no linkage to that marker is 0.05. If we use hundreds of markers to scan the whole genome, the chance that one or another of them will give a false positive result is clearly higher than if we use just a single marker. The question of how much higher is quite difficult statistically. Following Lander and Kruglyak (1995), the results of a whole genome linkage trawl can be categorized as:

- highly significant evidence for linkage (lod score > 5.4)
- significant evidence for linkage (lod score > 3.6)
- suggestive evidence for linkage (lod score > 2.2)

These thresholds are chosen to give chances of 0.001, 0.05 and 1, respectively, of finding such a high lod score once in a whole-genome linkage scan on the null hypothesis of no true linkage. Scores in the lower categories carry little weight until independent studies have replicated them.

Affected sib pair linkage analysis is an extremely robust method. There are no built-in assumptions that might be proved wrong. However, it has low power to identify factors that confer only a weak susceptibility to disease (*Table 13.4*). Studies of many complex diseases during the 1990s using affected sib pairs produced very few positive results. Either most susceptibility factors have effects too weak to be picked up by studying a few hundred sib pairs (the typical size of study), or perhaps there is very extensive heterogeneity, with each individual factor being operative in only a few families. Even when a significant result was obtained, the chromosomal region it defined was usually too large to provide a manageable list of candidate genes. This led researchers to turn to an alternative approach, association.

Association studies to identify susceptibility factors

Consider Bob and Carol (*Figure 13.6*). They each have T2D, in part because they both inherited a susceptibility allele on chromosome 9 from their shared great-

Table 13.4 – Numbers of affected sib pairs needed to detect a disease susceptibility factor

Relative risk of disease due to this locus	5x	3x	2.5x	2x	1.5x
Probability of allele sharing by affected sibs	0.634	0.556	0.536	0.518	0.505
Number of affected sib pairs needed to detect effect	94	559	1366	5379	67805

Affected sib pairs are powerful for detecting factors that raise the risk by a factor of more than 3. The poor track record of affected sib pair analysis suggests that most risk factors have a smaller effect than this. Data from Risch and Merikangas (1996).

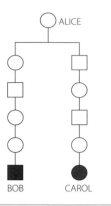

Figure 13.6 – Bob and Carol both inherited a susceptibility allele for T2D from their great-great-great grandmother Alice.

great-great grandmother Alice. They will share the segment of chromosome 9 that carries Alice's susceptibility allele, and so they will also each have the same allele for the various non-pathogenic SNPs that are located on that segment. It will be quite a small segment. During prophase I of meiosis there are an average of 60 crossovers per cell in males and 90 in females. An average chromosome might be split into three to six segments. A segment 10 cM long has a 90% probability of surviving one meiosis without being broken up by recombination, but only a $(0.9)^{10} = 0.35$ chance of remaining intact through the ten meioses that separate Bob and Carol.

Bob and Carol probably did not know they were related. They each have 32 great-great-great grandparents. Even if they were both enthusiastic family historians, it is unlikely they would know about all 32 of them and would have identified all their many descendants. Extending this example, N generations ago a person had 2^N ancestors (*Figure 13.7*). Each ancestor in turn would have on average 2^N descendants if the population size remained constant. Going back even 20 generations (say, 500 years, to 1500), 2^{20} is over 1 million. Ultimately we are all related. The word 'unrelated' will be used here to mean people who do not share any great grandparent and are unaware of any other common ancestor. People who thought themselves unrelated nevertheless share small chromosome segments that are inherited from distant common ancestors. The more distant the ancestor, the smaller each shared segment will be, but the larger will be the number of people who share it.

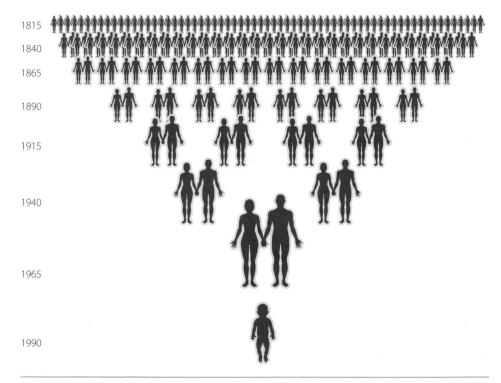

Figure 13.7 – *N* generations ago a person has 2ᴺ ancestors.
This number quickly exceeds the population of most countries a few hundred years ago. Even allowing for inbreeding and the isolation of communities, we are all related through distant common ancestors. (From an idea by Dr Bryan Sykes.)

Suppose one such ancestral segment contained an allele conferring susceptibility to diabetes. A collection of present-day unrelated diabetics would tend to share that chromosome segment. The allele is neither necessary nor sufficient to cause diabetes, so not every diabetic will have this segment, and some non-diabetic people will have it – but insofar as having the allele increases susceptibility, affected people are more likely than unaffected people to have that ancestral segment. Along with the susceptibility allele, they will share alleles of the SNPs that mark that segment. Looking for SNP alleles that are shared by cases more than by controls is the basis of association studies in complex disease. As *Box 13.3* shows, this approach is different in principle from the earlier linkage studies.

The HapMap project (http://hapmap.ncbi.nlm.nih.gov/) set out in 2002 to identify these shared segments. Initially, 270 individuals from four populations (white Americans of European descent, Yorubans from Ibadan, Nigeria, Japanese from Tokyo and Han Chinese from Beijing) were genotyped for over one million SNPs. Later extensions added in more SNPs and other populations. HapMap data show how each chromosome in each of us is a mosaic of ancestral blocks (see *Section 13.4* for more detail). The blocks vary in size, but average around 5 kb. The precise number, size and identity of blocks depends on the statistical criteria adopted to define a block, but the overall structure is clear (*Table 13.5*).

BOX 13.3

Linkage versus association

Linkage is a relationship between loci. It is a specifically genetic phenomenon. Looking at the data in *Table 9.1*, the *D1S252 locus* is linked to the dyschromatosis *locus*.

Association (in a genetic context) is a relationship between phenotypes or alleles. A particular marker allele, not the marker locus, is associated with a disease. The association is with the disease (the phenotype) not with a disease susceptibility locus that might have high-risk and low-risk alleles.

Linkage does not imply a population-wide association. Looking at the genotypes in *Figure 9.7*, although the *D1S2345* locus is linked to the dyschromatosis locus, no single allele of *D1S2345* is associated with dyschromatosis in all three families. However, within each family, a particular allele is associated – allele 4 in family 1, allele 7 in family 2, and allele 2 in family 3. These alleles are found in the majority of affected members of the respective families, though not in the recombinant individual IV-5 in Family 2.

Association is a purely statistical phenomenon, and not specifically genetic. An association between a genetic variant and a disease may have several causes:

- the variant may directly confer susceptibility to the disease
- the variant may be on the same shared ancestral chromosome segment as a variant that directly causes susceptibility
- if the population studied is not homogeneous with random mating (see *Section 10.2*), but contains subgroups that are relatively isolated from one another, the variant may happen to be more frequent in a subgroup in which the disease is also more frequent, for some unrelated reason. Such *population stratification* must be guarded against in association studies.

A database of all reported associations between diseases and genetic markers is maintained by the National Institute on Aging (the Genetic Association Database, http://geneticassociationdb.nih.gov/cgi-bin/index.cgi).

Table 13.5 – **Statistics of haplotype blocks**

Population	YRI	CEU	CHB+JPT
Average no. of SNPs per block	19.9	24.3	24.4
Average length of blocks (kb)	4.8	5.9	5.9
Fraction of genome spanned by blocks (%)	86	84	84
Average no. of haplotypes per block	5.12	3.63	3.63
% of chromosomes having haplotypes present in ≥5% of population	91	95	95

Note that the blocks in Africans are smaller and more diverse than those in the other populations. This is in keeping with the hypothesis that sub-Saharan African populations are older: there has been more time for repeated recombination to break up the blocks. Some parts of the genome do not give a clear block structure. YRI, Yorubans from Ibadan, Nigeria; CEU, white Americans of European ancestry; CHB, Chinese from Beijing; JPT, Japanese from Tokyo. Data from the first HapMap report, International HapMap Consortium (2005).

Research to define complex disease susceptibility factors has enjoyed an immense flowering over the last few years, based on three developments:

- the HapMap project has defined the ancestral chromosome segments across the genome
- high-resolution SNP chips allow a person to be genotyped for up to 1 million SNPs in a single operation
- researchers and funding agencies have recognized that successful studies require large sample sizes; this has prompted the formation of large consortia, able to recruit and genotype a thousand or more cases and controls for each disease.

As a result of these developments, hundreds of genome-wide association studies (GWAS) have been undertaken, involving innumerable diseases and traits (*Figure 13.8*). An up-to-date catalog is maintained by the US National Human Genome Research Institute (www.genome.gov/gwastudies/). The results of these approaches in Alzheimer disease and Type 2 diabetes are described in the next section. In *Section 13.4* we will take a more general look at the promise and limitations of association studies in complex disease.

13.3. Investigations of patients

For Alzheimer disease and T2D, the two diseases described in Cases 25 and 26, the scope for genetic advice is currently quite limited. For these conditions, as for most multifactorial diseases, genetic investigations are not part of current protocols for managing patients. However, investigations of people like Bill

Figure 13.8 – **An overview of genetic susceptibility factors identified by genome-wide association studies.**
The diagram gives an impression of the range of conditions explored by GWAS over the period 2006–2010, and the many susceptibility loci identified. Data from Hindorff *et al*. Available at www.genome-gov/gwastudies [accessed August 2010].

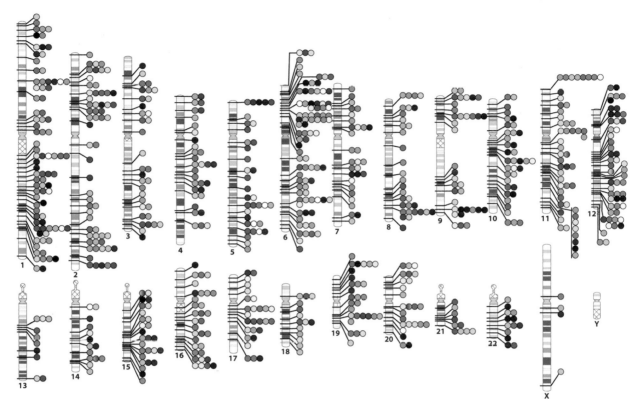

○ Acute lymphoblastic leukemia	● Cutaneous nevi	● Liver enzymes	● QT interval
● Adhesion molecules	● Dermatitis	● LP (a) levels	● Quantitative traits
● Adiponectin levels	● Drug-induced liver injury	● Lung cancer	○ Recombination rate
● Age-related macular degeneration	○ Eosinophil count	● Major mood disorders	○ Red vs.non-red hair
○ AIDS progression	● Eosinophilic esophagitis	● Malaria	● Renal function
○ Alcohol dependence	● Erythrocyte parameters	○ Male pattern baldness	● Response to antipsychotic therapy
○ Alzheimer disease	● Esophageal cancer	● Matrix metalloproteinase levels	○ Response to hepatitis C treatment
○ Amyotrophic lateral sclerosis	● Essential tremor	○ MCP-1	○ Response to statin therapy
○ Angiotensin-converting enzyme activity	● Exfoliation glaucoma	● Melanoma	○ Restless legs syndrome
● Ankylosing spondylitis	● F cell distribution	● Menarche & menopause	● Rheumatoid arthritis
● Arterial stiffness	● Fibrinogen levels	● Multiple sclerosis	● Schizophrenia
● Asthma	● Folate pathway vitamins	○ Myeloproliferative neoplasms	● Serum metabolites
● Atherosclerosis in HIV	○ Freckles and burning	○ Narcolepsy	● Skin pigmentation
● Atrial fibrillation	○ Gallstones	○ Nasopharyngeal cancer	● Speech perception
● Attention deficit hyperactivity disorder	● Glioma	● Neuroblastoma	● Sphingolipid levels
○ Autism	○ Glycemic traits	● Nicotine dependence	● Statin-induced myopathy
● Basal cell cancer	○ Hair color	● Obesity	● Stroke
○ Bipolar disorder	● Hair morphology	○ Open personality	● Systemic lupus erythematosus
● Bilirubin	● HDL cholesterol	● Osteoarthritis	● Telomere length
● Bladder cancer	● Heart rate	○ Osteoporosis	○ Testicular germ cell tumor
● Blond or brown hair	● Height	● Otosclerosis	● Thyroid cancer
● Blood pressure	● Hemostasis parameters	● Other metabolic traits	● Tooth development
○ Blue or green eyes	● Hepatitis	● Ovarian cancer	● Total cholesterol
● BMI, waist circumference	○ Hirschsprung's disease	● Pain	○ Triglycerides
○ Bone density	○ HIV-1 control	● Pancreatic cancer	○ Type 1diabetes
● Breast cancer	● Homocysteine levels	● Panic disorder	● Type 2 diabetes
● C-reactive protein	● Idiopathic pulmonary fibrosis	● Parkinson's disease	● Ulcerative colitis
● Cardiac structure/function	● IgE levels	● Periodontitis	● Urate
● Camitine levels	● Inflammatory bowel disease	● Peripheral arterial disease	● Venous thromboembolism
● Carotenoid/tocopherol levels	● Intracranial aneurysm	○ Phosphatidylcholine levels	● Vitamin B12 1evels
○ Celiac disease	● Iris color	○ Platelet count	● Warfarin dose
● Chronic lymphocytic leukemia	● Iron status markers	○ Primary biliary cirrhosis	● Weight
○ Cleft lip/palate	● Ischemic stroke	○ PR interval	○ White cell count
● Cognitive function	○ Juvenile idiopathic arthritis	● Prostate cancer	○ YKL-40 levels
● Colorectal cancer	● Kidney stones	○ Protein levels	
● Coronary disease	● LDL cholesterol	○ Psoriasis	
● Creutzfeldt-Jakob disease	● Leprosy	● Pulmonary funcl. COPD	
● Crohn's disease	● Leptin receptor levels	● QRS interval	

Yamomoto and **Zafira Zuabi** are now the mainstream of clinical genetic research. In this section we will look at the progress of investigations into the genetics of these two diseases. *Section 13.4* will set these examples into a more general framework to address the question at the head of this chapter – should we be testing for susceptibility to common diseases?

| CASE 25 | Yamomoto family | 333 | **346** | 389 |

- Family history of dementia
- ? Alzheimer disease
- Test for ApoE4?

When Bill Yamomoto talked with the geneticist, she confirmed his physician's statement that only early onset Alzheimer disease was strongly inherited. The condition in Bill's mother and aunt was the common late-onset form. Both forms are defined by the same post-mortem brain pathology, with abundant extracellular senile plaques and intracellular neurofibrillary tangles (*Figure 13.9*), but the late-onset form is not simply inherited. Bill pressed the geneticist about ApoE4. She confirmed that there is a statistical association with late-onset Alzheimer disease, and that this was valid in Japanese as well as in people of European origin. A number of studies had shown an E4 allele frequency of 0.25–0.3 in Japanese Alzheimer disease patients, compared to 0.10 in controls. However, she advised against testing. She showed him a statement on ApoE testing issued by a working group of the American College of Medical Genetics and the American Society of Human Genetics (1995) which concluded '... at the present time it is not recommended for use in routine clinical diagnosis nor should it be used for predictive testing'.

When Bill suggested this attitude was patronizing, she asked what he would do if the result was positive. 'Ask you what I must do to avoid developing the disease' he replied. 'But there's nothing I could tell you. There is no proven way of preventing Alzheimer disease, though there are drugs that may slow the progression. The best you can do is keep your mind active – but I would say that to anybody, regardless of their circumstances. And what would you do if the result was negative?' 'Celebrate!'. 'But you would be wrong – plenty of ApoE4-negative people go on to develop Alzheimer disease. The association is only statistical. It is not predictive for an individual.' The consultation did not reassure Bill about his risk, but it did persuade him that spending money on testing would not provide the reassurance he wanted.

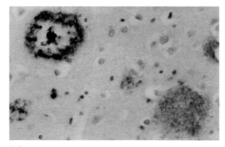
(a)

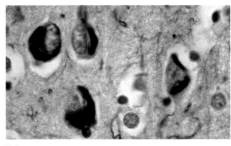
(b)

Figure 13.9 – The characteristic brain pathology of Alzheimer disease
(a) Amyloid plaques and (b) neurofibrillary tangles. Photos courtesy of Dr Simon Lovestone, Institute of Psychiatry, London.

A few percent of Alzheimer disease cases have onset before age 60. These early onset cases are often familial and often behave as mendelian dominant conditions. Those that do are amenable to standard linkage analysis and positional cloning. These approaches have identified three causative genes (*Table 13.6*).

Table 13.6 – Known causes of early onset Alzheimer disease

Gene	OMIM no.	Location	Number of recorded families	Product
APP	104760	21q21	78	Amyloid precursor protein
PSEN1	104311	14q24	362	γ-secretase subunit
PSEN2	600759	1q31	18	γ-secretase subunit

The total number of recorded families is from Bertram and Tanzi (2008). In total these causes explain only a tiny fraction of all Alzheimer disease; the great majority of cases are late-onset and non-familial.

The senile plaques in Alzheimer disease consist largely of β-amyloid protein. β-amyloid is derived from the amyloid precursor protein (APP) by proteolytic cleavage. APP is a 695 amino acid brain protein that is cleaved by the γ-secretase enzyme, producing $A\beta_{40}$ and $A\beta_{42}$ peptides. $A\beta_{42}$ is thought to be the pathogenic variant. γ-secretase is a complex of five polypeptides including the *PSEN1* and *PSEN2* gene products. The rare mendelian forms of Alzheimer disease have clearly implicated amyloid β-peptides in the pathology, although their exact role remains unclear.

Geneticists have much to offer members of families affected by early onset Alzheimer disease. They can try to identify a causative mutation in one of the known genes. If one is discovered, predictive testing can be offered, similarly to Huntington disease. A suitable protocol is described in the following chapter (*Box 14.2*). However, as Bill Yamomoto discovered, with the late-onset form we are still in the research phase and, at present, genetic services have nothing useful to offer. Family studies suggest that 60–80% of the variance in susceptibility is due to genetic differences between people, with a variety of environmental and lifestyle factors accounting for the remainder.

One risk factor was identified as early as 1993. The *APOE* gene on chromosome 19q13 encodes apolipoprotein E. Many variants of ApoE have been described (see OMIM 107741), but only three are common polymorphisms. *APOE**2, *3 and *4 are coding sequence variants producing ApoE proteins with either cysteine or arginine at positions 112 and 158 (*Table 13.7*). The gene frequencies have been studied in many populations. E4 is the ancestral allele, found in non-human primates, and it remains frequent in populations where foraging is still important. In settled agricultural populations the frequency of E4 is low.

ApoE4 is a risk factor for both coronary artery disease and late-onset Alzheimer disease among people living in Westernized environments. A large French study (Bickeboller *et al.*, 1997) found odds ratios for Alzheimer disease of 2.2

Table 13.7 – **The common apolipoprotein E variants and their gene frequencies in various populations**

	Residue 112	Residue 158	Spanish	UK	Chinese	Japanese	Native American	Khoi San
APOE*2	Cysteine	Cysteine	0.052	0.089	0.105	0.048	0.0	0.077
APOE*3	Cysteine	Arginine	0.856	0.767	0.824	0.851	0.816	0.553
APOE*4	Arginine	Arginine	0.091	0.144	0.071	0.101	0.184	0.370

Data from Corbo and Scacchi (1999).

and 11.2 for E4/E3 and E4/E4 genotypes, respectively, compared to E3/E3. E2 had an additional protective effect. Several different hypotheses have been proposed for the mechanism (see Zhong and Weisgraber, 2008). ApoE protein binds amyloid β-peptide, cholesterol, and many other molecules, with the different forms having different affinities. The E4 form enhances deposition of amyloid β-peptide. Neurons produce ApoE when stressed, and the E4 form is more subject to proteolytic cleavage, producing C-terminal fragments that may be toxic to mitochondria. Decreased mitochondrial function in neurons could lead to Alzheimer disease. *Figure 13.10* shows the multiple ways in which ApoE protein may be involved in the pathogenesis of AD.

ApoE4 is a major susceptibility factor for AD, but, as Bill Yamomoto learned, it accounts for only part of the genetic susceptibility. Attempts to identify other factors

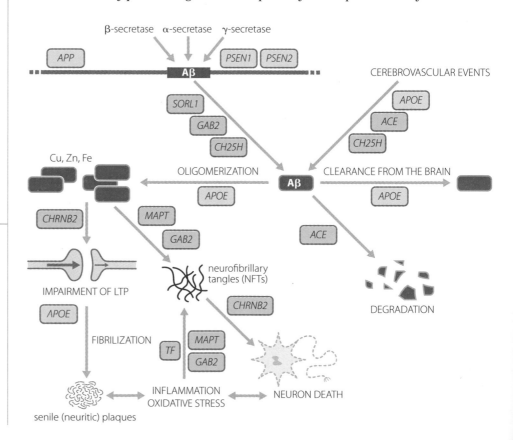

Figure 13.10 – Processes that may lead to Alzheimer disease.
Note the multiple stages where ApoE protein may be involved. The possible roles of other AD candidate genes (confirmed, green, or suggested, blue) are indicated. LTP long term potentiation. Reproduced from Bertram and Tanzi (2008) with permission from Nature Publishing Group.

have met with very limited success. Early studies used linkage analysis, mostly of affected sib pairs as described in *Section 13.2*. Using the Lander–Kruglyak criteria (*Box 13.3*), no investigation has found a *highly significant* result. Among *significant* or *suggestive* results, chromosomal regions implicated in one genome-wide trawl have seldom been replicated in others. Early association studies similarly produced conflicting results that could seldom be confirmed in replication studies. Bertram and Tanzi (2008) list and discuss ten candidate genes that have at least some support from meta-analyses of published findings. However, the new generation of large-scale genome-wide association studies, involving thousands of subjects, have definitely identified several factors (*Table 13.8*).

Table 13.8 – **Confirmed genetic susceptibility factors for late-onset Alzheimer disease**

Gene symbol	Gene name	OMIM number	Chromosomal location	Odds ratio
APOE	Apolipoprotein E	107741	19q13.2	3.57
CLU	Clusterin (Apolipoprotein J)	185430	8p21	0.85
EXOC3L2	Exocyst complex component 3-like 2	–	19q13.32	1.18
BIN1	Bridging integrator 1	601248	2q14.3	1.13
PICALM	Phosphatidyl inositol-binding clathrin assembly protein	603025	11q14	0.87

The top 5 results from www.alzgene.org/TopResults.asp [accessed 6 July 2010].

All these findings lead one to ask, what should we tell the patients? The answer is, not much. A measure of the ability of a test to identify cases is the AUC (area under the ROC curve – see *Section 13.4* for details). AUC values range from 0.5 (no predictive value) to 1.0 (complete prediction). The AUCs from two studies cited by Seshardri *et al.* (2010) were 0.826 and 0.670, respectively, based on age and sex alone. The difference between the two studies is presumably due to the younger average age and greater range of ages of cases in the first study (69 ± 9 years) compared to the second (80 ± 6 years). Incorporating the *APOE* genotype increased these figures to 0.847 and 0.702, respectively. Adding in *CLU* and *PICALM* added only 0.002 and 0.003 to the respective AUCs. In other words, knowing the *APOE* genotype adds little, and knowing the *CLU* and *PICALM* types virtually nothing, to predictions based on age and sex alone.

Several expert panels have advised against using ApoE or any other alleged risk factor for clinical purposes, most recently the European Federation of Neurological Societies in 2007. ApoE4 is neither necessary nor sufficient for Alzheimer disease. ApoE genotyping would not assist the diagnosis in a person with possible Alzheimer disease, and it would not usefully predict the likelihood of somebody developing Alzheimer disease. A British study concluded that the predictive power was too low to affect insurance underwriting, even for long-term care insurance (Warren,

1999). ApoE is quite properly tested as part of the investigation of dyslipidemias, and this raises the tricky question of whether patients should be told results that are irrelevant to their lipid problem and may be disturbing. Inevitably ApoE testing is also available over the internet. However, some research data suggest this is not a cause for moral panic. In one trial, some people in Bill Yamomoto's position welcomed APOE testing, and were not particularly disturbed when the result showed they were E4 positive.

| CASE 26 | Zuabi family | 334 | **350** | 389 |

- Woman aged 52 years, Zafira
- Overweight; sedentary lifestyle; insatiable thirst
- Type 2 diabetes
- Test son

Diabetes mellitus, defined by hyperglycemia > 7 mmol/l fasting, > 11 mmol/l non-fasting, or a glucose tolerance test, is a heterogeneous condition. In addition to many minor types, the two major types are:

- Type 1 (T1D) – a sudden onset disease in young people, the result of an autoimmune attack on the pancreatic β-cells, and not associated with obesity
- Type 2 (T2D) – normally with adult onset, associated with obesity and physical inactivity, without autoimmune features, and resulting from a combination of inadequate secretion of insulin and resistance to its effects; this is the type in Case 26

These two separate diseases both involve genetic susceptibility and environmental factors. For T2D, evidence for environmental factors comes from the alarming recent increases in prevalence, and from intervention studies showing the efficacy of weight control and exercise in reducing progression from a pre-diabetic to a full diabetic state. Evidence for genetic factors comes from family and twin studies, and from the ethnic variations in prevalence. λ_S is 3–6 and many studies have reported higher concordance in monozygotic compared to dizygotic twins. A positive family history confers an increased risk; 15–25% of first-degree relatives of T2D patients develop impaired glucose tolerance or overt diabetes. The prevalence varies greatly between different ethnic groups, even when members of the groups live intermingled in multiethnic communities.

The world faces an epidemic of T2D. In the USA, the prevalence doubled between 1990 and 2005. In 2007, 23.5 million adults in the USA (10.7% of the adult population) had T2D, costing the economy an estimated $174 billion. These figures, and similar trends from many other countries, have stimulated intensive efforts to understand the causes of T2D. *Figure 13.11a* shows the self-reinforcing pathogenic cascade that produces the hyperglycemia and increased free fatty acids of T2D, while *Figure 13.11b* shows the complicated events controlling insulin signaling.

As regards genetic causes, early linkage studies identified a mendelian subset that accounts for 1–2% of cases. Collectively called MODY (maturity onset diabetes of youth), these forms affect all ages and are not associated with obesity or inactivity. MODY can be caused by mutations in any of six or more genes, and identifying the cause is important because different forms respond well to different drugs. Apart from identifying MODY, early studies of T2D using either linkage or association were largely inconclusive. However, the new generation of large-scale genome-wide association studies has been successful in identifying many susceptibility factors (*Figure 13.12*).

(a)

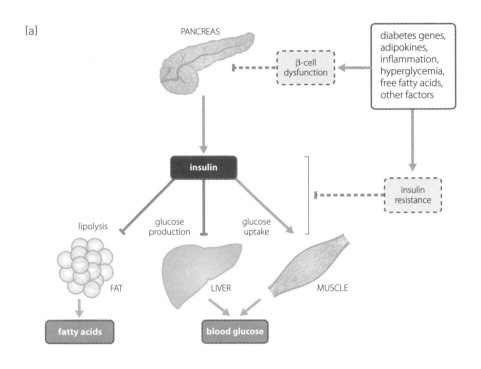

(b)

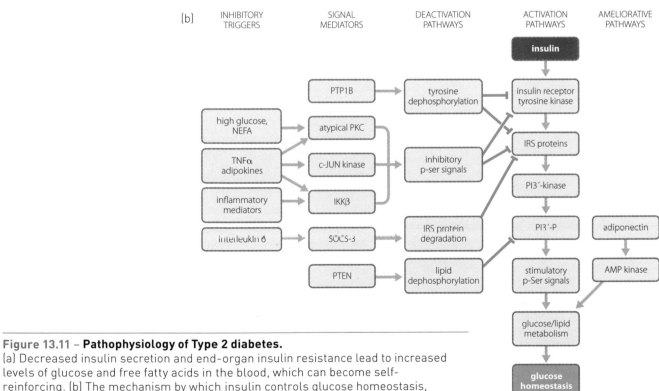

Figure 13.11 – Pathophysiology of Type 2 diabetes.
(a) Decreased insulin secretion and end-organ insulin resistance lead to increased levels of glucose and free fatty acids in the blood, which can become self-reinforcing. (b) The mechanism by which insulin controls glucose homeostasis, and factors influencing it. NEFA, non-esterified fatty acids; TNFα, tumor necrosis factor α; PTP1B, phosphotyrosine phosphatase 1B; PKC, protein kinase C; IKKβ, NFκB inhibitory unit kinase (an activator of NFκB); SOCS-3, suppressor of cytokine signaling-3; IRS, insulin receptor substrate; PI, phosphoinositol. Both figures reproduced from Stumvoll *et al.* (2005) with permission from Elsevier.

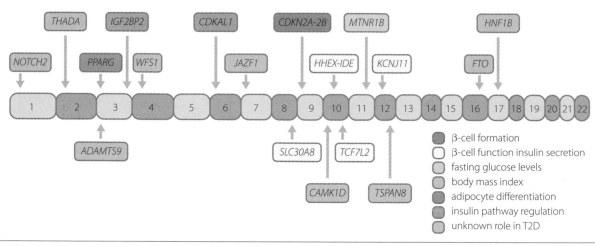

Figure 13.12 – Eighteen genetic susceptibility factors for Type 2 diabetes.
The figure shows the chromosomal locations of 18 genes in which variants have been associated with susceptibility or resistance to T2D. Their likely roles in the pathogenesis are shown by the color coding. Reproduced from Frazer *et al.* (2009), with permission from the Nature Publishing Group.

Several studies have examined the potential of all this new genetic knowledge to make a difference to diagnosis or management of T2D. At least six studies have used genotype data to try to improve the ability of routine clinical examination to predict the likelihood that somebody would develop T2D (*Table 13.9*).

The conclusion from these studies is that, as with Alzheimer disease, genotyping adds little value to predictions made using conventional clinical criteria plus family history. Taken in isolation, the genotypes are predictive of risk; when combined with clinical examination and family history they do slightly improve the prediction, but only very slightly. The study of Meigs *et al.* (2008) concluded that their 18 genotypes would result in, at most, 4% of their subjects being reclassified to a different risk category. As regards genetic advice, the Zuabi family is fairly typical. An overlapping set of problems – T2D, cardiovascular disease, coronary heart disease – cluster loosely in families. The metabolic syndrome is a clear predictor of risk, as are its individual components. While a strong family history predicts increased risk, there is little scope for specifically genetic advice: the general advice for every overweight and inactive person, regardless of family history, is to get some exercise and lose some weight. The many possible drugs are prescribed according to the physiology and not the genetics (except in MODY).

13.4. **Going deeper ...**

It has taken a long time to find reliable ways of detecting common disease susceptibility factors. The early linkage studies, mostly using affected sib pairs, were methodologically impeccable, and would have provided definitive answers if only the susceptibility factors had been stronger. The disappointing outcome of this phase of research showed that most factors were either too weak to be detected with feasible numbers of subjects, or maybe too heterogeneous. The data in *Table 13.4* showed how impossibly many sib pairs would be needed to detect modest effects by linkage. The same paper that produced those figures

Table 13.9 – **Does genotyping improve the ability to predict whether somebody will develop Type 2 diabetes?**

Clinical indicators	AUC from clinical indicators	Susceptibility loci genotyped	AUC using combined clinical and genetic data	Reference
BMI, plasma glucose level	0.68	*PPARG, CAPN10*	0.68	Lyssenko *et al.* (2005)
Age, sex, BMI	0.82	*GCK, IL6, TCF7L2*	0.82	Vaxillaire *et al.* (2008)
Age, sex, BMI	0.78	18 established loci	0.80	Lango *et al.* (2008)
Age, sex, BMI	0.66	18 established loci	0.68	van Hoek *et al.* (2008)
Age, sex, family history, medical history, physical examination, blood sample	0.90	18 established loci	0.901	Meigs *et al.* (2008)
Age, sex, BMI, family history, liver enzyme levels, smoking, measures of insulin secretion and action	0.74	16 established loci	0.75	Lyssenko et al. (2008)

The AUC statistic measures the predictive power of a test; the higher the value, the better the prediction; see *Section 13.4* for an explanation of this statistic. The 'established loci' used in the last four studies largely overlapped the 18 shown in *Figure 13.12*. BMI, body mass index.

also showed that such effects should be detectable by association studies using much more manageable sample sizes. This helped prompt a move from linkage to association studies. An additional motivation was the increased feasibility of identifying the actual causative variant. Whereas affected sib pair mapping defines shared regions of 10 Mb or more, far too large to search for sequence variants, association studies identify shared ancestral haplotype blocks only a few kb long, and readily searchable. Early work concentrated on candidate regions, defined either by previous linkage work or by the presence of a candidate gene. High-resolution SNP chips, on which 500 000 – 1 000 000 SNPs could be genotyped in a single operation, opened the way for GWAS. Nevertheless, it was necessary to decide which of the more than 10 million SNPs in the databases to test. This was where the HapMap project made its essential contribution.

Haplotype blocks and tag SNPs

As described earlier, the HapMap project showed how our genomes could be represented as a series of short haplotype blocks, typically of the order of 5 kb long. Blocks are regions where there has been very little recombination over the generations, and recombination hot-spots mark the boundaries between blocks. Typically there are 20–25 SNPs in a block. If each of 20 SNPs has two alleles, there are 2^{20} or 1 048 576 possible haplotypes. But in fact, as *Table 13.5* showed, for most such segments, only 4–6 different haplotypes are reasonably common.

This must be evidence of shared ancestral segments. It means that any particular segment in most humans is derived from only 4–6 ancestors. It does not mean we are all descended from the same 4–6 cavemen. The next chromosomal segment will also be derived from only 4–6 ancestors, but they will be different ancestors from the previous ones.

There is a small problem here, because the data from a SNP chip consist of *genotypes*; for example, a person might have G/C, A/A and A/C at three adjacent SNPs. But we want to know the *haplotypes*, and this depends on knowing whether that person's two haplotypes are GAA/CAC or GAC/CAA. This is the problem of *phase*. The best solution is to type the person's parents, and many of the HapMap samples did consist of trios of two parents and offspring. But this is an expensive option – three samples must be genotyped to define four haplotypes (once the two haplotypes in the offspring have been identified, the two non-transmitted haplotypes in the parents can also be deduced). More often, genotype data on an individual are phased using computer programs that pick out the most likely combination of haplotypes, based on existing knowledge of the frequency of the various haplotypes in that population.

Within a haplotype block, markers show *linkage disequilibrium* (LD) – that is, particular alleles of different SNPs in the block tend to go together. Knowing which allele is present at one SNP allows a prediction (an 'imputation') of the alleles at other SNPs in the block. It is not necessary to type every SNP in a block to tell which of the 4–6 alternatives a person has. Genotyping two or three carefully chosen SNPs ('tag SNPs') will usually suffice (*Figure 13.13*). There are

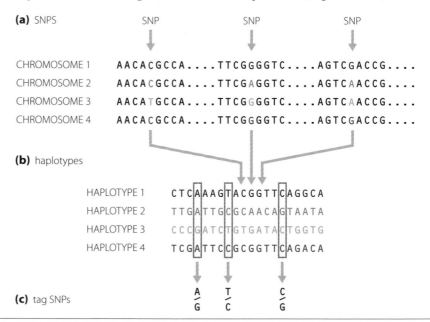

Figure 13.13 – Tag SNPs identify haplotype blocks.
(a) The same haplotype block in four different people. Scattered across the block are 20 SNPs. Three of them are shown. (b) A summary of genotypes at all 20 SNPs, omitting the invariant sequences between SNPs. (c) Typing just three tag SNPs serves to identify which of the four alternative haplotypes a person carries. Reproduced from The International HapMap Consortium (2003) with permission from Nature Publishing Group.

some limitations. Blocks are not uniform regions of perfect LD, separated from adjacent blocks by complete absence of LD. The structure is much more complex and subtle. LD is a quantitative measure that can have any value from 0 (no LD) to 1 (alleles at the two loci are always perfectly correlated), and blocks must be defined statistically as regions of enhanced LD. Some chromosome regions show strong uniform blocks, but many are much less clear cut, and in some regions there is no clear block structure (see *Table 13.5*). Thus tag SNPs do not give a perfect representation of all the variation across a chromosomal segment, but they do identify most of the variation most of the time.

We can begin to imagine describing somebody's genome by using tag SNPs to compile a list of which of the 4–6 alternative blocks is present at each chromosomal location. The relevance of this to mapping susceptibility factors is that if we compiled such a list from each of a number of people affected with our favorite disease, we might quite easily be able to spot which ancestral blocks they shared. Shared blocks would be strong candidates for containing ancient common variants that conferred susceptibility to the disease. In reality, the general procedure in GWAS is not to try in the first place to phase the raw data or identify haplotype blocks. Instead, the genotypes are checked directly for any association between an allele of a tag SNP and the disease in question. If a statistically significant association is found and confirmed in independent datasets, then the relevant haplotype block can be examined in more detail.

Avoiding false positives in a genome-wide association study

When a test looks for association with any of 500 000 SNPs, an extremely stringent P value must be used to identify true associations. Purely by random chance we would expect 25 000 SNPs (5% of the total) to each show nominally significant results with a raw P value of 0.05. Typically, GWAS use a threshold P value of 5×10^{-8}. This in turn means large samples are needed. It is also important to match cases and controls very carefully, as slight inadvertent differences between the two groups can easily introduce spurious associations. Is it sufficient to use people from the same ethnic group and country as controls, or should they be from the same locality? Many populations do exhibit fine-scale structure, as expected because local people are more likely to be part of the same extended family. Mismatching is suspected if there are many differences between allele frequencies in cases and controls.

One solution to the matching problem is to use internal controls. The Transmission Disequilibrium Test (TDT) uses the non-transmitted chromosomes of the parents as controls. The study sample consists of cases and their two parents. For testing association with a particular allele of a marker, only parents who are heterozygous for that allele are considered. It is irrelevant whether or not the parent is affected. The test simply compares how often the heterozygous parent transmitted the allele in question, rather than his other allele, to the affected case (*Figure 13.14*). Significance is assessed using a simple χ^2 test. GWAS usually rely on a case–control design – experience suggests that matching for ethnicity and country of origin is generally sufficient to avoid spurious results. However, the TDT can be useful in follow-up studies of candidate SNPs, at least for early-onset diseases where parents are readily available.

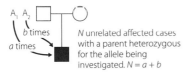

N unrelated affected cases with a parent heterozygous for the allele being investigated. $N = a + b$

if allele A_1 is associated with susceptibility we would expect A_1 to be transmitted to the affected person more often than A_2

test statistic: $(a–b)^2/(a+b)$

Figure 13.14 – The Transmission Disequilibrium Test.
The test statistic has a χ^2 distribution.

Making clinical use of GWAS data

Having identified a susceptibility factor, we might wish to use it as a test to help define the genetic susceptibility of a person for the relevant disease. Various measures of test performance were described in *Box 11.1*. As discussed in *Section 11.3*, there is usually a trade-off between sensitivity and specificity. The ability of a test to discriminate between people who will and will not develop the disease depends on the details of that trade-off. It is usefully summarized in the quaintly named receiver operating characteristic (ROC) curve (*Figure 13.15*). The important feature is the area under the curve (AUC, sometimes called the c-statistic). This can be seen as measuring the extent to which the test will correctly categorize a pair of people, one of whom will, and the other of whom will not develop the disease. An AUC of 0.5 (the straight diagonal line in the figure) implies a purely random performance, no better than tossing a coin. An AUC of 1.0 implies a perfect test. This statistic was used in *Section 13.3* to describe the performance of various tests predicting susceptibility to Alzheimer disease and T2D. We saw that genotyping for all known susceptibility factors added very little to predictions based purely on clinical examination and family history. The same is true for most other complex diseases.

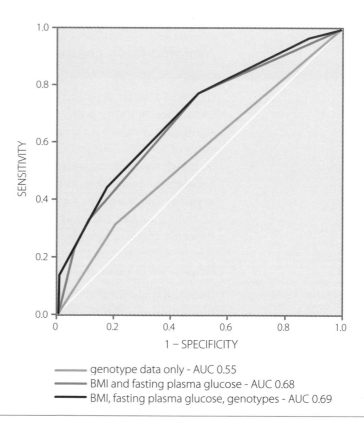

genotype data only - AUC 0.55
BMI and fasting plasma glucose - AUC 0.68
BMI, fasting plasma glucose, genotypes - AUC 0.69

Figure 13.15 – An ROC curve for predictions of Type 2 diabetes.
Sensitivity (true positive rate) is plotted against 1–specificity (false positive rate). The ability of a test to predict disease, in this case T2D, is measured by the AUC. The greater the AUC, the better a test is. Modified from Janssens and Khoury (2010) with permission from Wolters Kluwer Health.

Why have GWAS told us so little that is clinically useful?

The specific examples of Alzheimer disease and T2D are typical of the great majority of complex diseases. GWAS have been technically very successful; they have identified hundreds of confirmed susceptibility factors, but their low clinical utility has been a major disappointment.

Association studies look for shared ancestral variants. They depend on the Common Disease – Common Variant hypothesis – the idea that most common disease susceptibility factors are ancient common variants. But any variant that has survived in a population for many generations cannot be highly pathogenic (exceptions might be variants that are only pathogenic in combination with some aspect of modern Western lifestyles, such as smoking or abundant high-fat food; or variants that matter only in post-reproductive life; or perhaps variants that offer some compensating advantage). Thus it is not surprising that most of the factors identified in GWAS have odds ratios well below 1.5. However, this does leave a major problem of 'missing heritability'. For most complex diseases, all the known genetic susceptibility factors, taken together, explain very little of the overall heritability, as estimated from family or twin studies. Several possible explanations have been advanced.

Most susceptibility factors are copy number variants, not SNPs – as described in *Section 2.4*, there are hundreds of copy number variants in normal genomes, ranging from a few hundred base pairs to megabases in size. Common copy number variants account for more of the nucleotide differences between two normal people than do SNPs. They are fewer in number than SNPs, but larger in size. Rare copy number variants are the cause of many syndromes (see Case 13, Meinhardt family and *Disease box 13*). Many of the common variants include genes, and it seems plausible that they might influence disease susceptibility. There arc indeed examples of common copy number variations that have phenotypic effects. However, modern SNP chips assay for copy number variants as well as SNPs, and scoring for these has not identified the missing heritability.

Most complex diseases are truly polygenic – GWAS of 1000 or so cases and controls are well powered to detect susceptibility factors giving an odds ratio of 1.5 or more. We can assume that the great majority of all such factors have been identified for all the well-studied diseases. However, there is much less power to detect weaker risk factors. Those that have been detected have been the result of a fortunate combination of genotypes in the study subjects. Many other factors with similar low odds ratios will have escaped detection. On this view, the missing heritability lies in the combined effect of hundreds of weak susceptibility factors. Some statistical evidence supports the existence of many weak factors, and some researchers would like to conduct studies with 100 000 cases and controls to find them. Others question the value of knowing about them.

Most currently identified factors are not the actual susceptibility factor – GWAS use tagging SNPs to identify ancestral chromosome segments. Somewhere on the segment there should be the real causative variant, but it is not generally the SNP that initially identified the segment. There may not be a perfect correlation between presence of that SNP and presence of the causal variant. Some segments may carry the SNP but not the causal variant, and *vice versa*. The true causal variant may therefore show a stronger association with the disease than the SNP did. Identifying the actual causative variants has been a big challenge in complex disease research, requiring time-consuming functional studies of candidate variants. Only a few have so far been identified. Some have argued that these experiments are looking in the wrong place, and that the true causative variants may be anything up to a megabase away (see Cirulli and Goldstein, 2010). Whether or not that is true, we will have a much clearer picture of the extent of true missing heritability once we can move from associated SNPs to causal variants.

Most susceptibility is due to rare variants with large effects – most GWAS can only detect effects of alleles with a frequency of at least 5%. The Common Disease – Common Variant hypothesis holds that most susceptibility is due to combinations of such common alleles. But this may be wrong. For most mendelian diseases there is extensive allelic heterogeneity. Hundreds of different mutations can be found among individuals with most mendelian diseases, at least those that are the result of loss of function of a gene. Similarly, genome sequencing in tumors is revealing an immense diversity of individually rare variants. Why should complex diseases be different? On this view, the missing heritability will be found by abandoning association studies, and sequencing whole genomes, or selected genes, in large panels of cases and controls. A variety of mutations will be found, but all affecting certain pathways, and they may have much higher odds ratios than the factors identified through GWAS. This theory is currently being tested by large-scale projects using next-generation sequencing. Cirulli and Goldstein (2010) consider some of the possibilities.

Most susceptibility is due to gene–gene and gene–environment interactions – everyday disasters are usually the result of unlucky combinations of individually innocuous factors. One person driving too fast round a corner meets somebody else doing the same, and it is raining and the road is slippery, and one driver is trying to tune his radio and not paying as much attention to the road as he should. Maybe medical disasters are the same – each individual case is the result of a specific one-off combination of variants, none of which in isolation would have caused disease. Suppose a particular combination of two SNP alleles conferred a strong susceptibility to a disease, but neither individually has any effect. SNP A is present in 50% of people, SNP B in 2%. If somebody is affected and has both variants, his sib has a 1 in 4 chance of having the same combination, and the heritability, as assessed by λ_s will be high. In the general population, SNP A will be associated with disease risk, but only weakly. Comprehensive testing, even for two-way interactions, in the huge datasets generated by the latest GWAS requires huge computer resources; testing for more complex, and maybe more realistic, interactions is even harder, except for limited sets of candidate loci. Limited studies to date have not uncovered evidence of important interactions, but the possibility must remain that they exist.

So should we be testing for susceptibility to common diseases?

An answer to the question at the head of this chapter has been given in an interesting and important paper (Ashley *et al.*, 2010). Clinicians examined a middle-aged American man, checked his family history and worked out his risks for a whole range of conditions based on their findings. A large team then sequenced the man's entire genome and used an impressive array of bioinformatic tools to see how far his risk for each disease had changed in the light of his genome sequence. The most striking conclusion from all this technical virtuosity is how little clinically useful information emerged. His risk for a few diseases had gone up, for a few it had gone down, but the only substantial risk was for heart disease because of his family history. Somewhat more interesting results came from an analysis of pharmacogenetic variants, but again nothing revolutionary.

So in mid-2010 the answer to our question is clearly 'no'. Private companies currently offer testing direct to consumers over the internet. As long as their advertising is honest and does not claim clinical utility for their tests, people should be free to buy tests to satisfy their curiosity, but this is essentially a recreational pursuit. This could change. The risk estimates in the paper of Ashley *et al.* (2010) were based on SNPs identified by GWAS. As we have seen, these are mostly very weak indicators of risk. The game could change if new approaches identify the missing heritability. Equally, genome-wide studies of epigenetics might provide stronger predictions, based on patterns of DNA methylation and histone modifications that are fixed in an individual but probably not inherited from the parents (see *Chapter 7*). We are only at the beginning of understanding the genetic architecture of common complex diseases. Thus it would be premature in the present state of knowledge to devote public resources to testing healthy people for susceptibility to common diseases. Not only can we not identify most of the susceptibility, but even if we do know a significant factor, such as ApoE in Alzheimer disease, we may not be able to do anything about it. The vision of moving from a diagnose-and-treat to a predict-and-prevent model of healthcare remains distant. A workshop of the NIH and Centers for Disease Control (Khoury *et al.*, 2009) has set out some of the steps that would be needed to start bridging the gap. Today's medical students will find out how soon the vision will become reality.

DISEASE BOX 13

Autism

Since the first description of early infantile autism in the 1940s the range of disorders included under the heading of 'autistic spectrum disorders' has widened. Around 1 in 150 children in the USA have a diagnosis of autistic spectrum disorder, around 1 child in 1000 has a severe form. By definition, children with autism must manifest delays in 'social interaction, language as used in social communication, or symbolic or imaginative play' with 'onset prior to age 3 years', according to the Diagnostic and Statistical Manual of Mental Disorders. Children with classic autism, which can sometimes present with regressive features around 18 months of age, generally have impairment of:

- social interaction, including poor eye contact, failure to develop age-appropriate peer relationships and to seek to share activities
- communication development, including delay or total lack of spoken language or use of repetitive language and lack of imaginative or imitative play
- behavior manifested by inflexibility of routines, obsessions and repetitive and stereotypical patterns of activity

Whilst children with classic autism usually require special educational provision and remain dependent for all their lives, those individuals at the milder end of the spectrum are often diagnosed later in childhood or adult life and live relatively normal lives.

Autism illustrates many of the problems that beset genetic analysis of psychiatric and behavioral characters. While definitions such as that quoted above ensure that clinicians mean the same thing when they use the word 'autism', such definitions are essentially arbitrary and do not necessarily describe a biological entity. Classic autism shades through Asperger syndrome into 'normal' personality variants without any natural boundaries (see *Box figure 13.2*). The sex ratio for classic autism in multiple studies has been around 4M:1F – but we all accept that 'normal' boys are more likely than girls to spend hours obsessively playing solitary computer games and to be socially inept. There are numerous cytogenetic and monogenic disorders where autism or autistic features are frequent; these include Rett syndrome, Fragile X syndrome and duplications of chromosome 15q11–13. A few percent of children whose primary diagnosis is autism turn out to have one or other of these conditions, but the great majority do not. Evidently autism is a pattern of behavior that can have many different causes.

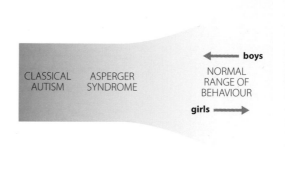

Box figure 13.2 – Autistic spectrum disorders merge into normal behavior with no natural boundaries.

No environmental factors have been identified as major causes of autism. Early reports of abnormal parenting, with 'refrigerator mothers' were not substantiated by more careful studies, and despite the publicity it has received, no serious study has implicated the MMR (measles – mumps – rubella) or any other vaccine. By contrast, many observations point to important genetic determinants. The sibling recurrence risk (after the birth of a child with classic autism) is 6–8%, so that λ_s is 20–50 (depending on definitions). This is among the highest sibling risks for a common complex disease (compare with *Table 13.2*). For second degree relatives the risk is sharply lower at around 0.18%. Concordance is much higher among monozygotic than dizygotic twins (70–82% versus 0–10%, depending on the criteria). The fall-off between MZ and DZ twins, and between first and second degree relatives, is much sharper than in most complex diseases. This might be for either of two reasons:

- genetic susceptibility might depend on specific combinations of an unusually large number of genes
- susceptibility might be largely due to new mutations; these might be conventional sequence changes, copy number variants or epimutations.

It would be nice to know which of these explanations is correct, because they have diametrically opposite implications for genetic research into autism. The first explanation would mean that studies need to be done on an extremely large (and expensive) scale to detect associations. The second implies that the association approach will never work; the best approach would be sequencing (including bisulfite sequencing) of candidate genes in a panel of affected individuals.

Genetic investigation has followed the usual routes. Twelve whole genome linkage scans were reported between 1998 and 2004. Using the Lander–Kruglyak criteria (*Box 13.2*) there were no highly significant lod scores, and just one significant score, 3.74 for chromosome 2q. Three GWAS were reported in 2009. A number of candidate genes have been more or less convincingly identified. Several have roles in synaptic function, or in establishing connectivity between different brain regions. The Autdb database (www.mindspec.org/autdb.html) has a comprehensive list of candidate genes, and Abrahams and Geschwind (2009) provide a review and lists of loci. Mutation screens suggest that the causes of autism are very heterogeneous: each gene is mutated in only a tiny proportion of all cases tested. A promising development has been the identification of copy number variants in 7–10%

of patients with autism. Interestingly, the same variants are often associated with several different neuropsychiatric problems, including autism, schizophrenia and mental retardation. Deletions at 1q21.1, 15q11–13, 16p11 and 16p12, and duplication at 22q11–13 have been repeatedly observed. In some cases the variant is also present in an apparently normal parent. The affected patients often have additional copy number variants or mutations. A picture is emerging in which combinations of mutations or copy number variants cause a neurodevelopmental vulnerability that may manifest as different conditions, perhaps depending on the particular combination (Girirajan *et al.*, 2010).

Research into psychiatric and behavioral phenotypes involves all the same problems as research into any complex disease, but with the added difficulty that diagnostic labels are arbitrary. Autism is typical: the word describes a type of behavior that may have all sorts of different causes in different individual cases. Researchers try to define 'endophenotypes' to target more homogeneous groups – that is, characters that are part of the overall phenotype but that may lie closer to the underlying gene action. The choice of possible endophenotypes is wide, making confirmation studies and meta-analysis more difficult. In the meanwhile it is important in individual cases to investigate the possibility of one of the known monogenic or cytogenetic causes, to draw a detailed family pedigree recording cases of autistic spectrum disorders, and to give recurrence risks based on empiric data.

For information on autism see www.nimh.nih.gov/publicat/autism.cfm. For up-to-date information on GWAS see the online Catalog of Published Genome-Wide Association Studies (Hindorff *et al.*; www.genome.gov/gwastudies). Websites of the UK and US support groups are www.nas.org.uk/ and www.autism-society.org.

DISEASE BOX 13 – continued

13.5. **References**

Abrahams BS and Geschwind DH (2009) Advances in autism genetics: on the threshold of a new neurobiology. *Nat. Rev. Genet.* **9**: 341–355.

American College of Medical Genetics / American Society of Human Genetics Working Group on APOE and Alzheimer disease (1995) Statement on use of apolipoprotein E testing for Alzheimer disease. *JAMA*, **274**: 1627–1629.

Ashley EA, Butte TJ, Wheeler MT, *et al.* (2010) Clinical assessment incorporating a personal genome. *Lancet*, **375**: 1525–1535.

Bertram L and Tanzi RE (2008) Thirty years of Alzheimer disease genetics: the implications of systematic meta-analyses. *Nat. Rev. Neurosci.* **9**: 768–778.

Bickeboller H, Campion D, Brice A, *et al.* (1997) Apolipoprotein E and Alzheimer disease: genotype-specific risks by age and sex. *Am. J. Hum. Genet.* **60**: 439–446.

Cirulli ET and Goldstein DB (2010) Uncovering the roles of rare variants in common disease through whole-genome sequencing. *Nat. Rev. Genet.* **11**: 415–425.

Eckel RH, Grundy SM and Zimmet PZ (2005) The metabolic syndrome. *Lancet*, **365**: 1415–1428.

Frazer KA, Murray SS, Schork NJ and Topol EJ (2009) Human genetic variation and its contribution to complex traits. *Nat. Rev. Genet.* **10**: 241–251.

Girirajan S, Rosenfeld JA, Cooper GM, *et al.* (2010) A recurrent 16p12.1 microdeletion supports a two-hit model for severe developmental delay. *Nat. Genet.* **42**: 203–209.

Hindorff LA, Junkins HA, Hall PN, Mehta JP and Manolio TA. A Catalog of Published Genome-Wide Association Studies. Available at: www.genome.gov/gwastudies.

Janssens ACJW and van Duijn CM (2008) Genome-based prediction of common diseases: advances and prospects. *Hum. Molec. Genet.* **17**: R166–R173.

Janssens ACJW and Khoury MJ (2010) Assessment of improved prediction beyond traditional risk factors: when does a difference make a difference? *Circ. Cardiovasc. Genet.* **3**: 3–5.

Khoury MJ, McBride CM, Schully SD, *et al.* (2009) The scientific foundation for personal genomics: recommendations from a National Institutes of Health – Centers for Disease Control and Prevention multidisciplinary workshop. *Genet. Med.* **11**: 559–567.

Lander E and Kruglyak L (1995) Genetic dissection of complex traits: guidelines for interpreting and reporting linkage results. *Nat. Genet.* **11**: 241–247.

Lango H, UK Type 2 Diabetes Consortium, Palmer CN, *et al.*(2008) Assessing the combined impact of 18 common genetic variants of modest effect sizes on type 2 diabetes risk. *Diabetes,* **57**: 3129–3135.

Lyssenko V, Almgren P, Anevski D, *et al.* (2005) Genetic prediction of future type 2 diabetes. *PLOS Med.* **2**: e345.

Lyssenko V, Jonsson A, Almgren P, *et al.* (2008) Clinical risk factors, DNA variants and the development of Type 2 diabetes. *New Engl. J. Med.* **359**: 2220–2232.

Meigs JB, Shrader P, Sullivan LM, *et al.* (2008) Genotype score in addition to common risk factors for prediction of Type 2 diabetes. *New Engl. J. Med.* **359**: 2208–2219.

Risch N and Merikangas K (1996) The future of genetic studies of complex human diseases. *Science,* **273**: 1516–1517.

Seshardri S, Fitzpatrick AL, Ikram MA, *et al.* (2010) Genome-wide analysis of genetic loci associated with Alzheimer disease. *JAMA,* **303**: 1832–1840.

Stumvoll M, Goldstein BJ and van Haeften TW (2005) Type 2 diabetes: principles of pathogenesis and therapy. *Lancet,* **365**: 1333–1346.

The International HapMap Consortium (2005) A haplotype map of the human genome. *Nature,* **437**: 1299–1320.

van Hoek M, Dehgan A, Witteman JCM, *et al.* (2008) Predicting type 2 diabetes based on polymorphisms from genome-wide association studies: a population-based study. *Diabetes,* **57**: 3122–3128.

Vaxillaire M, Veslot J, Dina C, *et al.* (2008) Impact of common type 2 diabetes risk polymorphisms in the DESIR prospective study. *Diabetes,* **57**: 244–254.

Warren V (1999) *Report of Work Group on Genetic Tests and Future Need for Long-term Care in the UK*. Continuing Care Conference, London.

Zhong N and Weisgraber KH (2008) Understanding the association of Apolipoprotein E4 with Alzheimer disease: clues from its structure. *J. Biol. Chem.* 284: 6027–6031.

Useful websites

The Alzheimer Research Forum provides an authoritative and up-to-date source of much information, including, in the Top Results page, a league table of genetic susceptibility factors identified by meta-analysis of published findings: www.alzgene.org

13.6. **Self-assessment questions**

(1) Which of the following would provide the strongest evidence for involvement of genetic factors in susceptibility to heart attacks?
(a) A raised incidence of heart attacks among sibs of index cases.
(b) Increased concordance of like-sex compared to opposite-sex twin pairs.
(c) For index cases who were adopted, an increased incidence among the biological, but not the adoptive, relatives.
(d) The observation that children tend to resemble their parents in healthy or unhealthy eating habits.

(2) Two unrelated women each suffer from a complex disease where family, twin and adoption data suggest that genetic susceptibility is important. The disease is twice as common in men as in women. Anne is the only affected person in her family; Betty's brother and son are also affected. For each of the following four comparisons, decide whether the risk is:
(a) higher
(b) lower
(c) the same
(d) impossible to predict from these data

(1) The risk of Anne's or Betty's next child being affected, compared to the risk to the offspring of an affected man.
(2) The risk of a son of Anne being affected, compared to the risk to a daughter of hers.
(3) The risk of a son of Betty being affected, compared to the risk to a daughter of hers.
(4) The risk Anne's next baby will be affected compared to the risk to Betty's next baby.

(3) A mutation arises on a chromosome bearing a particular haplotype of markers. What would be the half-life (in generations) of the association between the mutations and a marker located, (a) 1 cM and (b) 5 cM away?

(4) In the 1950s the statistician Ronald Fisher argued that the known association between smoking and lung cancer did not mean that smoking

caused lung cancer. He suggested that incipient lung cancer causes an irritation in the lungs that drives people to smoke; or alternatively that people with a certain nervous constitution have a tendency both to develop lung cancer and, independently, to take up smoking. How would you prove him wrong?

(5) Locus A has three alleles, A*1, A*2 and A*3 with gene frequencies 0.5, 0.4 and 0.1, respectively. The linked locus B has three alleles B*1, B*2 and B*3 with gene frequencies 0.6, 0.3 and 0.1 respectively. Which of the following would be evidence of linkage disequilibrium?
(a) The frequency of the haplotype A*1, B*1 is 0.30.
(b) The frequency of the haplotype A*2, B*2 is 0.14.
(c) The frequency of the haplotype A*3, B*3 is 0.03.
(d) The frequency of the haplotype A*3, B*2 is 0.01.

(6) Which of the following is evidence for linkage disequilibrium between cystic fibrosis and the linked *KM19* DNA polymorphism?
(a) In a comparison of ten populations, the one with the highest prevalence of CF also had the highest frequency of *KM19* allele 2.
(b) *KM19* allele 2 is found on 91% of chromosome 7s carrying CF but only 25% of those not carrying CF.
(c) The *CFTR* and *KM19* loci both map to chromosome 7q31.2.
(d) In family studies, the *CFTR* and *KM19* loci show close linkage.

(7) In a bean-bag containing a very large number of black beans, one bean in 100 is red. Eyes shut, you put in your hand and take out a bean. If you are given ten tries, what is the chance you will pick out at least one red bean? Now apply this argument to a search for susceptibility genes. You test 1000 markers, each with 4 alleles, for association with a disease you are studying. What P value for an association will be significant at the 5% level? Would the answer be the same if instead of testing for association, you tested 1000 markers distributed across the genome for linkage?

(8) One million SNPs are tested in a panel of 500 affected people and 500 controls. SNP 629 380 has two alleles that are present at frequencies of 50% each in the controls. What is the threshold number of affected people who must have SNP allele 1 for this to show significant association with the disease?

(9) At a disease susceptibility locus the relative risk of disease for genotypes 1–1, 2–1 and 2–2 is 4:2:1. Calculate the expected proportion of affected sib pairs who are both 1–1, both 2–1 or one each 1–1 and 2–1 if the parents are:
(a) 1–1 × 2–2
(b) 1–1 × 2–1

CHAPTER 14 | What services are available for families with genetic disorders?

Learning points for this chapter

After working through this chapter you should be able to:

- Understand how genetic services are organized and what clinical geneticists and counselors do
- Describe the value of diagnosis and counseling for patients and parents
- Describe the common pediatric indications for referral to a genetic clinic
- Describe the process of syndrome diagnosis
- Describe the common adult indications for referral to a genetic clinic
- Give examples of problems with puberty or reproduction that may be appropriate for genetic referral and investigations
- Give examples of common teratogens and the problems they cause
- Describe the main methods of prenatal diagnosis, their uses and risks
- Describe the approaches that are being made to management and treatment of genetic diseases

14.1. Case studies

There are no new cases for this chapter, which will instead draw on all the previous cases used throughout the book

14.2. Science toolkit

The provision of genetic services varies considerably but almost all countries with well-developed healthcare systems now have specific provision for individuals and families with, or at risk of, genetic disorders. Such services are usually provided by specialists in genetic medicine (or other specialists with an interest in genetic disorders), often in conjunction with trained genetic counselors or nurses, and supported by genetic laboratories.

Genetic medicine can be distinguished from most other specialties in that it provides services to patients of all ages affected with disorders of any body system, and their families. Clinical geneticists offer diagnosis and counseling to people affected with disorders that may have a genetic cause **and** to apparently healthy, but at-risk, individuals. They have specialist knowledge of rare disorders including natural history and complications. They can offer screening, monitoring, prevention of complications (anticipatory care) and therapies, or can advise on who can undertake this care. They are a major source of information to families and support groups, and to other professionals in health and social care and in education. Research and development of new services are an integral part of this fast-moving specialty.

Common reasons for referral to a genetic clinic are given in *Box 14.1*. Typically when a patient or family is referred to a genetic medicine department by a primary care physician or another specialist, they are seen in an outpatient clinic although some inpatients are seen for urgent consultations, particularly when there are pregnancy complications or after the birth of a baby with abnormalities. Prior to the consultation, contact is often made with the family to obtain details of previous medical investigations, to record the family history and to get copies of relevant notes. Textbooks still have a place as important information resources to consult before a clinic, especially when the patient is known to have a rare disorder, and excellent books are listed in *Section 14.5*.

A consultation starts with the construction of a pedigree (see *Chapter 1*), followed by the taking of a detailed history of the medical condition in the affected person(s),

---

Common reasons for referral to a genetic clinic

Common pediatric indications for referral

- Abnormalities of growth: overgrowth and short stature (including skeletal dysplasias)
- Neurodevelopmental problems +/– seizures
- Isolated learning disability
- Multiple malformations +/– learning disability
- Single malformation, e.g. cleft lip/palate, congenital heart defect, renal anomaly
- Family history of Duchenne muscular dystrophy, cystic fibrosis, sickle cell disease
- Disorders identified through screening such as inborn errors of metabolism
- Sensory abnormalities, especially of vision and hearing
- Inherited skin disorders

Common adult indications for referral

- Family history of cancer, especially breast, ovary and bowel
- Family history of a cancer-predisposing syndrome such as neurofibromatosis type 1 or type 2, or von Hippel-Lindau syndrome
- To investigate the possibility of Marfan syndrome
- Family history of cardiomyopathy or cardiac rhythm disorder
- Family history of neurodegenerative disorders such as Huntington disease
- Family history of later onset neurological or neuromuscular diseases such as myotonic dystrophy or inherited ataxias
- Family history of monogenic vision or hearing disease such as retinitis pigmentosa (OMIM 312600, 268000, etc.) or inherited late onset deafness
- Family history of other monogenic disorders such as adult polycystic kidney disease (OMIM 173600) or familial hypercholesterolemia
- Reproductive genetic issues

and then a physical examination. In individuals with dysmorphic conditions, detailed measurements are taken to verify clinical impressions, e.g. wide-spaced eyes, short fingers and low-set ears, and compared against appropriate centile charts. Photographs may be taken for record purposes; it is often difficult to describe subtle facial or other body differences in words. Investigations may then be ordered. It is important to inform patients about any implications that the results of tests may have for them and for other relatives, and to reassure them that if a DNA sample is stored that it will not be used for any purpose other than diagnosis, unless further consent is sought. It may be possible at the first appointment to make a diagnosis on clinical grounds, or a follow-up appointment may be needed after results of investigations have been received. The clinical geneticist will usually write a summary letter for the patient after the consultation, with copies to the referring doctor and other specialists. If no diagnosis is made, particularly in children with a dysmorphic disorder, a review appointment may be arranged for a year or two later when new conditions may have been delineated or diagnostic technology has improved. This was the case for the Meinhardt family (Case 13) in *Chapter 4* where SNP arrays eventually revealed the cause of Madelena's problems.

The importance of a diagnosis

As the cases in the text illustrate, family history, clinical observations, and examination and investigations are the first steps in establishing a diagnosis. However, clinical geneticists also depend heavily on access to databases and to the medical and scientific literature, particularly for diagnosis of very rare disorders and for information about rare features and complications. They need to find out where research is taking place and whether new treatments are being developed.

Patients and their families whose conditions are undiagnosed can feel isolated and there are numerous studies which have described the importance of a diagnosis both for patients and their families and also for clinicians and others involved in their care. Some of the benefits of making a precise diagnosis in a baby with birth defects include:

- providing accurate information about the condition (its natural history and its prognosis) to parents and professionals involved in the care of the baby
- influencing the management of the baby, e.g. it may direct further investigations or screening for complications
- facilitating accurate genetic counseling, especially with regard to recurrence risk and possibilities for prenatal diagnosis
- making it easier for families to access support from other sources, e.g. lay support groups, social services (benefits), the education system
- helping research into normal and abnormal morphogenesis.

Risk assessment and genetic counseling

Genetic counseling involves much more than giving out recurrence risks – but an indispensable start is to get the recurrence risks right. Those giving risks need to have enough understanding of the science and the methods for risk calculation to be able to justify a quoted figure, even if they did not calculate it themselves.

- *For mendelian conditions* the increasing availability and success of mutation testing have made this part of counseling much easier over the past decade. Where risks are based just on the pedigree, the main difficulties come with serious dominant and X-linked conditions where new mutations are frequent. In these cases Bayesian methods are important tools (see *Box 14.2*). Counselors (including clinicians offering counseling) need to have enough understanding of Bayesian methods to be able to follow and justify a calculation, whether or not they themselves normally do the calculations.
- *For chromosomal conditions* such as trisomies, recurrence risks are empiric risks. Where a parent carries a balanced abnormality (as with Ellen Elliott in Case 5) cytogenetic colleagues should be consulted about the risks of the various unbalanced outcomes. Although each case is a one-off, cytogeneticists can give guidance based on the geometry of meiotic pairing, for example in the tetravalent in a carrier of a reciprocal translocation.
- *For complex diseases* risks are empiric. The most important point is to use data that are up to date (risks change with changing incidences) and relate to the appropriate ethnic group.

Genetic counseling is essentially an information-giving and communication process. The widely accepted definition of genetic counseling (American Society of Human Genetics, 1975) states that genetic counseling is:

"a communication process which deals with human problems associated with the occurrence, or the risk of occurrence, of a genetic disorder in a family. This process involves an attempt by one or more appropriately trained persons to help the individual or family to:

(1) comprehend the medical facts, including the diagnosis, probable course of the disorder, and the available management;
(2) appreciate the way heredity contributes to the disorder, and the risk of recurrence in specified relatives;
(3) understand the alternatives for dealing with the risk of recurrence;
(4) choose the course of action which seems to them appropriate in view of their risk, their family goals and their ethical and religious standards, and to act in accordance with that decision; and
(5) make the best possible adjustment to the disorder in an affected family member and/or the risk of recurrence of that disorder."

Reproductive genetics

Many genetic centers were founded to offer services to prospective parents wishing to know their risks of having a child affected with a genetic disorder and because of emerging techniques for prenatal diagnosis. This is still the case for many centers, but for others much of the clinical work is carried out in obstetric departments, with samples being sent directly to genetic laboratories, and only

BOX 14.2

An introduction to Bayesian calculations in genetics

This method of combining probabilities was invented in the 18th century by the Reverend Thomas Bayes. It has turned out to be very useful for calculating genetic risks. It starts with a **prior probability** – how likely is a hypothesis in the first place? It then allows you to bring in relevant evidence supporting or opposing the hypothesis (conditional likelihoods) and to combine these to obtain an overall or posterior probability. To apply this method:

(1) Set out each possible mutually exclusive hypothesis that you are testing. Cover all possibilities, so that one or other of your alternatives must be true. Usually there are just two alternatives – individual X either is or is not a carrier of this disease – but sometimes there are more (you might want to calculate the probabilities that X is aa, Aa or AA).

(2) Assign a prior probability to each. In genetics these are usually the mendelian 1 in 2, 1 in 4, etc. probabilities. They must add up to 1.

(3) Considering your first additional piece of evidence, for each alternative outcome in turn, write down the likelihood of having made that observation *if that alternative were the true one*. These are the conditional likelihoods. They do not necessarily add up to 1.

(4) If there are other relevant observations that are completely independent of the first one, repeat step 3 for each such observation.

(5) When the list is complete, multiply the numbers down each column of the table. The results are called joint probabilities.

(6) Since the final probabilities for each of the possible hypotheses must add up to one (i.e. one of them must be true), you must scale the joint probabilities so that they sum to 1. Do this by dividing each one by the sum of all the joint probabilities. The result is the final probability of each hypothesis, in the light of the prior probability and all the additional observations.

To illustrate it, here is how to calculate the risk that the healthy sister of a child with cystic fibrosis is a carrier. The steps are color coded.

Hypothesis – sister is:	AA	Aa	aa
Prior probability:	¼	½	¼
Conditional: she's unaffected:	1	1	0
Joint probability	¼	½	0
Final probability	¼ / (¼+½+0) = ⅓	½ / (¼+½+0) = ⅔	0

1. Set out the alternatives. As the child of two carrier parents she could be AA, Aa or aa.
2. The prior probability is just the mendelian 1:2:1 probability.
3. This is the tricky bit. Remember, each conditional likelihood is the likelihood of the observation, *given that the particular hypothesis is true*. If she is AA then she will definitely be unaffected (likelihood = 1). Similarly if she is Aa. If she is aa there is no chance she would be unaffected (obviously you could introduce variable penetrances here, which is a major use of the method).
4. Multiply down each column.
5. Divide each joint probability by the sum of all joint probabilities, to make them sum to 1.

The *Guidance* for this chapter's *Self-assessment questions* give some more examples and discussion of Bayesian calculations. Bayesian approaches to questions of probability are attractive because they correspond to the way we decide whether or not to believe something in everyday life. As mentioned in the guidance for *SAQ1* of *Chapter 9*, you may well believe your friend if he tells you that he missed a lecture because he overslept, but not if he tells you it was because he had been abducted by aliens. You assess the overall credibility of his story in the light of its prior probability. Thus Bayesian calculations are a form of quantitative common sense.

complex cases being referred to the genetic clinic. Common reproductive issues which may trigger a referral to a genetic clinic are described below.

Recurrent miscarriage

It has been estimated that 10–15% of all clinically recognized pregnancies end in a miscarriage. Recurrent miscarriage is defined as the loss of three or more pregnancies. There are many possible causes; more than one contributory factor may underlie the recurrent pregnancy losses which affect 1% of all women. Only a proportion of women presenting with recurrent miscarriage will have a persistent underlying cause for their pregnancy losses. Maternal age and previous number of miscarriages are two independent risk factors for a further miscarriage. All couples with a history of recurrent miscarriage should have peripheral blood karyotyping performed. In approximately 3–5% of such couples one of the partners is found to carry a balanced structural chromosomal anomaly. The most common types of parental chromosomal abnormality are balanced reciprocal or Robertsonian translocations. In a future pregnancy there is a 5–10% chance of an unbalanced translocation and prenatal diagnosis can be offered (RCOG, 2003).

Primary amenorrhea

Primary amenorrhea is the absence of menstrual periods often in association with the lack of other signs of puberty in a woman. Usually baseline hormonal investigations and often genetic tests will have been carried out by a gynecologist before referral to a genetic clinic. Diagnoses to be considered include the following.

- Turner syndrome. This disorder usually presents in infancy or childhood with short stature (see **Case 9, Isabel Ingram** in *Chapter 2*), but some women are not diagnosed until they present with primary amenorrhea in their teenage years. The main features, in addition to short stature and gonadal dysgenesis, are cardiovascular and renal malformations, although not all patients have these problems. Around half the patients with Turner syndrome have a 45,X karyotype with the rest having a structural abnormality of one X chromosome, or a mosaic karyotype comprising a 45,X cell line plus one or more other cell line(s) including 47,XXX, 46,XX and 46,XY.
- Congenital absence of the uterus and vagina. These patients lack Mullerian derivatives but they can have normal ovaries and so may have normal pubertal changes except for menstrual periods. There is a high incidence of associated abnormalities of the kidneys, cervical spine, limbs and heart. Most cases are sporadic.
- Androgen insensitivity syndrome (AIS). This disorder, previously known as testicular feminization syndrome, is associated with a 46,XY karyotype and mutations in the androgen receptor gene on Xq11. Girls with AIS are phenotypically normal females at birth and they can present with inguinal herniae containing testes, or later as young adults with primary amenorrhea.
- Gonadal agenesis/dysgenesis. Around 20% of XY females have mutations or deletions of the *SRY* gene but the cause is unknown in the majority who often have a uterus and streak gonads.

- Hypogonadotrophic hypogonadism. The causes that are known are genetically heterogeneous. Treatment is by hormonal induction of puberty and maintenance and for a few there are fertility induction treatments.

Precocious puberty

This is defined as the appearance of signs of pubertal development at an abnormally early age. Generally for girls this is before 8 years and for boys before 9 years of age, but there are variations between populations; better nutrition and obesity are causing a drift towards earlier puberty. In most cases the cause is unknown and is not associated with any other abnormalities. If it is considered that final height will be very much reduced, or if puberty is extremely early, then medical treatments can be given to halt pubertal changes until a more acceptable time. Rare genetic causes include:

- congenital adrenal hyperplasia (21-hydroxylase deficiency) in males (see Case 19, Stott family for further discussion)
- McCune–Albright syndrome (OMIM 174800), a disorder comprising polyostotic fibrous dysplasia of bone and patchy skin pigmentation and which is due to a somatic activating mutation of the *GNAS1* gene in a mosaic form.

Infertility

Infertility is defined by the failure to conceive after 12 months of unprotected intercourse. It is beyond the scope of this book to consider all causes but genetic causes must be borne in mind, particularly those associated with male infertility.

- Klinefelter syndrome (47,XXY) has a prevalence of 1/600 – 1/800 male births and often presents in adult life with infertility. Boys enter puberty normally but by mid puberty the testes are smaller than normal and testosterone production is decreased and there is azoospermia.
- Congenital bilateral aplasia of the vas deferens (CBAVD; OMIM 277180) causes obstructive azoospermia and is usually due to mutations in the *CFTR* gene. Such males have a much higher incidence of the partially functional alleles, e.g. R117H or 5T splice variant, but the other allele may be a common CF mutation such a delta-F508 (p.F508del), so if such patients undergo sperm extraction procedures a child may be at risk of CF if the mother is also a carrier.
- Microdeletions or structural abnormalities of the Y chromosome. Up to 15% of males with azoospermia have deletions of azoospermia factors on Yq. Such deletions may result from homologous recombination between large repeat sequences.
- 46,XX males. This condition is usually due to a translocation of the *SRY* gene into the X chromosome, a cryptic cell line containing a Y, or mutations in genes in the pathway downstream of *SRY*.
- Kallmann syndrome (OMIM 308700). This disorder affects around 1 in 8000 males (and 1 in 40 000 females). Kallmann syndrome comprises hypogonadotrophic hypogonadism and anosmia (lack of a sense of smell). Inheritance is either X-linked due to mutations in the *KAL-1* gene or less

frequently autosomal dominant or recessive due to mutations in several other genes.

Consanguinity

This was considered in detail in *Chapter 10.* How to calculate the proportion of genes relatives share is shown in *Box 10.3.* In practice, couples who are related as cousins and planning to have children, and who come from communities where consanguinity is a customary practice, rarely request referral to a genetic clinic, although those from communities where this practice is uncommon sometimes do. More often referral follows the birth of an affected child.

- The empiric data usually given, where there is no family history of recessive disease, is that the birth prevalence of serious congenital and genetic disorders diagnosed by 1 year in unrelated parents is 2.0–2.5%, and for children of first cousin parents the risk is double that at 4.0–4.5%. For children of second cousins the risk is 3.0–3.5%. However, in some communities the risks are higher because a couple may be more closely related due to multiple consanguineous marriages in previous generations.
- The Birmingham birth study (Bundy and Aslam, 1993) found that the prevalence of recessive disorders in Northern European children, where only 0.4% of parents were related, was 0.28%, whereas in British Pakistani children, where 69% of parents were related, the prevalence of recessive disorders was 3.0–3.3%.

Teratogens

A common reason for referral in pregnancy to a genetic clinic is concern about the possible effects on a baby of maternal illness, of exposure to drugs and other substances, and to infections.

Maternal illness.

- Diabetes. Diabetic mothers have an increased risk of miscarriage and their infants have around a 6–9% risk of major congenital malformations. With excellent diabetic control these risks can be reduced, but even in very well controlled women the risks remain elevated compared to non-diabetic women. The main abnormalities seen include cardiac defects, neural tube defects and abnormalities of the skeletal system.
- Phenylketonuria. Previously, women with PKU had severe learning disability and rarely reproduced, but the introduction of effective screening programs and dietary treatment means that such women are now normal and are having babies. Unfortunately, many adolescents and young adults do not comply with recommendations about maintaining appropriate dietary control. An untreated woman has a very high risk of having a baby with microcephaly, growth retardation and congenital heart defects, and so it is very important to encourage women with PKU who are planning a pregnancy to resume strict dietary control.
- Epilepsy. Around 0.4–0.7% of pregnant women have epilepsy and many require anticonvulsant medication (see below). The risk of the medication has to be weighed against the risk of morbidity and mortality of the

seizures to both the mother and child. There is a suggestion that even without exposure to anticonvulsants there may be a slightly increased risk of abnormalities in infants of epileptic mothers.

- Maternal genetic disorders. In pregnancy, in addition to the risk of the child inheriting the condition from a parent, the mother's genetic disorder may confer added effects on both the child's and the mother's health. Examples include: the risk of severe polyhydramnios (excess liquor) and the severe effects of the congenital form of myotonic dystrophy where the child inherits the condition from the mother; and pregnancy in achondroplastic women which can result in severe respiratory compromise in the mother and the effects of prematurity in the baby due to the need for early delivery.

Drugs. These can be divided into drugs prescribed for maternal illnesses and so-called recreational drugs, and a few examples are given below.

- Anticonvulsants. There is emerging evidence that the risks to the infant from exposure to anticonvulsant drugs in pregnancy include both structural abnormalities and cognitive effects. It should be emphasized that the majority of exposed infants have no abnormalities but there is a definite increase, around two to three times, over the background risk for non-exposed children. Although specific abnormalities seem to be linked to certain drugs (e.g. cleft lip and palate and nail hypoplasia often arise following exposure to phenytoin, and neural tube defects may follow exposure to valproate), it is impossible to predict what effects might occur in an individual child, although if a woman has had one child with fetal anticonvulsant syndrome, and she remains on the same medication at the same dose, the sibling recurrence risk is estimated at 39–55%.
- Warfarin crosses the placenta and if a fetus is exposed, particularly in the second half of the first trimester of pregnancy, there is a high risk that the baby will have severe skeletal effects, such as chondrodysplasia punctata, which manifests as short limbs with stippled epiphyses, and hypoplasia of the nasal bone.
- Exposure to many other drugs has been linked to specific abnormalities in infants including heart disease, particularly Ebstein anomaly of the tricuspid valve, in babies exposed to lithium, central nervous system and heart defects and abnormalities of the first arch in babies exposed to retinoids, and choanal atresia, hypoplastic nipples and scalp defects in babies exposed to carbimazole.
- Alcohol – fetal alcohol syndrome is a well described condition which is easy to diagnose if there is a clear history of maternal alcohol ingestion and if the baby exhibits the typical behavior of withdrawal symptoms such as poor feeding, constant crying and jitteriness and clinical features such as low birth weight, microcephaly, short palpebral fissures and a long and flat philtrum. However, this information is often not available, which means that it has been very difficult to estimate risks of fetal alcohol syndrome in populations, but it is known that the incidence varies in different populations and social groups. Both chronic exposure throughout pregnancy and episodes of binge drinking are associated with

fetal alcohol syndrome and higher intakes associated with worse effects. Many countries now have government recommendations that pregnant women should abstain completely from alcohol in pregnancy.

- Cocaine is known to induce vascular constriction and this is thought to be the basis of the observed increases in miscarriage and placental abruption that are found in women abusing cocaine and the problems in their babies such as limb deficiencies, intestinal atresia and intracranial hemorrhage.

Infections in pregnancy.

- Chickenpox – varicella is generally a mild illness in childhood but if a pregnant woman is one of the 10% of non-immune adults there is a risk, if she is exposed, of congenital varicella in her baby including damage to the brain and eyes, skin scarring and limb hypoplasia. The risk if she is exposed at less than 13 weeks gestation is low but is significantly higher after maternal infection later in pregnancy. The woman may also be at risk herself of a severe pneumonia. Guidelines and recommendations have been drawn up for various scenarios (RCOG, 2007).
- Rubella is also a mild illness in childhood and adult life, but congenital rubella can be a devastating condition. Maternal infection at 8 weeks' gestation results in severe effects in 90% of exposed babies, but this falls to around 10% by 20 weeks and very low risks thereafter. Features include growth retardation, learning disability, cataract, deafness and heart defects. Many countries now have immunization programmes for children.
- Other infections associated with fetal effects include cytomegalovirus (a member of the herpesvirus family where primary infection *in utero* is associated with growth retardation, microcephaly, hepatosplenomegaly, jaundice and thrombocytopenia) and toxoplasmosis caused by the parasite *Toxoplasma gondii* acquired by eating contaminated foods. Transmission is mainly in the second and third trimesters and babies can develop hydrocephalus, intracranial calcification, seizures and chorioretinitis.

Dysmorphology

In the 1960s, David Smith from the USA first used the term 'dysmorphology' to describe the study of human congenital malformations and patterns of birth defects. Dysmorphology is one of the subspecialties within genetic medicine dealing with patients who have congenital malformations (terms used in dysmorphology are defined and illustrated in *Box 14.3*) and syndromes. As well as the benefits for families in making a precise diagnosis as outlined above, the study of malformation syndromes can also help to identify mechanisms underlying normal development.

To make a syndrome diagnosis, the steps followed are essentially the same as for other clinical situations, i.e. history, examination, investigations and synthesis. However, a different emphasis is placed on several aspects compared to other clinical situations.

BOX 14.3

Terminology used in dysmorphology

Malformation: a morphologic abnormality that arises because of an abnormal developmental process (a primary error in morphogenesis), e.g. cleft lip.

Malformation sequence: a pattern of multiple defects resulting from a single primary malformation, e.g. talipes and hydrocephalus can result from a lumbar neural tube defect.

Malformation syndrome: a pattern of features, often with a unifying underlying cause, that arises from several different errors in morphogenesis ('syndrome' from the Greek 'running together').

Deformation: distortion by a physical force of an otherwise normal structure.

Disruption: destruction of a tissue which was previously normal.

Dysplasia: abnormal cellular organization within a tissue resulting in structural changes, e.g. within cartilage and bone in skeletal dysplasias.

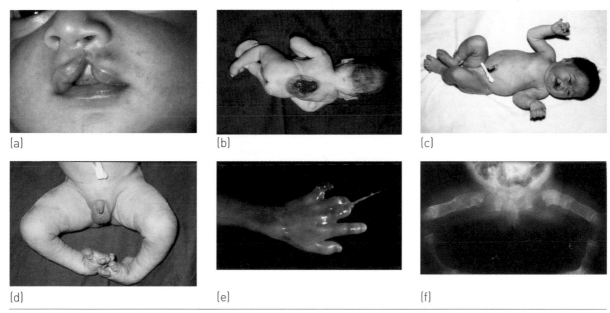

(a) (b) (c)

(d) (e) (f)

Box figure 14.1 – Clinical photographs of the main types of dysmorphic features.
(a) Cleft lip, a **malformation** representing failure of fusion of components of upper lip. (b) Meningomyelocele, talipes and hydrocephalus, a **malformation sequence** due to failure of closure of the neural tube and consequent effects. (c) Trisomy 13, a baby with a **malformation syndrome** consisting of holoprosencephaly, midline cleft lip and palate, polydactyly and heart defects. (d) Talipes, abnormal position of the feet, a **deformation** due to extreme lack of liquor *in utero*. (e) Amniotic bands, **disruption** of a normal hand by constriction with strands of amnion leading to amputation and secondary fusion of finger tips (syndactyly). (f) Femur bones with multiple fractures and abnormal modeling due to osteogenesis imperfecta, a skeletal **dysplasia**.

History

This concentrates particularly on:

- family history – this is usually taken in the form of a pedigree, noting such details as consanguinity or a possible mendelian pattern of inheritance
- past obstetric history – multiple early miscarriages may suggest one of the parents may carry a balanced chromosome abnormality for example

- maternal health – some maternal diseases such as diabetes or SLE may confer a higher risk of fetal abnormality; as described above, mothers with epilepsy, particularly those on anticonvulsant medication, may have a 2–3 fold increased risk of fetal abnormality
- maternal use of vitamin supplements and drugs – check if any of these are likely to be teratogenic
- pregnancy history – it would be relevant to know, for example, whether abnormalities were detected on a scan, whether any invasive procedures were carried out, and whether there was any problem with liquor volume.

Observation

This requires the following to be taken into account:

- posture and tone – some diagnoses can be suggested by observing a child prior to examination: the characteristic flexed posture of the fingers in trisomy 18, for example, or a very hypotonic posture in Prader–Willi and Down syndromes
- movements and behavior patterns – these are very characteristic in some syndromes: a girl with Rett syndrome will have repetitive hand movements (see *Disease box 7*) and individuals with Smith–Magenis syndrome (OMIM 182290) may hug themselves
- facial expressions – these may be typical in some syndromes: an individual with myotonic dystrophy has a mask-like face with poor facial movement, and the happy smiling face of an individual with Angelman syndrome is unmistakable
- personality – characteristic personality can be observed in patients with certain syndromes such as Williams syndrome where there is a friendly and talkative manner.

Physical examination

This should include documentation of:

- height and weight – this should be plotted on an appropriate growth chart; parental height should be taken into consideration
- proportions – these can be altered in certain conditions, e.g. achondroplasia or Marfan syndrome
- measurements of head circumference, facial features and other body parts where appropriate – these can be plotted onto charts for normal ranges and for specific conditions
- major and minor abnormalities – document carefully all abnormalities; where minor anomalies are concerned, be aware of what is abnormal and what is just part of normal variation, e.g. with minor 2/3 toe syndactyly.

It is often useful to document major and minor anomalies by taking photographs if the patient and/or parents permit. One has to be sensitive about asking for clothes to be removed for photographs, especially in older children, as this is not always necessary. It is, however, useful to remove as much 'clutter' as possible and avoid patterned backgrounds. Sequential photos of children at different ages are especially helpful in studying the evolution of phenotypes.

Some distinctive features uncovered by physical examination and observation may just be family characteristics. Taking a look at the rest of the family in person or from family photographs can be helpful.

Investigations

Many different types of investigation are used in syndrome diagnosis including the following.

- Cytogenetic studies. In many cases a routine karyotype will suffice but where a microdeletion syndrome is suspected the appropriate FISH test should be requested. Mosaic chromosome disorders may not be detectable on lymphocyte chromosome analysis and skin chromosome tests may be needed. Chromosome breakage studies may be indicated in some patients, particularly in those who are small, have microcephaly and other features such as radial aplasia and café-au-lait patches which suggest the diagnosis of Fanconi syndrome (OMIM 227650). In many laboratories there is now routine use of newer techniques such as MLPA and array CGH/SNP arrays. It is envisaged that these tests will soon replace routine karyotyping.

- Molecular genetic tests. There are databases which can be used to identify laboratories offering testing for specific monogenic disorders. Unfortunately testing may not be available on a service basis at the present time for many rare conditions.

- Metabolic testing. Testing for disorders of metabolism involving amino acids, organic acids, mucopolysaccharides and peroxisomes should be considered in patients with symptoms such as hepatosplenomegaly, coarse facies, joint stiffness, severe hypo- or hypertonia, early onset seizures or deterioration of consciousness.

- Infection screening can be helpful where congenital infection is suspected from the history or from clinical signs such as a rash, hepatosplenomegaly or cerebral calcification.

- Radiological investigations. X-rays are of paramount importance in the diagnosis of skeletal dysplasias. Radiographs of the hands and feet can be particularly useful. CT scans are useful to look for intracranial calcification; otherwise MRI scans provide more information and do not expose patients to radiation.

- Pathology/autopsy. Pathology investigations are useful for defining the full extent of abnormalities. With fetal pathology it is important to take into account the gestation of the fetus and the possibility of traumatic abnormalities sustained during delivery.

- Other miscellaneous investigations may be needed for specific disorders, e.g. Hb electrophoresis for the X-linked α-thalassemia-mental retardation syndrome (ATRX, see *Disease box 2*) and testing for leucopenia and retinal pigmentation in Cohen syndrome (OMIM 216550).

- Expert opinions. Dysmorphic syndromes can involve all body systems and it is impossible for any one person to be an expert in all areas so it is often necessary to refer for a specialist opinion.

Synthesis

- Ask some basic questions such as 'Are we dealing with a single malformation or multiple malformations?', 'Is the child likely to have a multiple anomaly syndrome?', 'Are there deformations that might tie in with the pregnancy history?', 'Does the family history help?'.

- When chromosomal syndromes have been ruled out and a single gene cause is strongly suspected, consider possible syndrome diagnoses in broad categories or 'syndrome families' including:
  - skeletal dysplasias
  - overgrowth syndromes
  - low birth weight and proportionate dwarfism syndromes
  - Prader–Willi-like and obesity syndromes
  - Angelman/Rett-like syndromes
  - Noonan-like syndromes
  - neurocutaneous and vascular syndromes
  - ectodermal dysplasias and other skin disorders
  - distinct MCA/mental retardation syndromes with a 'gestalt'
- Think whether you have seen a similar pattern before. Personal experience is helpful and people get better and more experienced at dysmorphology over time. You may be able to recognize a 'gestalt' which is familiar to you from a previous case or from literature you have read.
- Seek help from the literature. There are numerous textbooks and journals that can be of help to the dysmorphologist. *Gorlin's Syndromes of the Head and Neck* (2010) is a particularly comprehensive text.
- Search various databases. There are several available for dysmorphic syndromes including the London Dysmorphology Database and POSSUM. If a search is made using features which are very distinctive a reasonable 'shortlist' of possibilities may be produced.
- Seek help from colleagues. Share information and photographs/images with other colleagues within a department and specialists in the field. Present distinctive cases at dysmorphology meetings or use some of the emerging online 'Networks of experts'.

Following the diagnosis

Clinical diagnosis should be confirmed with a diagnostic test if available. Even experienced dysmorphologists should consult with colleagues to see if they agree with the diagnosis. Further consultation with parents is usually needed to explain the child's problems and to have a full discussion about the implications. Appropriate screening investigations should be arranged if the condition is associated with particular complications and, if needed, referral should be made to appropriate social services and support groups.

What if the diagnosis remains unknown?

A child should not be labeled as having a particular dysmorphic syndrome unless the physician is absolutely sure about it. It is far more difficult to remove an incorrect diagnosis than to attach one in the first place. Where a syndromic diagnosis is still likely but not apparent at the first consultation, it is important for the child to be followed up and re-evaluated at a later stage when new syndromes may have been delineated or more investigations might be available. Where patients have very distinctive features, either representing a 'new' syndrome or showing unusual features of one already described, it is can be helpful to document the findings in the literature.

Genetic testing

Like any other clinician, a clinical geneticist will call on a wide range of tests, many of which are not specifically genetic. Making a diagnosis can involve all the usual clinical skills and tests. Here we restrict ourselves specifically to genetic tests.

Diagnostic testing

This can involve chromosomal, biochemical and DNA analysis.

- *Chromosome analysis* is indicated in babies with multiple congenital malformations, in patients of any age with a combination of mental retardation and dysmorphism, and for otherwise unexplained infertility, recurrent miscarriages or intersexual states. The methods are described in *Chapter 2.*
- *Biochemical analysis* is indicated when certain symptoms and signs occur, such as enlarged liver and spleen, early onset seizures, neurological deterioration and coarsening of facial features.
- *Molecular testing* is useful when there is a strong suspicion, but not certainty, of a specific mendelian condition. As explained in *Section 5.4*, testing must be targeted, ideally at a specific mutation, but at least at one or two specific genes.

In general, diagnostic testing does not raise the same ethical issues as predictive testing, but clinicians need to be sensitive to possible implications for other family members.

Carrier testing

This is used for autosomal and X-linked recessive conditions, and also for balanced chromosomal abnormalities. It would normally be carried out at the request of the patient, and for a reason beyond mere curiosity. Counseling should always be part of the process, though when testing is done as part of a population screening program, pre-test counseling is likely to be quite minimal. Children should not be tested unless there is an immediate benefit to the child.

Predictive testing

This is used for late-onset conditions such as Huntington disease and familial cancers. It needs to be done within the context of a full clinical genetics service and to follow detailed written protocols that define in advance the response to each possible outcome. *Box 14.4* shows a protocol for predictive testing for Huntington disease.

Prenatal testing

This can be carried out at several stages of pregnancy.

- *Chorion villus biopsy* is performed at 10–12 weeks of gestation under ultrasound guidance (*Figure 14.1*). Either a transabdominal or

BOX 14.4

Protocol for predictive testing for Huntington disease

Various nationally agreed protocols differ in minor respects, but all require multiple counseling sessions. The following, reproduced from Tibben (2002) with permission from Oxford University Press, is typical. The patient is encouraged to bring a spouse, friend or supporter to each session.

Counseling session 1:
Sociodemographic details
Confirmation of family and clinical data
Assessment of impact of Huntington disease and test results
Assessment of knowledge of Huntington disease and of predictive testing
Reasons for requesting prediction
Neurological examination

Counseling session 2 (a month or more after session 1):
Assessment of psychological, personality and social resources, using standardized instruments
Further counseling and discussion of the disclosure session; agreement of the date of this session
Nomination of professional support
Signing of consent form
Taking of blood sample

Laboratory work:
The blood sample is split into two and sent to the laboratory on two different days, to minimize any risk of sample mix-up
The laboratory uses PCR to estimate the CAG repeat sizes on both copies of chromosome 4

Counseling session 3 (within 2 weeks of session 2):
Disclosure of test results

Follow-up 1:
2 days – 1 week, normally by telephone

Follow-up 2:
3 months

Follow-up 3:
12 months

Only a small proportion of people at risk eventually take the predictive test. Follow-up support is important for people whose test result is negative, as well as for those found to carry the disease allele. Genetics centers often maintain registers of families with Huntington disease (and other conditions where the risk extends beyond the nuclear family). These are administrative tools to provide a point of long-term contact for family members. In Manchester, for example, 1374 at-risk individuals in 514 extended Huntington disease families have volunteered to be included in the register, and they are each contacted once a year to check on any problems and advise them of any relevant new findings.

transcervical route may be used. The chorion is the outermost of the fetal membranes, and the sampling instrument should not penetrate the amniotic cavity. Once removed, the material needs expert dissection under the microscope to pick fetal material free of contaminating maternal tissue. Villi can be used for DNA extraction or for rapid cytogenetic analysis of dividing cells already present. Such short-term cultures need to be confirmed with longer term cultures. Mosaicism detected in villi is difficult to interpret: retrospectively it often turns out

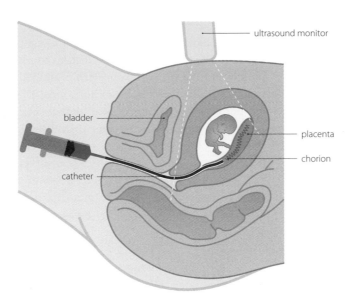

ultrasound monitor

bladder

placenta

chorion

catheter

Figure 14.1 – Chorion villus biopsy.

to have been confined to the placenta. For DNA testing, results should always be compared to a control sample of the mother's blood DNA, to ensure that the test result reflects the fetal genotype.

Chorion villus biopsy carries around a 2% risk of causing a miscarriage. There is a significant learning curve for the procedure, and it is always best to rely on an obstetrician who has already performed many such procedures.

- *Amniocentesis* is performed at 14–20 weeks of gestation (*Figure 14.2*) and carries a 0.5–1.0% risk of causing a miscarriage. Amniotic fluid

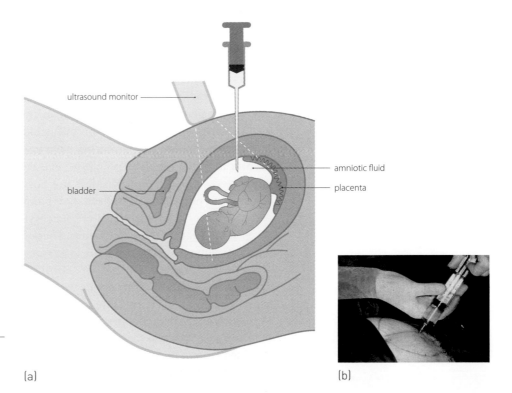

ultrasound monitor

amniotic fluid

placenta

bladder

Figure 14.2 – Amniocentesis.
(a) Diagram of procedure. (b) Withdrawing amniotic fluid.

(a)

(b)

consists mainly of fetal urine and washings from the lungs. It can be analyzed biochemically, or fetal cells can be isolated from the fluid and cultured for cytogenetic or molecular analysis. Biochemical analyses include testing for AFP, a protein produced by the fetal liver: a high level indicates that the fetus has a hole, most likely an open neural tube defect, but possibly an abdominal wall defect. There is an extensive literature on the interpretation of biochemical findings. Culture of cells from amniotic fluid for cytogenetic analysis takes around 2 weeks to obtain good quality preparations. Amniotic fluid is a poorer source of DNA than chorionic villi, because there are fewer cells. Newer techniques that do not require cell culture, such as QF–PCR (quantitative PCR with fluorescence-labeled primers) to detect specific trisomies, are increasingly being introduced into practice.

- *Analysis of fetal cells or DNA in maternal blood* has often been suggested as a non-invasive method of prenatal diagnosis. Many reports have shown that fetal cells are often detectable in the maternal blood. Typically there is about one fetal cell per milliliter of maternal blood. These rare cells could in principle be used to screen for a long list of anomalies, but the tests are not reliable enough for routine clinical use. A large multi-center study (NIFTY study, Bianchi *et al.*, 2002) attempted to determine fetal sex and to check for aneuploidy by interphase FISH of fetal cells in 3502 maternal blood samples. Among women carrying a singleton male fetus, at least one cell showing an X and a Y FISH signal was found in 41%; the false positive rate was 11%. For aneuploidy the detection rate was 74% with 0.6–4.1% false positives.

Because of these disappointing results, attention has moved to detecting free fetal DNA in the maternal circulation. Plasma from pregnant women contains free DNA, of which 3–6% is of fetal origin. The concentration of free DNA is much higher than the amount contained in the rare fetal cells. Fetal DNA is detectable from week 7, maybe earlier, and its concentration rises through pregnancy. The fetal DNA consists mainly of fragments <200 bp in length. Its origin is unknown, but is most likely to be placental (in which case confined placental mosaicism could be a problem, as with the chorion villus biopsy).

Highly sensitive PCR protocols have been used to sex the fetal DNA or to check for paternally inherited mutations. Because of the large excess of maternal DNA, it is not possible to test for inheritance of maternal mutations. An alternative approach has been described, where 12 cases of aneuploidy were successfully detected in a total of 18 cases using high-throughput shotgun sequencing (Fan *et al.* 2008). The highly fragmented cell-free DNA is extracted from maternal plasma and sequenced to generate millions of short DNA sequences from random genomic locations. By comparing these sequences with the known human genome sequence, it is possible to work out how many sequences have been derived from each chromosome. By comparing the total number of sequences obtained from a cell-free DNA sample with the number obtained from a normal genomic DNA sample, very small increases (less than 3%) in the amount of chromosome 21 can be detected in the cell-free DNA sample if the fetus carries an additional chromosome 21. The Royal College of Obstetricians and Gynaecologists' Scientific Advisory Committee have recently published a summary of progress in this field (RCOG, 2009).

- *Imaging* is discussed here because, when an anomaly is detected, it frequently leads on to a genetic test. It is the only thoroughly established non-invasive method for routine fetal testing. With each passing year imaging becomes more powerful and sophisticated. 3D and 4D imaging can now give really clear images of fetal structure and even facial features. A detailed fetal anomaly scan (different from the scans used to establish gestational age and check the number of sacs) is often done at around 18 weeks. A wide range of structural anomalies can be picked up and then investigated further, often by amniocentesis followed by cell culture and chromosome analysis, or by FISH analysis for specific disorders. For example, after detection of a heart defect, FISH analysis for 22q11 deletions may be performed. Imaging is also employed as a screening test to detect micro signs of Down syndrome; the most frequently sought sign is increased nuchal translucency, but other structural features such as absence of the nasal bone can increase the likelihood that a baby has Down syndrome.

Management and treatment of genetic disorders

Here we will discuss the principles of the three great hopes for general progress in treating genetic diseases: treatments based on an understanding of the gene function and pathways involved, gene therapy and cell therapy. Before getting into these, it is important to stress that, while the promise of these technologies lies in the future, there is already a lot that can be done here and now. The reputation of genetic disease for being untreatable is only partially deserved. Genetic patients, just like any others, have problems and symptoms that can be alleviated even if no radical cure is possible. Specific treatments based on an understanding of the abnormal function are available for a range of diseases. A number of examples are given in *Section 14.3*, and *Table 14.2* at the end of this chapter lists others.

Treatments based on understanding gene function and pathways
This is not a new area; dietary management and enzyme replacement therapies for some inborn errors of metabolism have been around for many years. But there is much excitement about the potential of using already approved drugs for new indications based on recent knowledge about the pathways in which certain gene products operate. For example, losartan is in a class of drugs known as angiotensin-receptor blockers and has been used for the treatment of hypertension. It is known to act by blocking the action of TGFβ. Patients with Marfan syndrome and mutations in fibrillin-1 have raised TGFβ signaling. Following studies in a mouse model of Marfan syndrome which showed beneficial effects of losartan, clinical trials in humans have now been started. A similar example concerns sirolimus, an mTOR signaling inhibitor, used in transplant medicine. Mutations in tuberous sclerosis genes result in constitutive activation of mTOR and so sirolimus

is being used in clinical trials in tuberous sclerosis (OMIM 191100) patients with angiomyolipomas in their lungs.

Another approach is exemplified by the recognition that utrophin is expressed at the muscle membrane in fetal life and that dystrophin is introduced alongside it. Thereafter utrophin is downregulated in the muscle membrane and its expression limited to the neuromuscular junction. In boys with Duchenne muscular dystrophy the gene that encodes dystrophin is mutated and no dystrophin is present in muscle, leading to devastating symptoms and early death. Studies of utrophin treatment in mdx mice which lack dystrophin have been promising and preclinical trials are underway with a utrophin upregulator, with the hope that clinical trials may start soon.

Gene therapy

The promise of gene therapy rests on the existence of well-established laboratory methods for getting genes into cells. It is surprisingly easy to get exogenous DNA into living cells in the laboratory, using any of a range of techniques (*Figure 14.3*). Broadly, these fall into physical methods and vector-dependent methods.

Physical methods include:

- *liposomes* – artificial membrane-bound vesicles that can fuse with cell membranes and release their contents into the cell;
- *receptor-mediated methods*, where the DNA is attached to the ligand for a cell-surface receptor which internalizes after binding the ligand;
- *electroporation*, where a short high-voltage pulse temporarily alters cell membranes such that they take up naked DNA from the medium.

Vector-based methods use engineered viruses that resemble the acute transforming retroviruses described in *Figure 12.4*. Compared to physical methods, these are often much more efficient at getting the foreign DNA into

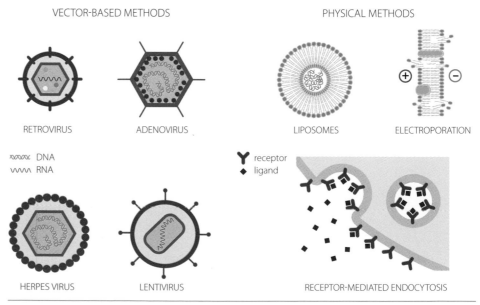

Figure 14.3 – **Methods of inserting an exogenous gene into a cell.**

a good proportion of the target cells. Many different viruses have been used. Factors governing the choice include:

- *capacity*: how long a piece of genetic material they can hold;
- *tropism*: some viruses preferentially infect certain types of cell;
- *ability to infect non-dividing cells*: retroviruses can only infect dividing cells;
- *integrating or non-integrating vectors*: integrating vectors such as retroviruses integrate the transferred gene into a chromosome of the host cell, ensuring that all daughter cells will carry a copy. Non-integrating vectors such as adenoviruses remain as extrachromosomal **episomes**, which will eventually be diluted out during cell replication. As we will see in the case of the Portillo family (Case 16, immunodeficiency) there are advantages and disadvantages to integration.

Depending on the nature of the condition it is designed to treat, gene therapy can have any of three aims:

Gene supplementation or augmentation. This aims to put a working gene into a cell that currently lacks it. This would be the aim of gene therapy for any loss of function condition, which includes many of the conditions covered in our *Case studies* (see below). Additionally it could be used to introduce a novel gene into a cell, usually for the purpose of creating a vulnerability in cells that one wishes to eliminate. Cancer cells might be made to express a novel antigen that would trigger a cytotoxic attack by the immune system, or an intracellular enzyme that would convert a harmless pro-drug into a toxic metabolite.

Gene silencing aims to prevent expression of a resident gene. This type of gene therapy would be required for diseases caused by gain of function or dominant negative mechanisms. In most cases the silencing would need to be specific for the mutant allele, leaving expression of the normal allele unaltered. Gene silencing might also be used to prevent expression of viral genes in an infected cell.

Gene repair aims to correct a malfunction in an endogenous gene, rather than silence or replace it. Proposals for gene repair rely on highly targeted homologous recombination or mismatch repair to patch specific defects in a gene. Alternatively the repair might be at the expression level, for example, by manipulating splicing to cause skipping or retention of specific exons of a gene.

Any of these methods might be applied *ex vivo*, on cells taken from the patient which, after modification, will be returned, or *in vivo* by injecting or otherwise introducing the therapeutic construct into the patient's body. Equally, one could in principle treat either somatic or germ-line cells. Germ-line gene therapy has an appealing finality to it compared with somatic therapy – the problem is dealt with once and for all – but is generally regarded as ethically unacceptable. In truth, the technical obstacles to germ-line therapy are far greater than for somatic therapy, and it is quite hard to think of circumstances where germ-line therapy would be useful even if it could be done (*Figure 14.4*).

Cell therapy

The obstacles to mending damaged tissues and organs by supplying new cells are the limited life and replicative potential of most cells, and the rejection of foreign

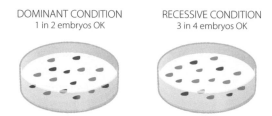

DOMINANT CONDITION
1 in 2 embryos OK

RECESSIVE CONDITION
3 in 4 embryos OK

Figure 14.4 – The limited usefulness of germ-line gene therapy.
The targets for germ-line therapy would most likely be embryos created by *in vitro* fertilization. Typically IVF might result in 5–10 embryos of which 1–2 are selected for implantation. A genetic test would identify which embryos would require the therapy. Depending on the mode of inheritance, either 1 in 2 or 3 in 4 embryos could be used without the need for any therapy.

cells. Although, of course, *organ* transplantation has been used successfully for decades, including for treating genetic diseases (e.g. kidney transplantation for polycystic kidney disease), *cell* transplantation usually relies on a small number of transplanted cells taking root and multiplying. This requires the use of **stem cells**.

It is believed that every tissue is maintained by a small number of stem cells. These cells have the potential to divide asymmetrically to produce another stem cell and a derivative cell that can go on to form the functioning cells of the tissue (*Figure 14.5*). Different stem cells differ in the range of cell types they can produce. **Embryonic stem cells** are totipotent. They can produce every cell type of the adult body. Perhaps when we understand much more about how to grow, maintain and differentiate them we will be able to grow organs and tissues

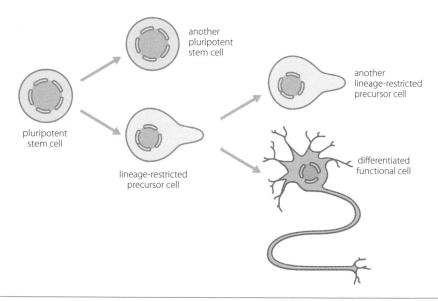

another
pluripotent
stem cell

another
lineage-restricted
precursor cell

pluripotent
stem cell

differentiated
functional cell

lineage-restricted
precursor cell

Figure 14.5 – Stem cells are capable of both self-renewal and differentiation into multiple lineages.
Stem cells in the embryo can produce every cell of the adult body; other stem cells are more restricted in the range of cell types they can produce.

to order from embryonic stem cells. Maybe this will be possible, maybe it will not. At present we don't know – but the potential is so alluring that laboratories throughout the world are devoting immense efforts to trying to find out.

Embryonic stem cells can only be obtained by destruction of a very early embryo (*Figure 14.6*). There is currently much debate about the potential of non-embryonic stem cells. The science is difficult and uncertain. Isolating and identifying stem cells requires an exceptional degree of laboratory skill, and experiments to explore their potential are often very hard to interpret. On top of the scientific difficulties are political and religious agendas that promote certain interpretations of the experiments. It will be some years before the science is secure enough to force consensus on the facts. Of course, the science can never dictate the ethics, but we look forward to a time when all parties to the ethical arguments can at least start from an agreed base of facts.

Amid the uncertainty, one form of stem cell transplantation is already part of routine clinical practice. Cord blood contains stem cells that can reconstitute every type of blood and bone marrow cell (and maybe other types of cell too). It can be collected at every birth with no risk or pain to the mother or baby. Methods for extracting stem cells are well established. Banks of cord blood stem cells, frozen in liquid nitrogen, have been set up and are routinely used in the treatment of leukemia and other blood disorders, and for bone marrow reconstitution in cancer patients who have had aggressive chemotherapy.

Heterologous cell transplants like these (i.e. using cells derived from a different person) raise problems of rejection and, for immune system cells, of graft-versus-host disease. Autologous transplantation, using one's own stem cells, would avoid these problems. There are three ways in which autologous stem cells might be obtained.

- Some people advocate storing a sample of cord blood from every baby, in case it is needed decades later. This might, however, produce only a limited range of cell types.

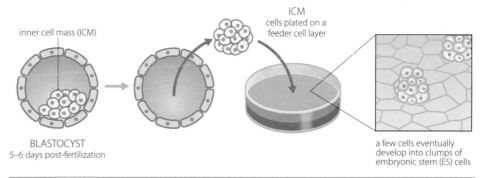

Figure 14.6 – Embryonic stem (ES) cells are derived from the 100–150 cell Inner Cell Mass (ICM) of an embryo at the blastocyst stage, 5–6 days post-fertilization. ICM cells are usually plated out on a layer of inactivated mouse fibroblasts as feeder cells. After removal from the blastocyst, ICM cells stop dividing and stop expressing stem cell markers. After some days one or two cells may resume growth and show re-expression of stem cell markers. These form clumps of cells from which the ES cells are obtained. ES cells have no exact natural counterpart in normal embryos.

- Improved methods and understanding may allow adult stem cells to be isolated from an uninvolved tissue of a patient, and made to transdifferentiate into stem cells for the appropriate tissue. Transdifferentiation (causing, say, a blood stem cell to change into a muscle stem cell) has been repeatedly reported, but there is controversy as to whether this is the true interpretation of the experiments. Reports differ about the multipotency and replicative potential of adult tissue-specific stem cells and, as with embryonic stem cells, these are often interpreted in the light of the speaker's personal ethical and religious standpoint.

- Most controversially, **therapeutic cloning** could be used to generate embryonic stem cells that have the patient's genotype (*Figure 14.7*). While it is questionable whether blood or other tissue-specific stem cells could be made to transdifferentiate, embryonic stem cells would not suffer this limitation. This proposal is the focus of intense ethical debate, with some groups and governments seeking to ban it, and others claiming it would be unethical *not* to try to develop a technology that could transform the lives of innumerable patients. Whatever one's views on the subject, it is important to distinguish therapeutic cloning from **reproductive cloning** – that is, attempting to produce a cloned baby. It is quite questionable whether a cloned blastocyst is a potential human being. It would probably be unable to develop into a normal baby even if it were implanted, because of defects in epigenetic reprograming. The great majority of cloned animal blastocysts produced in this way fail to develop, and those few that come to term are usually abnormal. Even

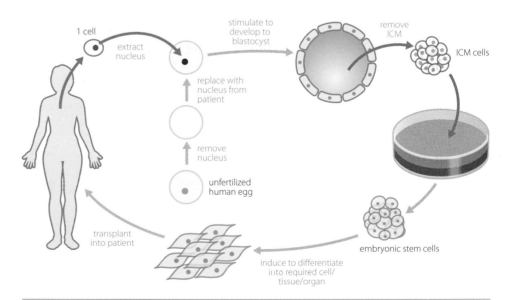

Figure 14.7 – Therapeutic cloning.
The aim of this procedure is to produce embryonic stem cells genetically identical to cells of the patient. It requires a supply of unfertilized human eggs, and entails destruction of any embryos produced. However, it is quite distinct from reproductive cloning, which aims to produce a cloned baby.

those animals that appear normal when young, like Dolly the sheep, usually die early. Embryonic stem cells, however, appear to have erased all previous epigenetic programming.

14.3. **Investigations of patients**

Table 14.1 summarizes the 26 *Case studies*. Rather than discuss each case separately, they are collected into groups for most of the discussion of what could be done.

Possibilities for prenatal diagnosis

Prenatal diagnosis could, in principle, be offered for almost all of the conditions described in the *Case studies*. The exceptions would be leukemia (an acquired condition), and Alzheimer disease and type 2 diabetes (complex diseases where genetic prediction is not possible). For most of the mendelian conditions it would

Table 14.1 – Summary of the 26 *Case studies* used in this book

Case	Family	Conditions where the problem affected development, so that treatment is necessarily symptomatic	Case	Family	Conditions where the problem is a continuing malfunction, where therapy might, in principle, aim to rectify the malfunction
3	Choudhary	Hearing loss	1	Ashton	Huntington disease
5	Elliot	Chromosomal anomaly	2	Brown	Cystic fibrosis
7	Green	22q11 deletion	4	Davies	Duchenne muscular dystrophy
8	Howard	Down syndrome	6	Fletcher	Leber's optic neuropathy
9	Ingram	Turner syndrome	11	Kavanagh	Sickle cell disease
10	Johnson	Marfan syndrome	12	Lipton	Fragile X
13	Meinhardt	Chromosomal anomaly	14	Nicolaides	Thalassemia
15	O'Reilly	Stickler syndrome	16	Portillo	X-linked severe combined immunodeficiency
17	Qian	Angelman syndrome	20	Tierney	Acute lymphocytic leukemia
18	Rogers	Prader–Willi syndrome	21	Ulmer	Tay–Sachs disease
19	Stott	Congenital adrenal hyperplasia	22	Vlasi	Phenylketonuria
			23	Wilson	Breast cancer
			24	Xenakis	Familial adenomatous polyposis
			25	Yamomoto	Alzheimer disease
			26	Zuabi	Type 2 diabetes

only be possible if the causative mutation had been previously identified – as we saw in *Chapter 9*, this was a particular challenge in the case of hearing loss.

Several of the chromosome abnormalities occurred *de novo* (in Cases 7, 8, 9, 13, 17 and 18). In these cases the recurrence risk is very low and in general the parents would be reassured rather than offered prenatal diagnosis in future pregnancies. For the *de novo* structural rearrangements (Cases 7, 13 and 17) germ-line mosaicism can never be ruled out, so there is a finite though small recurrence risk. If the parents were particularly anxious it would be appropriate to offer prenatal testing, but to point out that the chance of detecting a recurrence is probably smaller than the risk of losing the pregnancy because of the procedure. Of course, the two risks are not necessarily equally important, and families will make their own judgement of the relative weights to put on them. In our cases, of those six families only Anne Howard (Case 8, Down syndrome) was tested in her next pregnancy. In her case she and her husband decided to have tests partly because of the small increase in risk associated with her age and partly because they felt they would not be able give Helen all the attention she needed if they had another baby with Down syndrome.

For the other conditions, decisions about prenatal diagnosis would be governed by several factors:

- the legal and ethical framework in the country – in some countries prenatal testing is legal only for a defined list of conditions; in others it is left to negotiation between parents and clinician
- the practical availability of testing, including whether somebody else – the state or an insurance company – will pay for it
- the severity of the condition – for example, many people would not regard hearing loss as an indication for termination of affected fetuses
- the availability and effectiveness of treatment – demand for prenatal diagnosis of cystic fibrosis, for example, depends on views about the current and future prospects for treatment
- the age of onset of the condition – many people do not see late-onset conditions such as Huntington disease as appropriate for prenatal diagnosis
- the situation of the individual family – how well could they cope, emotionally, physically and financially with the birth of an affected child?
- the moral principles or religious beliefs of the individuals concerned – some people would not countenance a termination, whereas others would see it as the least bad option.

Current possibilities for treatment

None of the conditions discussed is untreatable, although most are incurable at present. In *Table 14.1* they have been split into those where the current problem is the result of things that happened, or failed to happen, early in development, and those where the problem is largely due to things happening, or failing to happen, here and now. For the first group treatment is necessarily symptomatic, while for the second, in principle, a more fundamental treatment or cure might be possible.

Phenylketonuria (Case 22 – Vlasi family) comes nearest to being curable at present. Once diagnosed, the baby is put on a low protein diet to minimize its intake of phenylalanine. Some protein is of course necessary, as is some phenylalanine. Phenylalanine is an essential amino acid, that is, one that humans cannot synthesize but have to obtain from dietary protein. Careful titration of the phenylalanine level is necessary. Too low a level of protein or phenylalanine will cause malnutrition, retarded growth, etc., while too high a level of phenylalanine will cause brain damage. Keeping a child on the diet is immensely demanding for the family, especially if there are unaffected siblings. Well-intentioned friends or neighbors may feel sorry for a child who seems to be being subjected to a crank diet, and may slip it surreptitious treats. Peer-group pressure to conform may be very hard for the child to resist. Special phenylalanine-reduced flour is available so that the child can have its own cakes and cookies.

In many countries it is recommended that patients should remain on the diet all their lives, because MRI has documented white matter changes in teenagers and adults who discontinued the diet. Clinically, the consequences of non-compliance are less severe in adults; however, as mentioned in *Figure 11.5*, a phenylketonuric woman definitely needs to go back on the diet during pregnancy, or else the high phenylalanine level in her blood will damage her baby's brain, even though genetically the baby is not phenylketonuric.

In the final section of this chapter other examples are given of inborn errors of metabolism that can be treated by dietary manipulation.

Congenital adrenal hyperplasia (Case 19 – Stott family) is one of the few genetic conditions that can be treated *in utero*. As explained in *Chapter 8*, the virilization of baby girls is the result of a feedback loop that over-stimulates the adrenal glands. If a couple have previously had an affected child, in subsequent pregnancies the mother is given oral dexamethasone, a glucocorticoid that can cross the placenta, to damp down the adrenal hormone production. This is started at the earliest possible stage of the pregnancy. If a subsequent fetal sex test shows that the fetus is male the treatment can be discontinued. Children with CAH are treated with steroids to ensure normal growth and development.

Acute lymphoblastic leukemia (Case 20 – Tierney family) in children is nowadays treated quite successfully (the disease in adults has a much worse prognosis); 75–80% of children can expect to survive 5 years without any recurrence, and in the best centers true cure (long term disease free survival) rates are 80% or better. The response to therapy is partly a question of the genetics of the leukemia cells – a variety of chromosomal rearrangements produce different chimeric oncogenes that influence prognosis – and partly a question of genetic polymorphisms controlling the pharmacokinetics (absorption, metabolism and clearance) and pharmacodynamics (response of the target) of the drugs used. Treatment response is measured by the level of residual disease after induction of remission. PCR of the specific chimeric oncogene is used to check the number of remaining cells with the leukemic genotype. In favorable cases this is 0.01% or less of the original level. Stem cell transplantation is also often used, especially in adult cases. The cells are derived from cord blood from unrelated infants (see above).

Jason Tierney (Case 20) had two prognostically favorable features, his *TEL–AML1* translocation, and his thiopurine methyltransferase deficiency. Although the latter caused initial problems, it also meant that his cells had received very high effective doses of the drug.

For the *late-onset conditions* in *Table 14.1* there is the hope of prevention. The risk of type 2 diabetes (Case 26 – Zuabi family) can certainly be greatly reduced by physical activity and weight control. People with familial adenomatous polyposis (Case 24 – Xenakis family) are strongly advised to have their colon removed; unfortunately there is still a risk of gastric and peri-ampullary tumors. An appropriate diet can reduce the risk of recurrence. Prophylactic mastectomy is one option for women who carry mutations in *BRCA2* (Case 23 – Wilson family); those with *BRCA1* mutations often also opt for oophorectomy. Regular enhanced surveillance is important for people at high risk of cancer. No interventions are currently known that reduce the risk of Huntington disease (Case 1 – Ashton family) or Alzheimer disease (Case 25 – Yamomoto family).

Treatment of most of the other conditions in *Table 14.1* is symptomatic.

Possibilities for gene therapy

In principle, gene therapy might be applicable to any of the conditions in the right-hand column of *Table 14.1* where the problem is a continuing genetic malfunction.

- For complex diseases (Alzheimer's, diabetes) any such therapy would not try to correct the initial genetic susceptibility because, as we have seen, the effect of any one gene is small. Possibly some point in a final common pathway of pathogenesis might present a suitable target, but in general gene therapy is an unlikely first line of attack with complex diseases.
- For the leukemia and cancers, any therapy would be directed at the neoplastic cells. Clinical trials have attempted to make neoplastic cells more immunogenic by expressing a foreign antigen on the cell surface.
- As a gain of function condition, Huntington disease would need a more sophisticated version of gene therapy than the remaining diseases in our list, all of which are caused by loss of function and might, in principle, be treatable by gene augmentation.
- As mentioned above, the easiest targets for gene augmentation are diseases where the exact level of expression of the introduced gene is not important, and a low level could be clinically useful. This makes cystic fibrosis, Duchenne muscular dystrophy, hemophilia and X-SCID the most appropriate targets.
- For Duchenne muscular dystrophy, the huge size of the gene and the difficulty of getting a foreign gene into a high proportion of muscle cells have so far frustrated attempts at gene therapy.

X-SCID is so far the one success story of gene therapy (Case 16 – Portillo family). In *Section 9.3* we mentioned that a second affected boy was born recently to a distant relative in the Portillo family. For this baby, the prospects are much brighter than for Pablo, who was born in 1989. There are two options:

- Bone marrow transplantation. As mentioned, provided this is done early the results are good. If a perfectly HLA-matched sib is not available, marrow can be used from a parent or a sib who shares one HLA haplotype with the affected baby, though the success rate is not as high. The marrow is first depleted of T cells to avoid graft-versus-host disease.
- Gene therapy. Pioneering work by Alain Fischer's group in Paris successfully cured 9 of 11 babies with X-SCID (*Figure 14.8*). Other groups have now achieved similar results. However, high optimism turned to gloom when two of the treated babies, and later a third, developed T cell leukemia. In two of the cases this was shown to be due to integration of the retroviral vector close to an oncogene, *LMO2*. The strong promoter used to cause high expression of the therapeutic *IL2RG* gene had the effect of up-regulating expression of *LMO2*. This is similar to the way the 8;14 translocation in Burkitt's lymphoma up-regulates the *MYC* oncogene by placing it next to the highly expressed immunoglobulin heavy chain gene (*Chapter 12*).

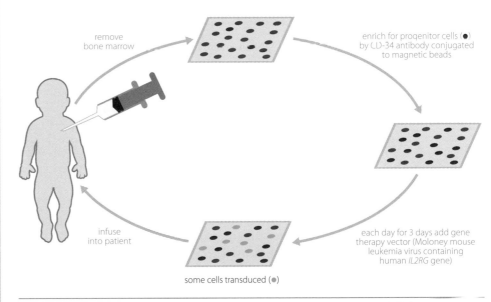

Figure 14.8 Gene therapy protocol for severe combined immunodeficiency.
The disease is caused by loss of function mutations in the *IL2RG* cytokine receptor gene. A retroviral vector was used to integrate a working copy of the gene into chromosomes of hemopoietic precursor cells. This gave them a selective advantage when re-infused into the patient, and they were able eventually to reconstitute T cell and NK cell function in 9 of 11 babies treated. Similar treatment was not successful in older patients with a partial malfunction of the gene.

After the initial shock, when trials of retroviral gene therapy were halted worldwide, some measure of optimism returned. The leukemia was brought under control. Without gene therapy these babies would have died. Where there is no alternative, the risk seems worth taking. Possibly some modification of vector design or the treatment protocol may lessen the risk. It remains true that the risk of this sort of insertional activation has moved up the list of potential problems of gene therapy using integrating vectors.

More recently, gene therapy has been used in clinical trials in London and Philadelphia in patients with a type of early onset severe retinal dystrophy, Leber's congenital amaurosis (blindness; OMIM 204100), associated with mutations in *RPE65*. An adeno-associated virus vector expressing RPE65 was injected directly into the retina in affected patients with a measurable restoration of some function in several patients.

Possibilities for cell therapy

Huntington disease and Alzheimer disease are high on the list of candidates for cell-based therapy. Regardless of the initial cause, in both cases it is loss of cells from specific brain regions that causes the clinical problems. The brain is an immunologically privileged site – that is, allografts (grafts from a different individual of the same species) are not usually rejected, although xenografts (grafts from a different species) often are. Animal studies have demonstrated the long-term survival of transplanted brain cells.

Preliminary trials have already been made of striatal cell transplantation in Huntington disease. A 6-year follow-up of one trial has been published (Bachoud-Levy *et al.*, 2006). Five Huntington disease patients received grafts into the striatum of fetal brain tissue. The tissue was obtained from the corresponding brain regions of 7.5–9 week aborted human fetuses – a developmental stage at which the brain contains suitable neuronal precursor cells. The results of this small trial showed real clinical improvement in some cases, and a temporary halt in the normal progression of the disease. By 6 years the normal decline was again evident. The transplanted cells can (sometimes) replace the lost cell population, but not halt the neurodegeneration in the rest of the affected brain regions. Other trials have also been reported, though with less intensive follow-up, and further trials are in progress.

These trials give real hope that cell-based therapy for Huntington disease can eventually be developed. The greatest present limitation is the source of cells. Quite apart from the ethical problems of using tissue from aborted fetuses, the tissue must be used fresh and it cannot be properly characterized or grown up in the laboratory. Real progress depends on identifying stem cells that can be preserved, grown in the laboratory when required, and induced to differentiate in the appropriate way.

14.4. Going deeper ...

Most people's long term hopes for effective treatment for many genetic diseases rest on gene therapy or stem cell transplantation, although in fact treatments based on knowledge of the genetic and cellular mechanisms may prove to be equally effective and without so many associated risks.

Gene therapy

Hopes for gene therapy have followed a manic-depressive course over the past 20 years, with recurrent highs and lows. In the beginning many people thought it might be easy to transfer the techniques from the laboratory to the clinic.

As early as 1990 it was claimed that a child with combined immunodeficiency (an autosomal recessive type due to deficiency of adenosine deaminase, not the X-linked type described in Case 16) had been cured by gene therapy. In fact it was enzyme replacement therapy, used simultaneously with the attempted gene therapy, that was probably responsible.

The continuing problem with gene therapy is obtaining reasonably long lasting and reasonably high level expression of the introduced gene.

- First, a sufficient proportion of cells in the target tissue must be transfected. Retroviral vectors give the highest efficiency, but they can be used only on dividing cells and, as we saw with X-SCID, integration is a mixed blessing. Adenoviruses seemed to be promising non-integrating vectors, but high doses can cause inflammatory responses that, in the case of Jesse Gelsinger (see www.uvm.edu/~cgep/Education/Expert.html) were fatal. None of the physical methods detailed in *Section 14.2* can target a useful proportion of cells under realistic clinical conditions. Novel viral vectors may have the most promise.
- Next, a sufficiently high level of expression must be achieved. Because this is difficult, most work has focused on conditions where even a low level of expression should be beneficial. Cystic fibrosis and hemophilia are examples of diseases where 10% of the normal expression level would bring real clinical benefits.
- If high expression could be achieved, the next problem would be to control it. The hemoglobinopathies should be good targets for therapy – the genes are small and exceptionally well understood, and the conditions are hugely important. The problem is that the expression level of an introduced globin gene would need accurate control. Over-expression of an introduced β-globin gene might convert a patient's β-thalassemia into α-thalassemia.
- Stable expression has proved extremely difficult to achieve. Cells commonly use epigenetic mechanisms to shut down expression of transgenes. Non-integrating vectors are especially likely to cease working after a short time. This has led many researchers to focus on situations where long-term expression is not needed – killing cancer cells or virally infected cells, for example.

Despite all these problems, there is a huge ferment of research and development in gene therapy. Many ingenious systems have been demonstrated in laboratory proof-of-principle experiments. Dozens of companies are pursuing novel approaches. Hundreds of phase I clinical trials have been run, particularly for cancer and infectious disease rather than for mendelian conditions. Despite the problems, X-SCID remains a real landmark success and there is early promise of treatment for Leber's congenital amaurosis. Given the ever-growing number of methods we have for manipulating genes and their expression, it is hard to believe that nothing useful will be achieved over the next decade. Perhaps the main question is whether any achievement will be a generally applicable breakthrough, leading to gene therapy for a whole list of conditions, or whether it will be a series of disease- and cell-specific tricks that will be of great benefit to a few patients but leave the whole field little further forward.

Stem cell therapy

This has suffered from the same over-hype as spoiled the reputation of gene therapy in the 1990s. It is easy to paint a beguiling picture of tissues and organs grown to order in a brave new world – whether this will ever bear any relation to reality is quite another question. We still know very little about the real potential of embryonic stem cells or any other stem cells. The number of embryonic stem cell lines presently available is very small, which for such an intensively researched high profile subject illustrates just how difficult these techniques still are. Compared to the technical difficulties, legal obstacles will probably not be major factors impeding progress. Research will simply move to countries where it is not only permitted but strongly encouraged. If any of the promised clinical benefits are realized, pressure from patient groups to allow the technology will be politically irresistible. The supply of eggs may be a more significant factor.

While we wait for these new technologies to live up to the hype, it is too easy to overlook all that has already been achieved.

Diagnosis and counseling

These may be undramatic, but they can make a huge difference to the lives of families affected by genetic disease.

- A diagnosis is the cornerstone of clinical management. Without it clinical management is unfocused and complications not anticipated.
- When the diagnosis is of a lethal condition, e.g. trisomy 18, the most appropriate management is usually supportive care even if a structural malformation is present where surgery would normally be undertaken.
- Families will often consult many doctors and their child may be made to undergo multiple tests in search of a diagnosis. Getting to the right specialist is important.
- Establishing a diagnosis and providing information about a condition has real therapeutic value for many people even if there is no cure. Links can be made with support groups. The families have something to write on forms, and educational and social services are more readily provided.
- A diagnosis and counseling can help dispel the guilt and anger that can seriously impact the quality of life in families after the birth of a child with a malformation or disease. It is not enough simply to tell the parents that it wasn't caused by something one or other of them did. The professional skills of a counselor can help parents work through the natural reactions of shock, grief and anger.
- Counseling can relieve the burden of anxiety by dispeling exaggerated general estimates of recurrence risks and, especially in X-linked and recessive diseases, identifying family members who are at negligible risk. Contrary to popular belief, more people have good news and low risks given in genetic clinics than bad news and high risks.
- While counseling cannot abolish the real problems of living with an affected family member, it can help people focus on solutions rather than problems. Appropriate help can be given. Parents can be given a range of options for handling the recurrence risk.

Information resources and care pathways for patients with rare disorders

Patients with rare disorders often feel very isolated and indeed the majority of healthcare professionals they meet may know less about the disorder than the patients themselves. This is where support groups come in; most now have helpful websites, the groups also arrange support for newly diagnosed patients, organize meetings where families can share experiences, and promote research. A number of helpful online information resources have been developed focusing on rare conditions with sections for patients, professionals, researchers and industry. One of the largest is Orphanet (www.orpha.net) which has a base in every European country and is coordinated in France. It has extensive regularly updated summaries and reviews about rare diseases in addition to regional information about clinics and laboratories. GeneClinics (www.geneclinics.org) is based in the USA and has similar information about clinics and laboratories as well as useful reviews on a range of rare conditions.

In medicine now, most treatments and management plans for common conditions are based on evidence from published studies, but for rare disorders evidence-based guidelines are few and far between. This is mostly because studies to develop the evidence have not been done due to the rarity of the conditions and the general belief that genetic diseases are untreatable. However, a number of professional organizations and initiatives have now started to address this problem. While it is often not possible to reach the levels of evidence found in common diseases, there is benefit in drawing up guidelines for rare disorders based on expert opinion, and to initiate studies to develop better levels of evidence using recognized methodology.

Testing

Testing is a crucial part of the overall aim of allowing families affected by a genetic condition to live as normal lives as possible. This is well illustrated by a study by Modell *et al.* (1980) on families at risk of serious forms of thalassemia. Before prenatal diagnosis was available, when the birth of an affected child made a couple aware of their 1 in 4 risk of having further affected children, they virtually ceased reproduction. Most subsequent pregnancies were accidental and they sought termination of 70% of them. Prenatal diagnosis for this condition became available in 1975. At-risk couples then resumed normal reproduction, with fewer than 30% of pregnancies being terminated for thalassemia. The effect of prenatal diagnosis was to reduce the number of terminations and to enable at-risk couples to have normal families.

The real example described below of a family with Duchenne muscular dystrophy further illustrates how the increasing accuracy of both carrier testing and prenatal testing can allow couples to avoid termination of wanted pregnancies. *Figure 14.9* shows how the distribution of carrier risks for Duchenne muscular dystrophy among families known to one large genetics center has changed as new knowledge allowed more precise genetic testing.

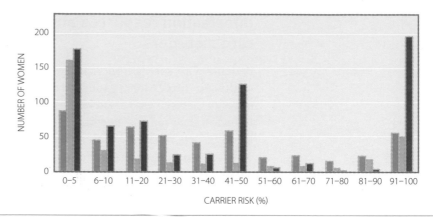

Figure 14.9 – Distribution of DMD carrier risks among women in families on the North West Genetic Register, Manchester.
Blue bars: risks based on pedigree and creatine kinase, before any molecular testing was available. Green bars: risk distribution in 1989 among women where the pedigree structure allowed gene tracking. Red bars: risks when direct mutation testing became available. The peaks at intermediate risks in the latter series are mostly from girls currently too young to test. Data courtesy of Dr Elizabeth Howard, St Mary's Hospital, Manchester.

Treatment

Treatment is available for a wide range of genetic diseases. Concentrating on the hopes for dramatic technologies such as gene and stem cell therapy distracts attention from the incremental but very real advances that have been made in treating a whole range of genetic diseases. We are indebted to an excellent brief article by Munnich (2006) for a list of some of these incremental advances; the article should be consulted for more details and references.

A central point made by Munnich is that patients do not suffer from their mutations, but from the functional consequences of those mutations. Often knowledge of the mutation or even the gene is irrelevant to treatment. We do not need to know whether a genetic patient's kidney failure is due to Alport syndrome (OMIM 301050), polycystic kidney disease or nephronophthisis (OMIM 256100) to know that a kidney transplant will greatly improve his life. We do not need to know which of the 100 possible genes has caused a child's deafness before we can consider the possible benefits of a cochlear implant. Even with Huntington disease, a famously 'untreatable' condition, life for the patient and his carers can often be improved by drugs such as neuroleptics and antidepressants, and attention to diet and the home environment.

In other cases a closer knowledge of the gene function, though not necessarily of the gene itself, is the key to treatment. *Table 14.2* lists some examples and particularly interesting cases include the following.

- Type I tyrosinemia (OMIM 276700) is a severe inborn error of metabolism that is especially prevalent in the Saguenay-Lac Saint Jean region of Quebec because of a founder effect. Referring to the diagram of tyrosine catabolism (*Figure 8.4*), the defective enzyme is downstream of the final step shown. The block results in accumulation of maleylacetoacetic

Table 14.2 – Examples of genetic diseases where symptoms can be ameliorated or sometimes abolished by treatments based on a knowledge of the malfunction, but not necessarily of the DNA sequence

Strategy	Example	Disease
Supply missing molecule		
	Insulin	Diabetes
	Growth hormone	Pituitary dwarfism
	Factor VIII	Hemophilia A
Replace defective enzyme		
	Acid beta-glucosidase	Gaucher disease
	Alpha-galactosidase	Fabry disease
	Alpha-glucosidase	Pompe disease
Dietary supplementation		
	High carbohydrate diet	Glycogen storage diseases
	Cholesterol	Smith–Lemli–Opitz syndrome
	Mannose	Carbohydrate-deficient glycoprotein syndrome 1b
	Biotin	Biotin-responsive carboxylase deficiency
	Pyridoxine	Pyridoxine-responsive homocystinuria
	Cobalamin	Cobalamin-responsive organic aciduria
	Alpha-tocopherol	Pseudo-Friedreich ataxia
	Creatine	Creatine synthesis deficiency
Dietary restriction		
	Low phenylalanine diet	Phenylketonuria
	Low protein diet	Maple syrup urine disease
	Low fat diet	Hypercholesterolemia
	Avoid phytanic acid	Refsum disease
Enhance residual enzyme activity		
	Fibrates	Fatty acid oxidation disorders
Remove a toxic product		
	Bleed regularly	Hemochromatosis
	Cysteamine	Cystinosis
Block a pathogenic process		
	NTBC	Tyrosinemia Type I
	Bisphosphonates	Osteogenesis imperfecta

Data from Munnich (2006).

acid, and overflow reactions then produce succinyl acetone. This abnormal metabolite inhibits production of porphobilinogen in the heme biosynthesis pathway. The result is a severe porphyria-like syndrome and death through liver failure or cancer. Type II tyrosinemia, by contrast, is a mild condition in which the first step in tyrosine catabolism is blocked (*Figure 8.4*). NTBC (2-(2-nitro-4-trifluoromethylbenzoyl)-1,3-cyclohexanedione) inhibits the enzyme, tyrosine transaminase, that is deficient in this mild form of tyrosinemia. It produces a **phenocopy** of Type II disease. Because of this block, there is no production of maleylacetoacetic acid, and the patient's disease is converted from the fatal Type I to the mild Type II disease.

- In carbohydrate-deficient glycoprotein disease type Ib (OMIM 602579) the underlying defect is an inability to isomerize fructose to mannose (deficiency of mannose phosphate isomerase). The symptoms of profuse diarrhea and severe liver disease are entirely due to lack of mannose. They can be completely rectified by oral mannose.

- Cystinosis (OMIM 219800) is an atypical lysosomal storage disease. The defect is not in a lysosomal enzyme, but in a lysosomal membrane transporter protein. Non-functioning of the transporter means that cystine is unable to get out of lysosomes. The accumulation produces symptoms including renal failure, pancreatic insufficiency, corneal erosions, central nervous system involvement and severe myopathy. Oral cysteamine is an effective treatment. Cystine consists of two molecules of cysteine linked by an S–S bridge (Figure 14.10). Cysteamine, given orally, enters lysosomes using a specific transporter. There it can displace one cysteine molecule from cystine to form a mixed cysteamine–cysteine

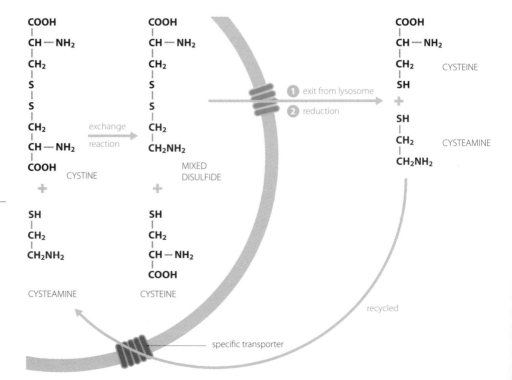

Figure 14.10 – Treating cystinosis with cysteamine. Cysteamine and the mixed disulfide are able to cross the lysosomal membrane, but cystinosis patients lack the specific transporter protein that in normal people allows cystine to exit lysosomes. Their symptoms are caused by accumulation of cystine in lysosomes.

disulfide, which is able to exit the lysosome, apparently using a lysine transporter. Once outside the lysosome, the mixed disulfide may be reduced, freeing the cysteamine to ferry another cysteine molecule out of the lysosome.

In other cases interventions are targeted more specifically at changing gene expression. Such treatments are mostly still experimental, for example:

- Symptoms of deficiency or abnormality of β-globin in sickle cell disease or β-thalassemia are milder in patients who continue to express some fetal hemoglobin during adult life (hereditary persistence of fetal hemoglobin, HPFH). Patients in whom production of the fetal γ-globin has been shut down as part of normal development may be stimulated to re-express the gene by treatment with hydroxyurea.
- The antibiotic gentamycin can induce mis-reading of mRNA by ribosomes, such that the ribosome occasionally ignores a stop codon. Gentamycin has been used to improve symptoms in cystic fibrosis patients who have a nonsense mutation. Clearly it would be catastrophic to cause ribosomes to ignore a high percentage of stop codons, but even a very small degree of read-through may allow significant clinical improvement in cystic fibrosis.
- The anti-epileptic drug valproate affects intron–exon splicing. Preliminary trials in spinal muscular atrophy (OMIM 253300, see Section 6.2) suggest valproate may prolong the life of affected infants. More targeted ways to modify splicing have been attempted in the dystrophin gene. The aim is to induce specific exon skipping so as to make frameshifting deletions frame-neutral and thus convert Duchenne muscular dystrophy into the milder Becker form (see Section 6.2). Oligonucleotides are custom-designed to match the relevant exon–intron junction. This approach falls more into the realm of gene therapy, with the usual problems of securing effective delivery and expression of the oligonucleotide.

The true story of one Manchester family (note that only the names have been changed) affected by Duchenne muscular dystrophy shows how the advances in genetics over the past three decades have improved their lives, even though a cure or effective treatment for the disease remains elusive.

- In 1977, a 3-year old boy Alan was diagnosed as having DMD, on the basis of clinical examination (problems running and climbing stairs, pseudohypertrophy of his calves), elevated serum creatine kinase and muscle histology.
- His mother Betty was referred to the genetics service. When the pedigree was taken (*Figure 14.11*, grey part), it showed that Betty had had two affected brothers, both wheelchair-bound in their early 20s and who had now died. Thus Betty and her mother Christine are obligate carriers. Betty had two sisters, Delia and Elly. Through Betty, Delia and Elly were invited to attend the genetic clinic and were counseled about their 50% risk of being carriers. Blood was taken for creatine kinase testing, but the results on Delia and Elly were not either high or low enough to significantly modify their carrier risks.

- In 1982 Delia, now married, was pregnant. She requested fetal sexing. Amniocentesis was carried out at 16 weeks. It took 2 weeks to get enough dividing cells for cytogenetic analysis. This showed the fetus was male. This wanted pregnancy was terminated by induced delivery at 18 weeks.
- In 1984 Delia was pregnant again, but miscarried at 10 weeks before any testing. Elly was now married but, having watched the traumas of her two sisters, was not willing to risk having children.
- By this time DNA markers had been defined that were linked to the *DMD* locus. Gene tracking (see *Chapter 9*) was used to estimate Delia's and Elly's carrier risks. Because all markers showed at least 5% recombination with the disease, two markers were used, one mapping proximal and the other distal to the disease locus. If a meiosis was non-recombinant for the two markers, there was only a very small risk that it would nevertheless be recombinant between the markers and the disease – only double recombinants would produce that result. If a meiosis showed recombination between the two markers, then no prediction could be made, but at least a false prediction would have been avoided. The result of the analysis (magenta lines in *Figure 14.11*) suggested that Delia had a >99% risk of being a carrier, while Elly's risk was very low, conservatively reported as 2%. Retrospectively, the risk that the fetus terminated in Delia's first pregnancy would have been affected was increased from 25% to 50%, which made Delia feel more confident that she had done the right thing. Elly now felt able to start a family.
- In 1985 Delia was pregnant for the third time. By now chorion villus biopsy was available (green lines in *Figure 14.11*). This was performed

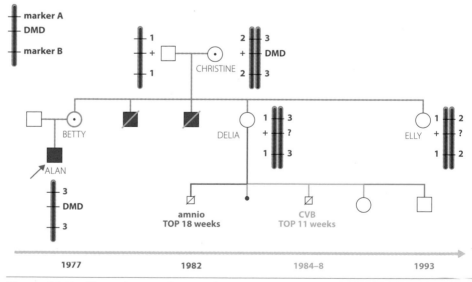

Figure 14.11 – How advances in genetics affected a family with Duchenne muscular dystrophy.
This is a real family; only the names have been changed. The colors show how the pedigree evolved over time. The black rules represent the results of gene tracking using two DNA polymorphisms, A and B that map either side of the disease locus. Allele numbers are arbitrary; + signifies the normal allele at the *DMD* locus. TOP, termination of pregnancy.

at 10 weeks. Rapid cytogenetic analysis showed the fetus was male. The pregnancy was terminated surgically at 11 weeks.

- In 1988 chorion villus biopsy in Delia's fourth pregnancy showed the fetus was female. She went on to deliver a normal healthy girl.
- In 1993 Delia was pregnant for the fifth time. By now the dystrophin gene had been cloned (blue lines in *Figure 14.11*). Testing Alan's DNA identified the family mutation, a frame-shifting deletion of exon 45 (see *Table 6.2*). Chorion villus biopsy was performed. Cytogenetic analysis showed a male fetus. Molecular testing for Y-specific sequences confirmed that the fetus was male, but exon 45 of the dystrophin gene could be PCR-amplified from the fetal DNA, showing it had not inherited the mutation. The pregnancy continued and Delia delivered a normal boy.

This family story illustrates several aspects of genetic services. First, how rapidly scientific advances can be delivered into clinical service; secondly, how options for individual family members can change even when the disease remains incurable, and thirdly, the importance of long-term follow up of families. Delia's daughter will soon wish to know her carrier status and options.

Finally we should perhaps consider some of the objections that have been raised against continuing progress in clinical genetics.

- *Helping people with genetic disease to live normal lives allows them to pass on their genes and shows an irresponsible lack of concern for future generations.* We dealt with this in relation to mendelian diseases in *Chapter 10*. In relation to complex diseases, this is really an objection to the whole of medicine – indeed to the whole of civilization. What is a civilized society but a collective attempt to prevent the operation of natural selection?
- *Offering prenatal diagnosis for a genetic condition devalues people with that condition.* Understandably, people living with spina bifida, achondroplasia or Down syndrome are highly sensitive to the suggestion that they should never have been born. The desire of parents for healthy children does indeed conflict with the need to respect the lives of people with disabilities. Each of us probably has our own point at which we would draw the line. The only general solutions to the conflict (allowing no choice or unfettered choice) are unacceptable to a majority of people in most countries. Perhaps the wisest course is to try as far as possible to circumvent the conflict by insisting that, whatever indications we may accept for termination of pregnancy, when an affected child is born we must value it as much as we would any other person and provide appropriate support and services to the family.
- *Curing certain conditions is another way of devaluing people with that condition.* This has particularly surfaced in relation to cochlear implants for deaf children. If these are done on a very young child they can be quite successful in terms of enabling the child to understand speech. Most hearing people would not question the benefit of enabling a deaf child to hear, but many people in the deaf community see it otherwise. They contend that attempting to cure deafness is tantamount to trying to undermine their culture.

This is similar to the question whether people in small linguistic isolates should be educated in their own minority language or in the national language of their country. For an individual, learning the national language widens his opportunities, but it threatens the minority culture with extinction in two or three generations. Perhaps the best aim in cochlear implantation is to make the child bilingual, in signing and in spoken language. This is the policy in Sweden but in few other places. It is worth pointing out that most children with profound congenital hearing loss are born into hearing families and are not part of the deaf community in their formative years. The Swedish solution leaves them free to make their own decisions about where they belong when they are old enough to do so.

- *Advances in genetic testing and reproductive choice put us on a slippery slope.* The 'designer baby' catchphrase, so beloved of journalists, usually surfaces early in this discussion. It has been repeatedly used in connection with 'savior siblings'. These are babies born after *in vitro* fertilization, where embryos were selected to be HLA-compatible with an older child who has a serious disease that could be cured by a transplant of HLA-compatible cord blood stem cells. Allowing this selection, say the critics, opens the door to much more extensive selection of embryos for non-medical reasons.

  The absurdity of this objection can be seen by looking at *Figure 14.4.* Suppose Mr and Mrs Frank N. Stein decide they want a tall blue-eyed blonde boy with an IQ of 150. They go through the trauma and expense of IVF and end up with eight embryos in a dish. Four are female and are discarded. Blue eyes and pale hair are not simple mendelian characters, but they are usually recessive. Photographs of the parents do not show us blue-eyed blonde people, so we must assume they are at best heterozygous for these attributes. Thus only 1 in 4 of their embryos will fit their pigmentary aspirations. Out go three, leaving them with just one. What a pity it happens to grow into a man 160 cm tall with an IQ of 95!

The 'designer baby' example just quoted shows that there is very little mileage in embryo selection. However, if the gene therapy technique of *Figure 14.8* were applied to the embryos of *Figure 14.4*, the story might be very different. Suppose that one day in the future all the limitations of gene manipulation had been overcome, so that any desired genetic alteration could be achieved safely and with high efficiency. Perhaps babies really could be designed to order. Maybe ambitious parents could browse a catalog of desirable human characters and place their order. Moving further into science fiction territory, why stop at existing human characters? Like every new technology, this would bring risks as well as benefits. The ethical problems would be mind-boggling. But it is important to remind ourselves that this is science fiction and not everything in science fiction ever gets developed in reality – for example, we already know that time travel, as imagined by Hollywood, will never be developed. Unless every gene transfer into an embryo worked with 100% efficiency and 100% safety, attempts at multiple manipulation would run into the same problem of diminishing returns as embryo selection. And unless every one of the 100–150 cells in the inner cell mass of a blastocyst could be manipulated, the resulting baby might just be a low-level mosaic for the designed genotype. In short, while we must remain alert to new possibilities, moral panic about genetics is misplaced. For the foreseeable future, clinical genetics services will remain a small but important part of normal medicine, bringing great and ever-increasing benefits to those families needing them, while genetic science will increasingly become the foundation of much broader medical practice.

14.5. **References**

American Society of Human Genetics (1975) Genetic counseling. *Am. J. Hum. Genet.* **27**: 240–242.

Bachoud-Lévi A-C, Gaura V, Brugieies P *et al.* (2006) Effect of fetal neural transplants in patients with Huntington's disease 6 years after surgery: a long-term follow-up study. *Lancet Neurol.* **5**: 303–309.

Bianchi DW, Simpson JL, Jackson LG, *et al.* (2002) Fetal gender and aneuploidy detection using fetal cells in maternal blood: analysis of NIFTY I data. *Prenat. Diag.* **22**: 609–615.

Bundy S and Aslam H (1993) A five year prospective study of the health of children in different ethnic groups with particular reference to the effect of inbreeding. *Eur. J. Hum. Genet.* **1**: 206–219.

Fan HC, Blumenfeld YJ, Chitkara U, Hudgins L and Quake SR (2008) Noninvasive diagnosis of fetal aneuploidy by shotgun sequencing DNA from maternal blood. *Proc. Natl Acad. Sci. USA,* **105**: 16266–16271.

Modell B, Ward RH and Fairweather DV (1980) Effect of introducing antenatal diagnosis on reproductive behaviour of families at risk for thalassaemia major. *Br. Med. J.* **280**: 1347–1350.

Munnich A (2006) Advances in genetics: what are the results for patients? *J. Med. Genet.* **43**: 555–556.

RCOG (2003) Guideline number 17: The investigation and treatment of couples with recurrent miscarriage: www.rcog.org.uk/womens-health/guidelines [accessed 3 August 10].

RCOG (2007) Guideline number 13: Chickenpox in pregnancy: www.rcog.org. uk/womens-health/guidelines [accessed 3 August 10].

RCOG (2009) Scientific Advisory Committee Opinion paper 15: Noninvasive prenatal diagnosis using cell-free DNA in maternal blood: www.rcog.org.uk/ womens-health/guidelines [accessed 3 August 10].

Tibben A (2002) Genetic counseling and presymptomatic testing. In: *Huntington Disease*, 3rd edn, eds Bates G, Harper PS and Jones L. Oxford University Press, Oxford.

Recommended textbooks

Clinical Genetics. Oxford Desk Reference (2005). Firth HV and Hurst JA. Oxford University Press, Oxford.

Emery and Rimoin's Principles and Practice of Medical Genetics, 5th edn (2006). Rimoin DC, Connor JM, Pyeritz RE and Korf BR. Churchill Livingstone, Edinburgh.

Gorlin's Syndrome of the Head and Neck, 5th edn (2010). Hennekam RCM, Krantz ID and Allanson JE (eds). Oxford University Press, Oxford.

Management of Genetic Syndromes, 3rd edn (2010). Cassidy SB and Allanson JE. Wiley-Blackwell, Oxford.

Practical Genetic Counselling, 6th edn. (2004) Harper PS. Hodder Arnold, London.

14.6. Self-assessment questions

(1) A woman has a son with Duchenne muscular dystrophy. There are no previous cases in the family, there are no other children and the mother is an only child. She might be a carrier, or the boy might be a new mutation. Calculate the chance that she is a carrier. (See the *Guidance* for two ways of doing this important calculation.)

(2) This calculation uses the carrier risk, 2/3, calculated in the previous question. The woman has another child, a girl. Calculate the risk the girl is a carrier.

(3) The woman in *SAQ2* has two more children, both unaffected boys. Does this alter your estimate of her carrier risk? If so, use a Bayesian calculation to calculate her revised risk.

(4) A man comes from a large family in which an autosomal dominant condition is segregating. His mother is affected but he is healthy. The condition is 90% penetrant, so he might either not have inherited the disease allele or he might be a non-penetrant case. He marries. Calculate the risk that his first child will be clinically affected by the disease.

(5) Generalize the result of *SAQ4* for a condition with penetrance x, and calculate the maximum risk that such a person would have an affected child, if x could have any value.

(6) Your mother has Huntington disease. You are healthy at age 45. If half of people who have inherited the disease gene show symptoms by age 45, what is the chance that you have inherited the disease gene?

(7) Score each of the following statements as true or false:
(a) Empiric risks are used in counseling for non-mendelian diseases
(b) Empiric risks are based on mathematical simplifications
(c) Empiric risks embody no assumptions about genetic mechanisms
(d) Empiric risks are valid only for a particular population and time

(8) Outline proposals to develop gene therapy for (a) cystic fibrosis, (b) Duchenne muscular dystrophy, and (c) a rapidly growing brain tumor. In each case, consider the advantages and disadvantages of this condition as a target for gene therapy, the gene(s) and constructs you would use, which tissue or cells you would target and how.

Guidance on self-assessment questions

Chapter 1

SAQ 1, 2 and 3. Following the two questions as suggested in the text should lead you to a convincing answer. We are told that each disease is rare, so the chance of an unrelated person who marries into the family being a carrier (if the disease is recessive) is small.

Pedigree 3. Unlike every other pedigree in this book, this pedigree shows a real family. The disease is hemophilia A (OMIM 306700) and the family is Queen Victoria's. Queen Victoria is 1–2. The affected people are Leopold (II-1), Frederick (II-8), Leopold and Maurice Mountbatten (III-18, III-19), Rupert (IV-?), Alexis, Tsarevitch of Russia, murdered with his four sisters by the Bolsheviks in 1918 (IV-8), Waldemar and Henry of Prussia (IV-9, IV-11) and Alfonso and Gonzalo of Spain (IV-14, IV-19). V-1 is the present Queen Elizabeth II of Britain.

SAQ 4. This pedigree is ambiguous (you shouldn't be given one like this in an exam). Try each possible mode of inheritance. Don't be misled by the affected female, and don't jump to the conclusion that there is male to male transmission. An affected man has an affected son – but are you sure the son inherited his disease gene from his father? The risk for a child of IV-3 may depend on which mode of inheritance is correct.

Chapter 2

SAQ 1a. Consider events in oogenesis that could result in a missing X (egg fertilized by an X-bearing sperm) and events in spermatogenesis that could result in a sperm with either a missing X or a missing Y. Note that in reality, Turner syndrome is usually the result of anaphase lag rather than non-disjunction (see *Section 2.3*).

SAQ 2a. Use *Figure 2.8* to check whether the breakpoints are proximal (near the centromere) or distal (towards the telomere) on the chromosome arm. 2q22 is about one-quarter of the way down the long arm on chromosome 2 and 4q32 is about three-quarters of the way down the long arm of chromosome 4. Draw out the cross-shaped tetravalent formed when the two translocated chromosomes pair with their two normal counterparts. Draw it very roughly to scale, using different colors for the chromosome 2 and chromosome 4 sequences. Check that you are always pairing segments of matching color. Then draw out possible gametes. You could consider 3:1 segregation patterns as well as the 2:2 patterns shown in *Figure 2.17*.

Chapter 3

SAQ 2   CTCAAAAGCACGCTCCAGTTCCTCCAGCTG
            CAGCUGCAGGAACUGGAGCGUGCUUUUGAG

Remember that strands are anti-parallel but are always written in the 5′->3′ direction.

SAQ 3. Transcription starts at the start of exon 1. The first codon is the AUG initiation codon. Intron 1 starts at the end of exon 1.

SAQ 4. You could use a word processor to interleave and align the two sequences, or just compare them manually. Sequences present in the genomic DNA but absent in the mRNA are introns.

Chapter 4

SAQ 1a. First ask yourself, to get a 50 bp product, will the primers flank the underlined 50 nt sequence or will they lie inside it? Write in the complementary strand for the regions where your primers will anneal. Then put in all the 5′ and 3′ directions and remember that the primers will extend from their 3′ ends.

SAQ 4. Imagine you had one copy of each possible sequence n nucleotides long. There are 4^n such sequences, so the total length of all these would be $4^n \times n$. Look for a value of n such that this total $> 3\,000\,000\,000$. Of course, this exercise ignores the fact that the human genome is not a random sequence, and contains many repeated sequences – but it shows that a sequence does not need to be very long to be *potentially* unique within the human genome.

Chapter 5

SAQ 2. Hybridization is a property of single-stranded DNA. Double-stranded DNA doesn't hybridize to anything else.

SAQ 3. Remember that sequences must be read 5′ -> 3′. CTTAAG is not an *Eco*RI site. If you write in the complementary strand, you will notice that GAATTC, like most restriction sites, is palindromic – that is, it reads the same on both strands.

Chapter 6

SAQ 1. Ask whether each change would specifically cause a failure to transport chloride ions across apical cell membranes.

SAQ 2. Two of the changes are deletions of one or a few nucleotides. One change affects a splice site.

SAQ 3. A laboratory might report the last sequence variant as p.V29M but in fact it might very well affect splicing – it replaces the last nucleotide in exon 1, and a G at this position is part of the normal consensus splice site sequence.

SAQ 4. c.216C>G is a mis-sense mutation, p.172M – it creates an internal methionine codon. This is not an initiator codon: translation initiates at the first suitable AUG in the mRNA, and once initiated, further AUGs are just read as normal methionine codons.

Chapter 7

SAQ 1. Here is one possible pedigree. The condition is autosomal dominant and so it affects both sexes and the mutant gene can be transmitted by both sexes – but it is always non-penetrant when it is inherited from the mother.

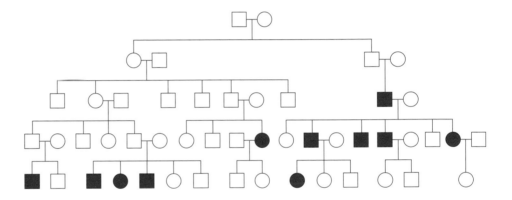

SAQ 6. This is the sequence recognized by the primer giving the 313 bp product in *Figure 7.14*. You can see all the sequences in the paper by Zeschnigk *et al.* (1997).

SAQ 7. There is an obligate crossover in every male meiosis between the Xp and Yp copies of the pseudoautosomal region. The crossover point might be proximal or distal to the location of the marker. You could try assuming that 50% of the crossovers are located between the centromere and the marker locus. In female meiosis crossovers within this region are quite uncommon.

Chapter 8

SAQ 2. Consider possible blocks in a multi-step pathway, or a block in post-translational processing (see *Section 8.4*).

SAQ 5. Eliza is homozygous for HLA-B27 and for HLA-DR4. You need to use the latter fact to work out the DR allele in each haplotype.

Chapter 9

SAQ 1. Although every meiosis may be recombinant or non-recombinant, only the meioses in the mother of the third generation are informative about this. The χ^2 result (3.6, 1 d.f.) is almost significant at the 5% level, while the lod score is well below the threshold for significance [L1 = $(\frac{1}{2})^{10}$; L2 = $(1 - \theta)^8 . (\theta)^2$; maximum lod score = 0.83 at $\theta = 0.2$]. The reason is that the lod score, but not the χ^2 test, takes into account the low prior probability of linkage. That is, given two loci picked at random, the chance they would show linkage is of the order of only 1 in 50 – they would probably be on different chromosomes, and even if they were on the same chromosome they might well be sufficiently far apart not to show linkage. Common sense tells us that we need to take the prior probability into account when deciding whether or not to believe something. For example, you may well believe your friend if he tells you that he missed a lecture because he overslept, but not if he tells you it was because he had been abducted by aliens. See Strachan and Read *Human Molecular Genetics* (Chapter 11 in the 2nd edn, available on the Internet, Chapter 13 in the 3rd edn.) for a brief explanation of how the lod score threshold includes the prior probability, or Ott, *Analysis of Human Genetic Linkage* for full details.

SAQ 2. Work out the haplotypes, starting with generation 2. The marker alleles have been chosen in this example to allow unambiguous haplotypes to be assigned to each individual. You can then identify which haplotype in individual II-1 is linked to the disease locus (remember we have been told that the disease is linked to this chromosomal region). When you examine the paternal haplotypes in generation III you can see that individuals III-3 and III-5 have inherited recombinant paternal disease-carrying haplotypes. The positions of crossovers show that the disease locus must map below marker A (from III-3) but above marker C (from III-5). III-6 has a recombinant maternal haplotype. The crossover might be anywhere between markers A and D. This recombinant does not provide any data for mapping the disease locus.

SAQ 4. The combination of deafness and diabetes is known sometimes to be caused by mutations in the mitochondrial DNA. NB Although it is sensible to attempt this sort of prioritization, when the causative gene is finally found, often it is not one of the more obvious candidates.

Chapter 10

SAQ 2. Remember that only people who are homozygous at one or other locus are affected; people who are heterozygous at two or more loci are unaffected. In reality, as explained, it would be unwise to rely on Hardy-Weinberg figures for such a rare recessive condition.

SAQ 3. You could try solving this by saying $p^2 + 2pq = 0.64$; substitute (1-p) for q, and you get a quadratic equation to solve for p. It can be done – but it is a lot easier to start by noting that $q^2 = 0.36$

SAQ 4. Treat the first part as a 3-allele Hardy–Weinberg problem, as in *Box 10.1*, with non-functioning, low functioning and normal alleles.

SAQ 5. Remember the difference between obligate carriers and possible carriers.

SAQ 6. Genetic counseling is non-directive.

Chapter 11

SAQ 4. You may be surprised that the odds ratios for the two cases are different:
- for variant A $(750 \times 500)/(500 \times 250)$
- for variant B $(75 \times 950)/(50 \times 925)$

  This is a point to bear in mind when interpreting the relative risk conferred by a variant. The more common a variant is, the more extreme the odds ratio (that is, the further away from 1, whether >1 or <1). Odds ratios approach the intuitive relative risk only for rare variants. Many SNPs in genome-wide association studies are common.

SAQ 5. Estimate the relative numbers by counting squares under the appropriate part of each curve. The curves have been drawn having equal total areas, but remember that the curve for NTD should really have 1/100 the area of the normal curve.

SAQ 6. The risk before any screening that a couple are both carriers is $1/40 \times 1/40 = 1/1600$. We need to calculate the sensitivity of a test such that when the partner tests negative, there is only a 1 in 1600 chance that this is a false negative. You can see from *Table 11.1* that this is not readily achievable.

Chapter 12

SAQ 1. In regard to Statement 8, although it is generally true that mutations in oncogenes are somatic and not inherited, there are a few exceptions. Inherited mutations in the *RET* oncogene are found in familial thyroid cancer. If a gene product has more than one function it may be simplistic to talk simply of loss or gain of function. Equally, the classification of genes into oncogenes and tumor suppressor genes is a very useful tool for thinking about the molecular pathology of cancer, but it has its limitations.

SAQ 3. If the chance of a mutation in one cell is μ and there are N target cells, the overall chance one cell will acquire a mutation is $N\mu$. This is equal to the penetrance in somebody who has inherited one mutation. $N\mu = 0.9$, $\mu = 2 \times 10^{-4}$, so $N = 4500$. The incidence of sporadic cases is $N\mu^2$. This calculation no doubt grossly simplifies the biological reality.

SAQ 4. Using the scoring system of *Table 12.4*, simply adding up points across each pedigree gives a 12% chance of a *BRCA1* mutation in family A and a 14% chance in family B. But all 12 points in family A come from the paternal side, while in family B the paternal side has 9 points and the maternal side has 5. If there is a *BRCA* mutation, it is most likely to come from the father, but the likelihood is only 9%. This is of course a rather contrived example.

Chapter 13

SAQ 1. The familial eating habits might be learned or genetic. Opposite sex twins are all dizygotic, while like-sex twins may be either monozygotic or dizygotic. The first three observations all suggest genetic factors. The adoption data give the cleanest separation of genetic from environmental effects, though the Barker hypothesis (see *Chapter 7*) would sound a caution against drawing dogmatic conclusions.

SAQ 2. Because the disease is commoner in men than in women, the risk is always higher for a son than a daughter of a given person. The logic of *Box 13.1* dictates that the risk is higher for a child of an affected woman than for a child of the same sex of an affected man. Because Betty has two affected male first-degree relatives she is likely to have a higher susceptibility than Anne, so the risk for her child is greater.

SAQ 3. If the recombination fraction is θ, after n generation a proportion $(1-\theta)^n$ remain associated.

SAQ 7. This is the multiple testing problem and a Bonferroni correction is appropriate. Sometimes it is hard to decide how many questions were asked. If a marker has n alleles, and you check each for association, is that one question, or n or $n-1$? The Bonferroni correction is over-rigorous if the questions are not fully independent. If you look not only for associations with individual marker alleles but also with multi-marker haplotypes, are those extra independent questions? If you use linkage analysis and you know that there are susceptibility loci somewhere in the genome, each negative result reduces the area of the genome where the susceptibility factor(s) must be hiding – so are tests of the few remaining areas independent? In short, the multiple testing problem is severe in complex disease studies and requires expert statistical insight.

SAQ 9. For the 2–1 × 1–1 parents the mendelian proportions among the sibs must be modified by the fact that you have selected pairs that were both affected. This is most easily done by a Bayesian calculation, with the mendelian proportions as the prior probability and the fact that both sibs are affected as a conditional:

Genotypes of sibs:	(1–1, 1–1)		(1–1, 2–1)		(2–1, 2–1)
Prior probability	¼		½		¼
Conditional likelihood (both affected):	16	:	8	:	4
Joint likelihood	4	:	4	:	1
Final probability:	4/9		4/9		1/9

For an explanation of this method see *Box 14.1*.

Chapter 14

SAQ 1. This is an important basic calculation in genetic risk estimation so we show it in detail. There are two ways of arriving at the answer, which applies to any X-linked recessive condition where affected males never reproduce.

(a) If the population contains equal numbers of males, who each have one X chromosome, and females who each have two, then one-third of all X chromosomes are in males. Equally, one-third of all DMD X chromosomes are in males. Any DMD X chromosome that is in a male will not be transmitted to the next generation, thus one-third of all DMD X chromosomes are lost each generation. If the disease frequency remains constant over the generations, this must be balanced by new mutations. Thus one-third of cases are new mutations, so the chance that the mother of an isolated case is a carrier is 2/3.

(b) An alternative method starts by calculating the probability that any woman, picked completely at random, is a carrier of DMD. Call this probability P. Suppose she has a daughter. The probability that the daughter is a carrier is made of three parts:

- She might be a carrier because her mother is a carrier and she has inherited her mother's mutated X. The probability of this is $P/2$.
- She might be a carrier because although her mother was not a carrier, the X she received from her carried a new DMD mutation. Call the mutation probability μ.
- She might be a carrier because the X she received from her father carries a new DMD mutation. Again the probability of this is μ.

The daughter's overall carrier risk is $P/2 + 2\mu$. But our original woman was selected completely at random; exactly the same logic could have been applied to her and her mother. The carrier risk of the mother and daughter must actually be the same (if it weren't, by repeating the exercise over enough generations, you could get the risk to either 0 or 100%, which would be absurd). Therefore $P = P/2 + 2\mu$, from which we see that $P = 4\mu$.

Now we have worked out the prior probability that a woman is a DMD carrier, we can return to the original question and do a Bayesian calculation of the carrier risk of the woman who has a son with DMD. Either she is a carrier or she is not. The calculation goes as follows:

Woman is:	a carrier	not a carrier
Prior probability:	4μ	$1-4\mu \approx 1$
Conditional: affected boy	$\frac{1}{2}$	μ
Joint probability:	2μ	μ
Final probability	$2\mu/3\mu = 2/3$	$\mu/3\mu = 1/3$

SAQ 2. The daughter's risk is half the mother's risk – there is a 1 in 2 chance she will inherit her mother's 'risk' X rather than the other one.

SAQ 3.

- *Method 1*: repeat the calculation of SAQ1, adding in an extra line of conditionals for the two unaffected boys. Given that she is a carrier, the chance of having two unaffected boys is 1 in 4. Given that she is not a carrier, it is 1–2μ, which is effectively 1.
- *Method 2*: start with her 2/3 carrier risk as your prior probability. In that case, this has already used the information that she has an affected boy, so the only conditional likelihoods are for the unaffected boys.

This illustrates the fact that it doesn't matter which pieces of information you put as prior probabilities and which as conditionals, just as long as you use each piece of information once and only once.

SAQ 4. First you need to calculate the chance that the man is a non-penetrant carrier. Use a Bayesian calculation. The prior probability is his mendelian 1 in 2 risk, the conditional is the fact that he is clinically unaffected. Having got his risk, the risk his son has inherited the disease gene is half the risk the father carries it. Then remember that even if the child inherits the gene there is only a 90% chance he will be clinically affected.

SAQ 5. The formula is $\frac{1}{2} \times \frac{(1-x)}{(2-x)}$. The answer, 8.6% risk for 59% penetrance, is surprisingly and reassuringly low. If a condition has low penetrance, this increases the risk the unaffected father may carry the disease gene, but at the same time it reduces the risk the child will be clinically affected if it does inherit the gene.

SAQ 6. The 'obvious' answer, 1 in 4, is wrong. Use Bayes to get the correct answer.

Glossary

3′ untranslated sequence – in a messenger RNA, the part downstream of the stop codon.

5′ untranslated sequence – in a messenger RNA, the part upstream of the translation initiation (AUG) codon.

Acrocentric – of a chromosome, having the centromere close to (but not at) one end. In humans, chromosomes 13, 14, 15, 21 and 22.

Acute transforming retrovirus – a small RNA virus, part of whose genome has been replaced by an activated oncogene (see *Figure 12.4b*).

Affected sib pair (ASP) method – a model-free method of linkage analysis that seeks chromosomal segments which pairs of brothers or sisters who have the same disease share more often than by chance (see *Table 13.3*).

Alleles – alternative forms of a gene.

Allelic heterogeneity – the situation where a clinical condition can be caused by any of several (often very many) different mutations within a certain gene. Characteristic of loss of function conditions (cf. **locus heterogeneity**).

Alternative splicing – alternative choices of which segments of an RNA primary transcript are retained in the mature messenger RNA (see *Figure 3.11*).

Amniotic fluid – the fluid surrounding a fetus, contained by the amnion.

Analytical validity – of a test, the extent to which it measures that which it claims to measure.

Anaphase – the phase of cell division (mitosis or meiosis) in which chromosomes or chromatids separate and are pulled to opposite poles of the cell.

Aneuploid – of a cell, not **euploid**; having missing or extra chromosomes.

Anneal – of complementary single strands of nucleic acid, to hybridize forming a base-paired double helix.

Anticipation – the tendency of a disease to become more severe, more frequent, or to start at an earlier age, in successive generations. Often an artifact of biased ascertainment.

Apoptosis – a specific mechanism by which a cell kills itself.

Association – the statistical tendency of two things to go together more often or less often than by random chance. The combination occurs at a frequency that is not equal to the product of the individual frequencies.

Assortative mating – choosing a mate who is genetically similar to oneself. Can be based either on having a similar phenotype or on being related.

Autosome – any chromosome that is not the X or Y sex chromosome.

Autozygosity mapping – mapping a recessive condition in inbred kindreds by finding a shared ancestral chromosome segment that is homozygous in all the affected people (see *Figure 9.8*).

Balanced – of a chromosomal constitution, having nothing extra or missing. Also used loosely of Robertsonian translocations, even though these lack part of the short arms of the acrocentric chromosomes involved.

Bias of ascertainment – collecting a sample that is statistically unrepresentative of the larger population.

Bisulfite sequencing – a method of identifying unmethylated cytosines in DNA; after treatment with sodium bisulfite they are converted to uracil, which is scored as thymine on sequencing (see *Figure 7.10*).

Bonferroni correction – a rigorous statistical correction for multiple testing, consisting of multiplying the *P* value for an observation by the number of different questions asked.

cDNA – complementary DNA; a DNA copy of messenger RNA made using reverse transcriptase. Human cDNAs represent only 1–3% of the genomic DNA but contain most (but not all) of the clinically relevant sequences. Unlike genomic DNA, cDNAs are tissue-specific.

Cascade screening – ascertaining gene carriers by systematic testing of the extended family of an affected person (see *Disease box 11*).

Cell cycle checkpoint – a regulatory interaction that prevents a cell progressing through the cell cycle unless certain conditions are met (see *Figure 12.8*).

Centromere – the point at which the sister chromatids of a replicated chromosome are joined, and the location of the kinetochore, to which spindle fibers attach during cell division. Marked by heterochromatin containing a special histone H3 variant, CENP-A protein.

Chimera – of a person, having cells derived from two different zygotes – a rare condition, the opposite of twinning. Of a gene, made by a chromosomal rearrangement that brings together exons of two different genes to form a novel gene. A common occurrence in cancer (see *Box 12.3*).

Chorionic villi – outgrowths of fetal origin on the external surface of the chorion, the outermost of the fetal membranes.

Chromatid – a single DNA double helix packaged into a chromosome. Chromosomes normally exist as a single chromatid, but when they are seen during cell division they consist of two sister chromatids joined at the centromere.

Chromatin – a general term for the DNA–protein complex of which chromosomes consist.

Chromatin disease – a disease caused by faulty regulation of chromatin structure (see *Disease box 2*).

Chromosomal instability – accumulation of structural and/or numerical chromosome abnormalities in abnormal (e.g. cancer) cells.

Coefficient of inbreeding – the probability that a person is homozygous at any given locus because of the inbreeding of his parents. Equal to half the coefficient of relationship of the parents.

Coefficient of relationship – the proportion of their genes that two people share by virtue of having identifiable common ancestors (see *Section 10.2*).

Common disease–common variant hypothesis – the hypothesis that most genetic susceptibility factors for common complex diseases are ancient variants that are common in the general population. The hypothesis underlying attempts to identify susceptibility alleles by association studies.

The contrary hypothesis is that susceptibility is due to a heterogeneous collection of recent mutations.

Comparative genomic hybridization – (CGH) – a technique for detecting sequences anywhere in the genome that are present in an abnormal number of copies (see *Figures 4.7* and *4.8*).

Compound heterozygote – a person with a recessive condition who has two different mutant versions of the relevant gene.

Congenital – present at birth; not necessarily genetic.

Consensus sequence – of a family of related sequences, the sequence having the most common nucleotide at each position (which may or may not be the most common actual whole sequence).

Conserved sequences – sequences that are unchanged or little changed in related species.

Copy number variant (CNV) – a form of DNA variation in which a certain sequence (which may be anything from a few bp to megabases) is present in differing numbers of copies in different individuals. The copies are usually present as tandem repeats, but may be dispersed. Many CNVs are non-pathogenic common variants.

Cousin – in genetics, used specifically to mean first cousin (q.v.).

CpG dinucleotide – a cytosine immediately upstream of a guanine in a DNA sequence. The target of DNA methylating enzymes, and hotspots for CpG→TpG mutations.

CpG islands – short chromosomal regions (typically less than 1 kb) where the usual genome-wide depletion of CpG dinucleotides has not taken place. See *Section 7.4* for their significance.

Cryptic splice site – a sequence in an exon or an intron that resembles a splice site but not sufficiently to be used as one; a mutation may change it so that it does get used as a splice site ('activating a cryptic splice site').

Denaturing – separating the two strands of a double helix by heat or high pH; also called melting.

Denaturing high performance liquid chromatography (dHPLC) – a method of testing a PCR product or other double-stranded DNA fragment for changes, compared to a reference fragment, by checking the speed with which it passes through a column.

Diagnostic test – a test that establishes the diagnosis in a patient affected by a disease (cf. a **predictive test**, a **screening test**).

Dichotomous character – a character such as a disease, that some people have and others do not (cf. **quantitative** or **continuous characters**, that everybody has).

Dideoxynucleotide (ddNTP) – a chemically modified nucleotide used in DNA sequencing to terminate growing DNA chains (see *Figure 5.2*).

Diploid – of a cell or organism, having two genomes. The normal condition of human somatic cells.

Dominant – a character is dominant if it is manifest in a heterozygote. Dominance and recessiveness are properties of characters, not of genes or alleles.

Dominant negative – a mutation where the product of the mutant allele interferes with the function of the normal product in a heterozygote.

Dosage-sensitive – of a gene, where different non-zero copy numbers have an effect on the phenotype.

Dot blotting – a hybridization test in which either the test DNA or the probe is spotted on to a solid support to immobilize it.

Downstream – on a nucleic acid strand, in the 3′ direction (of the sense strand in a gene).

Driver mutation – a mutation that contributes to the evolution of a tumor and is subject to positive selection during tumor development.

Dysmorphology – the study of congenital malformations and syndromes.

Embryonic stem cell (ES cell) – a totipotent stem cell obtained from the inner cell mass of a blastocyst (see *Figure 14.6*).

Empiric risks – risks defined by survey data, as distinct from risks worked out by applying genetic theory.

ENCODE Project – an international collaborative project (Encyclopedia of DNA Elements, www.genome.gov/10005107) that aims to identify all functions of human DNA (see *Section 6.2*).

Epigenetic – making heritable (from cell to daughter cell, or sometimes from generation to generation) changes in gene expression without changing the nucleotide sequence. Effected by DNA methylation and/or changing chromatin structure.

Epimutation – a mutation that causes an epigenetic change but not a DNA sequence change.

Episome – an extrachromsomal genetic element.

Euchromatin – chromatin with a relatively open structure in which genes can be active if suitable transcription factors and co-activators are present; the opposite of **heterochromatin**.

Euploid – of a cell, containing some number of complete chromosome sets, without any extra or missing chromosomes. The opposite of aneuploid.

Exome – the totality of all exons in a genome.

Exon – a segment of genomic DNA that corresponds to sequence in a mature mRNA. Exons include the 5′ and 3′ untranslated regions of a gene as well as the coding sequence.

Expression array – a microarray of oligonucleotides or cDNAs that will hybridize to individual mRNAs or cDNAs. When hybridized to bulk cDNA from a cell or tissue the pattern of hybridization reflects the repertoire of mRNAs in the source material (see *Sections 4.4* and *12.4*).

Familial – tending to run in families; not necessarily genetic.

Fetal exclusion test – a linkage-based method of telling whether or not a fetus is at risk of inheriting a late-onset dominant disease present in a grandparent, without doing a predictive test on the parent (see *Figure 9.10*).

First cousins – Jack and Jill are first cousins if one of Jack's parents is the sib of one of Jill's parents.

Fluorescence *in situ* hybridization (FISH) – *in situ* hybridization using a fluorescently labeled DNA or RNA probe (see *Figures 4.6, 4.14* and *4.15*).

Founder effects – an unusually high frequency of a particular allele or haplotype in a population that is descended from a small number of founders, one or more of whom happened to carry that sequence.

Fragile site – in a chromosome preparation, a region that appears relatively uncoiled and extended. Usually only seen under specific culture conditions, e.g. after treatment with bromodeoxyuridine or aphidicolin. Most fragile sites exist as non-pathogenic polymorphic variants. The FRAXA and FRAXE fragile sites (see *Disease box 4*) are unusual in being pathogenic.

Frame-shift mutation – a mutation that alters the reading frame of a coding sequence (see *Box 3.3* and *Section 6.2*).

Functional genomics – studying the functions of all the genes in a genome or all the genes expressed in a cell or tissue.

G-banding – a standard procedure in which chromosomes are treated so that they stain in a characteristic and reproducible pattern of dark and pale bands, as shown in *Figure 2.5*.

Gene conversion – a process in which a short stretch (typically 100 bp) of DNA sequence in a gene is replaced with similar but not identical sequence from another allele or gene. A recombination-like process but non-reciprocal – the donor gene is unchanged (see *Box 8.2*).

Gene frequency – the gene frequency of allele A_n is the proportion of all alleles of the A gene in a certain population that are A_n.

Gene pool – the totality of alleles at a particular locus in a certain population.

Gene tracking – using linked polymorphic markers to follow the segregation of a chromosomal segment through a pedigree. Used to follow a pathogenic mutation when, for any reason, it is not possible to check for the mutation directly by sequencing (see *Figure 9.9*).

Genetic drift – a change in gene frequencies between generations because of chance differences between the gene frequencies in one generation and the genes in the gametes that go to make the next generation. Only happens if the number of gametes is small, i.e. the breeding population is very small.

Genome – the totality of genetic material of an organism.

Genomic – of DNA, the DNA as it occurs in the cell nucleus, in contrast to cDNA.

Germ-line – the lineage of cells that are potentially transmissible to the next generation. In humans and other animals the germ-line separates from somatic cells very early in embryogenesis.

Germinal mosaic – a person who, owing to a mutation that occurred after they were conceived, has a mutant cell population in their germ-line, so that they can produce recurrent mutant gametes. A major pitfall in pedigree interpretation and risk estimation.

GWAS – genome-wide association study; a study in which SNPs spread across the genome are tested for association with a disease in a case-control study.

Haploid – of a cell or organism, having only a single genome (i.e. 23 chromosomes in humans).

Haplo-insufficiency – the condition in which a single functional copy of a gene is not sufficient to produce a normal phenotype, so that loss of function mutations in the gene produce a dominant character.

Haplotype – a set of closely linked alleles on a chromosome that is normally inherited as a block.

HapMap project – an international collaborative project that aims to catalog all the conserved ancestral chromosome segments in several different human populations (see *Section 13.4* and http://hapmap.ncbi.nlm.nih.gov).

Hardy–Weinberg distribution – the mathematical relationship between gene frequencies and genotype frequencies seen when no distorting factors are present. Seldom applies in humans to rare recessive conditions where many cases are due to consanguinity (see *Box 10.1*).

Heritability – the extent to which differences between people with respect to a character (in a particular population at a particular time) are due to the genetic differences between them. Heritabilities are correlation coefficients, symbolized as h^2 and taking values between 0 (no genetic influence) and 1 (wholly determined by genetic differences) (see *Section 13.2*).

Heterochromatin – chromatin that is highly condensed and genetically inactive. Found mainly at centromeres.

Heteroduplex – a DNA double helix containing mismatches (see *Figure 5.8a*).

Heteroplasmy – of a person, having two or more genetically different types of mitochondria.

Histone code – the idea that combinations of different covalent modifications of histones in nucleosomes determine the structure and activity of chromatin.

Homologous chromosomes – the two No. 1 chromosomes, etc. in a person. Homologous chromosomes contain the same array of loci but, unlike sister chromatids, they are not copies of each other. They may differ in small ways (minor DNA sequence differences) or sometimes in large ways (because of translocations, etc.).

Homozygous – having both alleles at a locus the same. The criteria used to assess identity may be more or less stringent, depending on the question being addressed.

Hybridize – of complementary single strands of nucleic acid, to anneal forming a base-paired double helix.

Informative meiosis – in linkage analysis, a meiosis where the genotypes allow it to be scored as recombinant or non-recombinant.

Intron – a segment of a gene that is part of the primary transcript but is excised by the splicing machinery and is not included in the mature mRNA.

Inversion – a structural abnormality in which part of a chromosome is in the wrong orientation compared to the rest (see *Figure 2.19*).

Karyogram – the correct term for a display of somebody's chromosomes, like in *Figure 2.9*. Usually loosely called a karyotype.

Karyotype – a person's chromosome constitution – also used loosely to describe a display of a person's chromosomes, as in *Figure 2.9*, etc.

Lepore – Lepore-type genes are chimeric genes produced by non-homologous recombination. Named after the hemoglobin β–δ chimeric gene that produces Hb–Lepore.

Library – in molecular genetics, a random collection of cloned fragments of a complex starting material (DNA or mRNA). The main types are genomic libraries and cDNA libraries (see *Box 4.4*).

Linkage – the phenomenon whereby loci that are close together on a chromosome tend to segregate together in families. The extent of the tendency (between random segregation and invariable co-segregation) measures the genetic distance in centiMorgans (between 0 and 50 cM) between the loci.

Linkage disequilibrium – a population association of particular alleles at two or more loci. Seen when the loci are closely linked and the alleles are features of a shared ancestral chromosome segment.

Locus – the position of a gene on a chromosome; a type of gene (as distinct from alleles, which are variant forms of the same type of gene).

Locus control region – a DNA sequence located many kilobases away from the transcription start site of a gene that controls the expression of a gene or group of genes (see *Section 3.4*).

Locus heterogeneity – the situation where a clinical phenotype can be caused by mutations at any one of several different loci, cf. **allelic heterogeneity**.

Lod score – the statistical measure of the significance of evidence for or against linkage. Equals the logarithm (base 10) of the odds that the loci are linked, with a given recombination fraction, rather than not linked (see *Section 9.2*).

Loss of heterozygosity – in cancer research, the observation that tumor DNA is apparently homozygous for a DNA polymorphism for which the normal DNA of the same patient is heterozygous. Usually the result of loss of a chromosome. If seen repeatedly, implies that the chromosome in question carries a tumor suppressor gene (see *Figure 12.7*).

Lyonization – X-inactivation (see *Figure 7.4*).

Lysosomal storage disease – an inborn error of metabolism where lysosomes are unable to degrade a certain type of material. As a result the material accumulates in lysosomes, leading to pathological effects.

Manifesting heterozygote – with an X-linked recessive condition, a female carrier who shows some clinical signs of the condition, most likely because by chance she has inactivated her good X in most cells of the affected tissue.

Mendelian – the manner in which genes and traits are passed from parents to their children. The four modes of mendelian inheritance are: autosomal dominant, autosomal recessive, X-linked dominant, and X-linked recessive. The term "mendelian" refers to Gregor Mendel (1822–84) who formulated the laws forming the foundation of classical genetics.

Meta-analysis – analysis of the combined data from a number of separate studies.

Metacentric – a chromosome that has its centromere in the middle (e.g. numbers 3 and 20).

Metaphase – the stage of mitosis or meiosis immediately before anaphase, when chromosomes are maximally contracted and aligned on the equatorial plane (metaphase plate) of the cell.

Methylation – attaching methyl (CH_3) groups to any molecule, but particularly used for converting cytosine in a CpG dinucleotide to 5-methyl cytosine as part of gene regulation (see *Figure 7.8*).

Methylation-sensitive restriction enzyme – a restriction enzyme such as *Hpa*II that will only cut unmethylated recognition sites (see *Section 7.2*).

Microarray – a solid support divided into a large number of cells in each of which a specific test sample or reagent has been anchored, allowing a large number of tests to be carried out in parallel. Microarrays of oligonucleotides, cDNAs, antibodies or tumor samples are widely used in genetic research.

Microdeletion – a chromosomal deletion that is too small (< 3–5 Mb) to be seen on a standard chromosome preparation; Detected by **fluorescence *in situ***

hybridization, comparative genomic hybridization, or **multiplex ligation-dependent probe amplification**.

Microsatellites – short tandem DNA repeats where the repeat unit is 1–6 nucleotides (tandem repeats with longer repeat units are called mini-satellites). Polymorphic microsatellites are one of the main types of DNA marker for linkage analysis.

Microsatellite instability – a property of tumors that are deficient in repair of DNA mismatches caused by replication errors. Compared to the normal DNA of the patient, tumor DNA contains new alleles of many microsatellites from all across the genome.

Mismatch repair – a protein complex, including the MSH2 and MLH1 proteins, checks newly replicated DNA for wrongly incorporated nucleotides, cuts them out and re-synthesizes that stretch of the DNA.

Modifier gene – a gene that modifies the phenotype of a mendelian condition whose primary cause is a different gene.

Monosomy – having one copy of one particular chromosome, but two of all the others (i.e. 45 in total for an autosomal monosomy).

Mosaic – having two or more genetically different cell lines. A person can be mosaic for a chromosomal variant or a single-gene change.

Multifactorial – a catch-all term to describe a character that is determined by many factors including several genes and environmental factors.

Multiplex ligation-dependent probe amplification (MLPA) – a method for simultaneously checking a large number (30–50) of short DNA sequences for copy number variations. Used especially for checking multi-exon genes for any whole-exon deletion (see *Figures 5.9* and *5.10*).

Next-generation sequencing – a collective name for different technologies that conduct millions of sequencing reactions in parallel, thereby generating vastly more sequence data per run than Sanger sequencing.

Non-parametric linkage analysis – linkage analysis that is based on the extent to which affected relatives share chromosomal segments, but does not depend on a specific genetic model for the cause of the phenotype (see *Section 13.2*).

Nonsense-mediated decay – a mechanism in cells that breaks down most mRNA molecules which contain a stop codon located more than 50 nucleotides upstream of the 3′-most splice site. Probably evolved to protect cells against dominant negative effects of truncated proteins (see *Figure 6.3*).

Nonsense mutation – a mutation that converts a codon for an amino acid into a stop codon (UAA, UAG or UGA in mRNA; TAA, TAG or TGA in the DNA).

Northern blotting – analyzing RNA by gel electrophoresis, transferring to a membrane and hybridizing to a labeled probe.

Nucleoside – a combination of a base and a sugar.

Nucleosome – the basic unit of chromatin, comprising 146 bp of DNA wrapped round a core consisting of two molecules each of histones H2A, H2B, H3 and H4.

Nucleotide – a combination of a base, a sugar and a phosphate.

Obligate carrier – a person whose pedigree shows that they must be a carrier of a recessive (autosomal or X-linked) condition. For X-linked conditions where new mutations are frequent, an obligate carrier must have affected or carrier relatives both in her own or a previous generation, and among her children or grandchildren. Having more than one affected child does not make a woman an obligate carrier because she might be a germinal mosaic.

Odds ratio – in a case–control study, the relative odds of a case and a control having a given variant (see *Box 11.1*).

Okazaki fragments – intermediates in DNA replication. As a replication fork moves along a double helix, one new strand growing in the $5'{\rightarrow}3'$ direction can grow continuously in the same direction as the movement of the fork, but the other is synthesized as a set of short (100–200 nucleotide) fragments that are later ligated together (see *Figure 12.3a*).

Oligonucleotide ('*oligo*') – a short piece of single-stranded DNA or RNA.

Oncogene – a gene that suffers gain of function mutations in cancer. Strictly applies only to the mutated version; the normal version is strictly called a **proto-oncogene**, but this distinction is often ignored.

One gene – one enzyme hypothesis – the hypothesis (defined by Beadle and Tatum in the 1940s) that the function of each gene is to direct synthesis of one specific enzyme. Now seen as only part of the story.

Passenger mutation – in tumorigenesis, a mutation that is the random result of the genetic instability of cancer cells, and which does not contribute to progression of the tumor.

Penetrance – the probability of a character being manifest, given a certain genotype. Penetrance is a property of a character or phenotype, not a gene or allele.

Pharmacogenetics – the study of single gene effects on the metabolism or action of a drug.

Pharmacogenomics – the genome-wide study of drug targets or drug effects.

Phenocopy – a phenotype that resembles a genetic phenotype, but is produced by non-genetic means.

Phenotype – the observable characteristic of a person (including the result of tests).

Pleiotropic – of a mutation, having effects on many systems.

Polygene – an unfortunate term sometimes used to describe the genes responsible for a polygenic character. Polygenes are not a different type of gene, they are ordinary genes that have variants which have a minor effect on some particular character. The same genes may have major effects on a different character.

Polygenic – in mathematical theory a polygenic character is determined by the combined action of an infinite number of genes, each of which has an infinitesimally small effect. In reality, polygenic effects can be due to just a handful of genes.

Population attributable risk (population attributable fraction) – of a cause of disease, the extent to which that particular cause is responsible for the overall incidence of the disease in the population.

Positional candidate – in identifying disease genes, a gene located in a chromosomal region identified by linkage as containing a disease gene.

Positional cloning – identifying a disease gene through linkage analysis followed by testing positional candidates for mutations; as compared to identifying the disease gene through investigation of the pathogenesis.

Positive predictive value – of a test result, the proportion of cases positive on the test that actually have the condition being sought (see *Box 11.1*).

Predictive test – a test that shows whether a currently healthy person is likely subsequently to develop a late-onset disease.

Pre-mutation – in diseases caused by expanded nucleotide repeats, an expansion that is not long enough to cause the disease, but is long enough to destabilize the repeat, so that later generations are affected (see *Disease box 4*).

Primary transcript – the initial RNA product of transcribing a gene. Contains all the exons and introns of the gene. The introns are cut out when the primary transcript is processed to form the mature mRNA.

Primer – in DNA synthesis, a short (10–40 nt) oligonucleotide that hybridizes to a single strand of DNA and that is then extended by DNA polymerase adding nucleotides to its 3′ end.

Prior probability – in Bayesian risk estimation, the initial estimate of how plausible each alternative hypothesis is.

Probe – a piece of single-stranded DNA labeled, for example, with ^{32}P or a fluorescent dye, that is used in a hybridization assay to test for the presence of a complementary sequence.

Prometaphase – late prophase of cell division. Cytogeneticists normally karyotype mitotic cells in prometaphase because the chromosomes are more extended than at metaphase and show the banding better.

Promoter – the DNA region immediately upstream of a gene on which the RNA polymerase complex is assembled to enable transcription of the gene.

Prophase – the first stage of mitosis or meiosis when the chromosomes are gradually condensing and becoming visible. Ends with the dissolution of the nuclear membrane.

Proteome – the complete set of proteins in a cell or tissue.

Proto-oncogene – the normal, unactivated version of an **oncogene**.

Pseudoautosomal region – the regions at the tips of the X and Y chromosome short arms that contain 2.6 Mb of homologous DNA and recombine in meiosis. Genes in this region show an autosomal pattern of inheritance. There is another short pseudoautosomal region at the tips of the long arms (see *Figure 7.5*).

Pseudogene – a non-functional copy of a gene. Pseudogenes are very common in the human genome.

QF-PCR – quantitative fluorescence-based PCR; used for rapidly checking a DNA sample for numerical chromosome abnormalities.

Quantitative character – a character like blood pressure that everybody has, but with varying magnitude. Sometimes called a continuous character, cf. **dichotomous character**.

Quantitative trait locus (QTL) – a locus that contributes to the phenotype of a quantitative character.

Random mating – a choice of mate unrelated to genotype; the opposite of **assortative mating**.

Real-time PCR – various methods by which the accumulation of a PCR product can be followed as the reaction proceeds. The basis of most quantitative PCR assays.

Recessive – a character is recessive if it is not manifest in a heterozygote. Recessiveness and dominance are properties of characters, not of genes or alleles.

Recombinant – a gamete produced by a person is recombinant for two loci if the two alleles that it carries came from different parents of the person.

Recombinant DNA – DNA produced by ligating together sequences derived from different sources – typically a human sequence of interest ligated into a vector.

Relative risk – the risk of a disease for a person with a specific genotype, or a specific relationship to an affected person, compared to the risk in the general population. Note that relative risks are quite distinct from absolute risks. A relative risk of 10 may be of no clinical significance if it only raises the absolute risk from 1 in 10 000 to 1 in 1000.

Reproductive cloning – a procedure that aims to produce a cloned baby (see *Section 14.4*).

Restriction endonuclease – an enzyme that cuts double-stranded DNA at a specific sequence, usually a 4- or 6-nucleotide palindrome.

Restriction fragment length polymorphism (RFLP) – a DNA polymorphism due to a nucleotide change that creates or abolishes the recognition site for a restriction enzyme (see for example, *Figure 5.15*).

Reverse dot blot – a **dot blot** where the probe rather than the test DNA is immobilized on the solid support. DNA **microarrays** are massively parallel reverse dot blots.

Robertsonian translocation – a special type of translocation in which two acrocentric chromosomes are joined close to their centromeres (see *Figure 2.20*).

ROC curve – receiver-operating characteristic curve; a graph of sensitivity vs. (1–specificity) of a test; the area under the curve is a measure of the discriminatory power of a test (see *Figure 13.15*).

RT–PCR – reverse transcriptase – polymerase chain reaction; a technique for making many DNA copies of an RNA. A common method for studying messenger RNA.

Screening test – a test used to select people at high risk from a population. Normally followed by a **diagnostic test** (see *Section 11.2*).

Second cousins – two people are second cousins if their parents are first cousins.

Sense strand – in a gene the strand of the double helix whose sequence corresponds to the sequence of the messenger RNA (the opposite of the template strand).

Sensitivity of a test – the proportion of people with the disease, etc. that is being sought, that the test picks up (see *Box 11.1*).

Sex-limited – a character that is seen in only one sex for anatomical or physiological reasons.

Sibs – brothers or sisters.

Signal peptide – the N-terminal dozen or so amino acid residues of a nascent protein that determine where it will be transported. Signal peptides are cleaved off once they have performed their function.

Single nucleotide polymorphism (SNP) – any polymorphic variation at a single nucleotide.

Single strand conformation polymorphism (SSCP) – a quick but fallible method for scanning a DNA fragment (up to 300 nt) for mutations (see *Figure 5.8b*).

Sister chromatids – the two chromatids of a chromosome as seen in a dividing cell. Sister chromatids are copies of each other, made during the preceding round of DNA replication.

Slipped-strand mis-pairing – a mistake in replication of a tandemly repeated sequence that results in the newly synthesized strand having extra or missing repeat units compared to the template.

SNP chip – a microarray of allele-specific oligonucleotides, used for genotyping many SNPs in a single operation. Can also be used to check for copy number variants.

Somatic mutation – a mutation in a cell of the body that will not be transmitted to offspring.

Southern blotting – analyzing DNA by restriction digestion, gel electrophoresis, transfer to a membrane and hybridizing to a labeled probe (see *Figure 4.5*).

Splice isoforms – alternative forms of a protein produced by alternative splicing of exons.

Stem cell – a cell that is capable both of self-replication and of giving rise to a variety of differentiated cell lineages (see *Figure 14.5*).

Stop codon – in a messenger RNA, a UAG, UGA or UAA codon that signals the ribosome to dissociate and cease extending the polypeptide chain; the corresponding sequence in a gene.

Submetacentric – of a chromosome, having a long arm and a short arm, e.g. most human chromosomes (the others are metacentric or acrocentric).

Tandem repeat – direct DNA sequence repeats that are adjacent to each other. Other types of repeats are inverted repeats (or palindromes) and dispersed repeats.

Telomerase – a ribonucleoprotein that can add TTAGGG units to the telomeres of chromosomes.

Telomere – the special structure that stabilizes the ends of chromosomes, comprising specific proteins complexed to tandemly repeated TTAGGG DNA sequences.

Template strand – in a gene, the strand of the double helix that base-pairs with the nascent RNA during transcription.

Teratogen – any agent that interferes with normal embryonic or fetal development.

Therapeutic cloning – a procedure that aims to produce embryonic stem cells genetically matched to a patient, in order to obtain cells or tissues for transplantation (see *Figure 14.7*).

***Trans*-acting** – of a genetic regulatory element, regulating a gene or genes that lie elsewhere in the genome (normally by making a diffusible regulatory product).

Transcription factor – a protein whose action is to facilitate transcription of a gene or genes by helping bring the RNA polymerase to the promoter.

Translocation – a structural abnormality in which two chromosomes swap non-homologous segments (see, for example, *Figure 2.14*).

Transmission disequilibrium test (TDT) – a test for association in the presence of linkage. Used in identifying disease susceptibility factors (see *Figure 13.14*).

Transposon – a 'jumping gene': a mobile genetic element that can move from one chromosomal location to another, either via excision or by making a mobile copy. They can be seen as a sort of intracellular virus. Transposons can be recognized by certain sequence features. About 50% of the human genome consists of transposons, but the great majority have accumulated mutations that destroy their ability to transpose.

Triploid – a cell or organism having three copies of the genome (in humans, 69 chromosomes). Normally lethal in animals including humans.

Trisomy – having three copies of one particular chromosome, but two of all the others, i.e. 47 in total. (see for example, *Figure 2.11*).

Trisomy rescue - the main mechanism producing uniparental disomy. A chance mitotic non-disjunction in a trisomic early embryo produces one cell with the correct chromosomal number, from which the whole baby develops (see *Figure 7.17*).

Tumor suppressor gene – a gene that suffers loss of function mutations in cancers.

Unbalanced – of a chromosomal abnormality, having extra or missing material, rather than just the correct material rearranged.

Uniparental disomy – having both copies of one chromosome pair inherited from the same parent. In isodisomy the two are copies of the same parental chromosome, in heterodisomy both chromosomes of that parent are present.

Unrelated – everybody is related if you go back far enough. In genetics, people are usually described as unrelated if they do not share any common great-grandparent.

Upstream – on a nucleic acid strand, in the 5′ direction (of the sense strand in a gene).

Vector – a DNA sequence into which a piece of DNA of interest can be ligated, allowing it to be introduced into cells and manipulated. Most vectors are engineered versions of natural plasmids or bacteriophages (see *Box 4.4*).

X-inactivation – the mechanism whereby in each cell of a person, genes on all but one of the X chromosomes are switched off, so that only one gene copy is active regardless of the number of X chromosomes present (see *Figure 7.4*).

Index

b after a page number means the entry appears in a box, f in a figure, g in the *Glossary*, t in a table. References to diseases have as far as possible been listed under the heading 'Syndrome'.